Functional
Training
with a Fork

Ronnie & Kathy Rowland

Innovators of the 7 Types of Functional Training

Library of Congress Cataloging-in-Publishing Data

Functional Training with a Fork/Ronnie and Kathy Rowland—first edition.

Copyright © 2015 by Ronnie and Kathy Rowland

All rights reserved. This book or any portion thereof may not be reproduced or used in any manner whatsoever without the express permission of the authors except for the use of brief quotations. We can be contacted at— functionaltrainingwithafork@gmail.com

This book was written to provide accurate information to the subject matter presented. It is published and sold with the understanding that the authors are not engaged in rendering medical, legal, or other professional services by publication of this work. Always consult your physician before beginning any exercise or nutritional program. This general information is not intended to diagnose any medical condition or to replace your healthcare professional. If medical assistance is required, the services of a physician should be sought.

First Printing, 2015

ISBN 978-0-692-50236-5

Printed in the United States of America

Ingram Content Group Inc.

1 Ingram Blvd.

La Vergne, TN 37086

Phone: 1-615-793-5000

ACKNOWLEDGMENTS

To Lenaya Raack, thank you for an extraordinary job editing our book.
You leaned out our book, making it functional for our readers.
We couldn't have done it without your patience and editing skills!
To Griselda M Design, thank you for your breathtaking graphic design
work. You are definitely an artist with a vision and easy to work with!
To our son Austin Rowland, thank you for giving us the freedom to write
Functional Training with a Fork!

CONTENTS

Introduction

Results 12
Our Children 16
Our Schools 16
The Fitness and Weight-Loss Industry 17

Chapter 1: The Functional Diet

Learn Your Genetic Limitations 24
The Functional Food Spectrum 25
Exercise Is Not Enough 27
Macronutrients 28
Sample Baseline Functional Diet 32
Ronnie's Functional Diet Plan 34
Kathy's Functional Diet Plan 35
Dessert 36
Protein 38
Healthy Carbs and Fats 40
Refined Sugar and Artificial Sweeteners 42
Sugar Alcohols 44
Alcohol 44
Mixing Carbs and Fats 44
Pre-Workout Meal 46
Timing Carbs 46
Timing Fats 47
The Best to Worst Fats 48
Basic Concepts of Losing Body Fat 51
Food Preparations 56
Visualization 59
Functional Heart 61
Extended Access to Fattening Foods 68
Stop Overeating 70
Shrinking Your Stomach 72
Yo-Yo Dieting 74
Take Responsibility 75
Food Pushers 76
Take Command 81
Support Groups 83
Quitters 84

CONTENTS

Chapter 2: Functional Training

Functionally Fit 92
Free Weights vs. Machines 95
Lower-Back Injuries 96
Building up the Transverse Abdominis 103
Building up the Glutes 106
Functional Sets, Active Release Techniques, and Gentle Static Stretching. . . 107
Overtraining. 109
Stress Kills 110
Healing the Brain with Functional Training 111
Driving a Motorized Vehicle 114

Chapter 3: The 7 Types of Functional Training

Summary of the 7 Types of Functional Training 117
7 Types of Functional Training In-Depth 121
   Slingshot Functional Training (SFT) 121
   Basic Functional Training (BFT) 124
   Advanced Functional Training (AFT) 126
   Highly Advanced Functional Training (HAFT). 132
   Group Functional Training (GFT). 138
   Post-Catastrophic Functional Training (PCFT) 141
   Rehabilitative Functional Training (RFT) 141

Chapter 4: Dysfunctional Training (DFT)

CrossFit® 145
Exercises Performed on Unstable Devices Such as a BOSU®ball 153
Improper Exercise Selection 155
Improper Functional Training Methods 157
Obsession 159

Chapter 5: Functional Muscle Fiber Training

Function of Type-2 Muscle Fibers 161
Function of Type-1 Muscle Fibers 163
Functional Muscle Toning 164
Functional Stretching and Functional Sets 165
Aggressive Static Stretching 170

CONTENTS

Chapter 6: Muscle Toning vs. Bulking

Training Myths 180
Bodybuilding 183
Struggling to Develop Muscle Tone 184
Proper Exercise Form for Males and Females 187
Bad Pain 190
Rest Time between Functional Sets 191

Chapter 7: Functional Cardio

Dysfunctional Cardio 196
Functional Cardio 199

Chapter 8: How the Immune System Functions

GMO and the Immune System 211
Hormones, Antibiotics, and the Immune System 215
Pesticides, Fertilizers, and the Immune System 217
Body-Fat Levels and the Immune System 224
Dysfunction Junction 225
Yo-Yo Dieting and the Immune System 228
Fiber and the Immune System 231
Probiotics, Prebiotics, and the Immune System 233
Heavy Metals, Antibiotics, and the Immune System 236
Amino Acids and the Immune System 238
Protein, Bone Density, and Kidney Function 241
Blood Sugar, Insulin, and the Immune System 243
Cholesterol and the Immune System 247
Cholesterol 251
LDL and HDL Cholesterol 253
The Causes of Heart Disease 253
Hormones and Cholesterol 258
Functional Training, Muscle Tone, and the Immune System 260
Dehydration and the Immune System 262
Water and the Immune System. 265
Excess Water Consumption 267
Water Sources. 268
Electrolytes and the Immune System 269
Functional Sex Improves Immune Functions. 272
Sleep and the Immune System 280
Drugs and the Immune System 281

CONTENTS

Vitamins, Minerals, and the Immune System 282

Chapter 9: Functional Hormone Replacement

Hematocrit and Estrogen Levels for Males and Females 290
Synthetic vs. Bioidentical Hormones 290
Insulin-Like Growth Factors 294
How to Properly Balance Female Hormones 295
The Women's Health Initiative Study. 300
Birth Control Pills 303
Preventing Hair Loss in Females 304
Testosterone and Breast Cancer 306
Women's Intimate Relationships and Hormones 308
How to Properly Balance Out a Man's Hormones 311
Low Estrogen in Males 313
Testosterone and Prostate Cancer 314
Men's Intimate Relationships and Hormones 316
Defensive Hormone Therapy 317
Emotional Connections 323

Chapter 10: Chronic Pain 327

Chapter 11: Hiring a Functional Personal Trainer 341

Chapter 12: How to Become a Functional Personal Trainer. 247

Chapter 13: Functional Managers in the Fitness Industry 255

Chapter 14: Be a Functional Gym Member 259

INTRODUCTION

Functional Training with a Fork is the most important health and fitness book ever written. **Functional Training with a Fork** is our expression for combining Functional Training with a Functional Diet. This book sets forth new standards for the health and fitness industry. It gives you a clear path to follow, as we take you step-by-step through the 7 types of Functional Training and the Functional Diet. **Functional Training with a Fork** is an education credential that ensures the highest standard for everyone involved in the health and fitness industry. Here is where you will not only find truthful information about exercise and nutrition, but self-awareness, hormone replacement, and your immune system. We believe it's important to explain what goes on behind the scenes so you can set goals for yourself that are both realistic and achievable. Otherwise, you are just going to end up frustrated.

People are more frustrated than ever because they can't find just one book that will guide them on how to lose body fat, build muscle tone, and improve their overall functionality. The maze of misinformation being handed out to the general public is keeping a lot of people from reaching their goals. This book isn't only going to help people regain control of their weight and health, it's also going to help give other personal trainers around the world some good information so they can help their clients succeed.

If you want to improve your life, we suggest that you begin reading this entire book as soon as possible. It was written in layman's terms to the best of our ability. **Functional Training with a Fork** explains from both a psychological and physiological standpoint what is involved in becoming happy, building self-confidence, and living a life of freedom. You will need to put down the phone, iPod, TV remote, or whatever it is that distracts you. Get your beverage of choice and go to a quiet room. Go somewhere comfortable and begin reading this book from start to finish. It's important that you finish the entire book. Only then will you gain the full knowledge on how to make positive changes in your life.

Functional Training with a Fork was written from years of hands-on experience working with various people from different genetic backgrounds. We have plenty of scientific and anecdotal evidence to back up what we teach. As long-time personal trainers, with more than 40 years of combined experience in gyms, we have witnessed real-life experiences and transformations. We currently work as a team at Gold's Gym in Aiken, S.C. We have combined our knowledge as male and female personal trainers to bring the best of both worlds to our clientele.

We absolutely love our jobs as personal trainers. We love people and want you to learn to love yourself, your exercise, and your diet. We are going to teach you time-tested secrets that are proven to work. By following the principles outlined in this book, you can become a much happier person. Happiness has less to do with obtaining things you don't have and more about making the things you do have more appealing.

This book will teach you how to become more attractive in your face and body through losing body fat and enhancing muscle tone. Your stress levels are going to lessen, and you will trade in your side order of fries for a side order of Functional Training. If you are currently feeling lonely, don't be surprised if you begin getting more attention. Expect to have fewer common aches and pains: You will live a more comfortable life and get a better night's sleep. You will see substantial improvements in your energy and functionality, allowing you to participate in more of life's pleasures. You will have a feeling of self-accomplishment by finishing what you started.

Functional Alert: When most people first get married all they want to do is eat and have sex. Over time a lot of people replace sex with food. We are going to show you how to avoid that tragedy!

It has been said that adult maturity is fully formed when a person reaches approximately 25 years of age. We disagree! Judgment and decision making cannot be fully reached until a person incorporates the principles found in **Functional Training with a Fork** regardless of their age. Mental clarity and mood will improve, allowing you to make more money and build more meaningful connections. You will begin noticing more of the little things that make a big difference in your day: for example, seeing your child's face light up or your pet rushing to greet you.
You will receive unexpected compliments about your looks that will brighten your day. You will improve monogamous relationships by enhancing your sex life. The negative impacts aging has on your body will become more manageable. Your family's future is going to be more secure because you and your children are going to have a better opportunity of living longer, more productive lives!

After six months of incorporating **Functional Training with a Fork**, you will begin to feel and look like a new person. You will never want to go back to living a dysfunctional lifestyle. When you clean up your diet, mind, and training program, you clean up your body. Then your body starts to function like it was designed to. You look different, feel different, and act differently. Your moods are different and a lot changes. This is why **Functional Training with a Fork** succeeds where other attempts at a lifestyle change often fail.

For many, all it takes to improve functionality is losing 10-20 pounds of body fat and adding 4-12 pounds of lean muscle. On the other hand, many find that gaining 10-20 pounds of body fat or losing 4-12 pounds of muscle is all it takes to experience detrimental changes in blood pressure, cholesterol, sugar levels, mobility, and appearance.

If you are obese or have health-related issues from a poor diet and a lack of Functional Exercise, we are going to show you how to make a permanent lifestyle change. It's what we do for a living! Two out of three adults in America are overweight and one-third of our population is now considered morbidly obese. In today's society, more people are dying of poor eating habits and a lack of proper Functional Exercise than all environmental factors combined. The estimated cost of treating obesity-related illnesses is around $210 billion a year.[1] Obesity has been quoted as a contributing factor to approximately 400,000 deaths in the United States each year.[2] Obese people have a much higher risk of deadly complications following surgery. Seeing people staying obese or eating highly toxic foods when they don't have to, is just unbearable for us. People who are not overweight, but have bodies that are not functioning properly on the inside, will also benefit from **Functional Training with a Fork**.

There will always be a few genetically gifted individuals whose bodies can withstand an enormous amount of abuse from living a dysfunctional lifestyle and be okay for most of their lives. They can eat greasy foods and sugar, and not exercise very much at all, and still live to be 90 years old. We believe many of these people could have lived to be around 120 years old had they taken better care of themselves. Unfortunately, most of us fall into the average-resilience category and die much earlier from living a dysfunctional lifestyle. In most cases, all of us should live to be around 100 years of age if we live right, but in today's society many are dying very young because of their poor lifestyles. There is such a thing as eating yourself into an early grave!
Ask yourself this question: How long do I want to live in good health?

Ronnie: *It's startling for some people to think they could live to be around 120 years old, but there are a few who do. Unfortunately, males with average genetics are not living past the age of 75 and females with average genetics are not living past the age of 80. This is because of their poor lifestyle (e.g., unmanaged stress, gluttony, hormonal imbalances, and a lack of Functional Training).[3] This means the person with average genetics is cutting his or her life span short by approximately 25 years, and it would be even more if we didn't have modernized medicine. Their later years are often filled with suffering due to medical conditions that could have been greatly delayed or avoided altogether! My wife and I love life and want to live as long as we can while being able to enjoy it. This book teaches you how to extend your time on earth. It also shows you how to escape various medical conditions that can take the joy out of life.*

We have been happily married for more than 20 years and it just keeps getting better. However, during the earlier years of our marriage we began to put on body-fat weight even though we were working out on a regular basis. There was nothing fun about it and it was beginning to put a strain on our marriage! Our weight gain was due to eating too much of the wrong kind of foods. Both of us know what it's like to be overweight and miserable, so we can sympathize with others who have weight problems. After being overweight for about two years, we decided to get our life back on track and have never looked back.

Today we both look and feel great. When we changed over to a functional lifestyle, some of our friends and family members couldn't understand why we spent so much time eating healthy foods and exercising. Now that we are older, we feel as good as we did 25 years ago and people think we look young for our age. Many of them have told us that if they could do it all over again they would have stayed in shape after graduating from high school. As people get older, the difference between those who take care of themselves and those who don't, becomes more obvious. We will never stop our functional lifestyle. The physical and mental benefits of **Functional Training with a Fork** are phenomenal!

Many people have been misled to believe that they will inevitably become depressed, overweight, lose the sexual intimacy that keeps relationships together, and have nothing to live for after they get past middle age. This is simply not true! People are finally beginning to learn that life can be just as good, if not better, as they get older. How? **Functional Training with a Fork!** The concepts found in this book allow you to age gracefully. Happiness will evolve into something completely different as you continue to mature, because you begin seeing things as they really are and learn how to deal with life in general.

Are you sick of being tired and overweight? Are you tired of feeling like you are going to fall asleep at work when it's only 9 am in the morning? We challenge you to invest in yourself by changing your lifestyle for one year to see what a difference **Functional Training with a Fork** makes in your overall functionality and appearance! If you say no, then we ask that you give it a test run for only 3 months to see if what we are telling you is truth or fiction. A lifestyle change is a big investment, so you need to make sure that the change you choose is a good fit for your body, both inside and out. This lifestyle change won't only affect you, it will affect your family and your community. A note to all parents: Today's kids are just as tough as kids of the past, but many of them are being programmed to become weaker. We feel that being a good parent means teaching our children the hard lessons in life.

We are living in a society that is losing its moral code and looking for entitlements: Too many people are becoming dishonest and feel that the world owes them something without giving anything in return. Personal goals through a lifestyle change can only be earned through hard work and a willingness to never quit. Success isn't going to chase you down; you have to make it happen! We believe a little hard work and struggle makes one stronger. The way we see it, people are inspired by two things:

what they want to be and what they don't want to be. If you are an open person with a willingness to listen and learn from objective material, then we know you can transform yourself and make a difference.

Results

Here are the results you can expect to achieve from using **Functional Training with a Fork**:

One month. After 1 month, most muscle soreness will begin to disappear. The first place you will begin seeing results is in the areas where you naturally carry the least amount of body fat. You will begin seeing some improvements in muscle tone.

Two months. After 2 months, you will see a noticeable difference throughout your entire body. By the end of the second month, you will notice an increase in energy levels and tightening in your abdominals. Your arms and legs will feel more toned. You will see the most improvement in those areas where you naturally carry the least amount of body fat; and if you continue following **Functional Training with a Fork** as outlined, you are on your way to a new body!

Three months. After 3 months, you will notice muscle definition in your shoulders and upper back along with a narrowing and tightening of your glutes and abdominals. Your biceps and triceps will become tighter, and people will often begin commenting on the changes you've made to your body in such a short time.

Six months. At 6 months, your entire body will have transformed. You will appear toned and need a new wardrobe! Your blood pressure, cholesterol, triglycerides, and sugar levels will be lower. Any depression and anxiety you may have will lessen. Your joints will ache less. Many of you will be able to lower or discontinue your prescription medications altogether with the consent of a physician. Your libido and cognitive abilities will improve due to increased blood flow and secretion of key hormones. You will make better decisions, and your mobility during everyday activities (including your sex life) will become significantly enhanced. You will also have an improved self-confidence and self-image and a renewed outlook on life.

One year. By devoting only one year to **Functional Training with a Fork**, you will have an appealing body that turns heads.

Two years. After 2 years, you will have the best body you can obtain according to your genetics.

Functional Training with a Fork also improves the function of your brain, sexual organs, heart, liver, kidneys, lungs, adrenals, pancreas, muscles, cartilage, skin, teeth, and, most important, your immune system, circulatory system, and lymphatic system by purging Dysfunctional Toxins that cause a lack of oxygen in the cells! It will also help prevent and even slow or reverse the progression of many medical conditions. Some medical conditions such as type-2 diabetes, high cholesterol, and high blood pressure have been labeled as incurable by some. **Functional Training with a Fork** has crushed that theory time and time again!

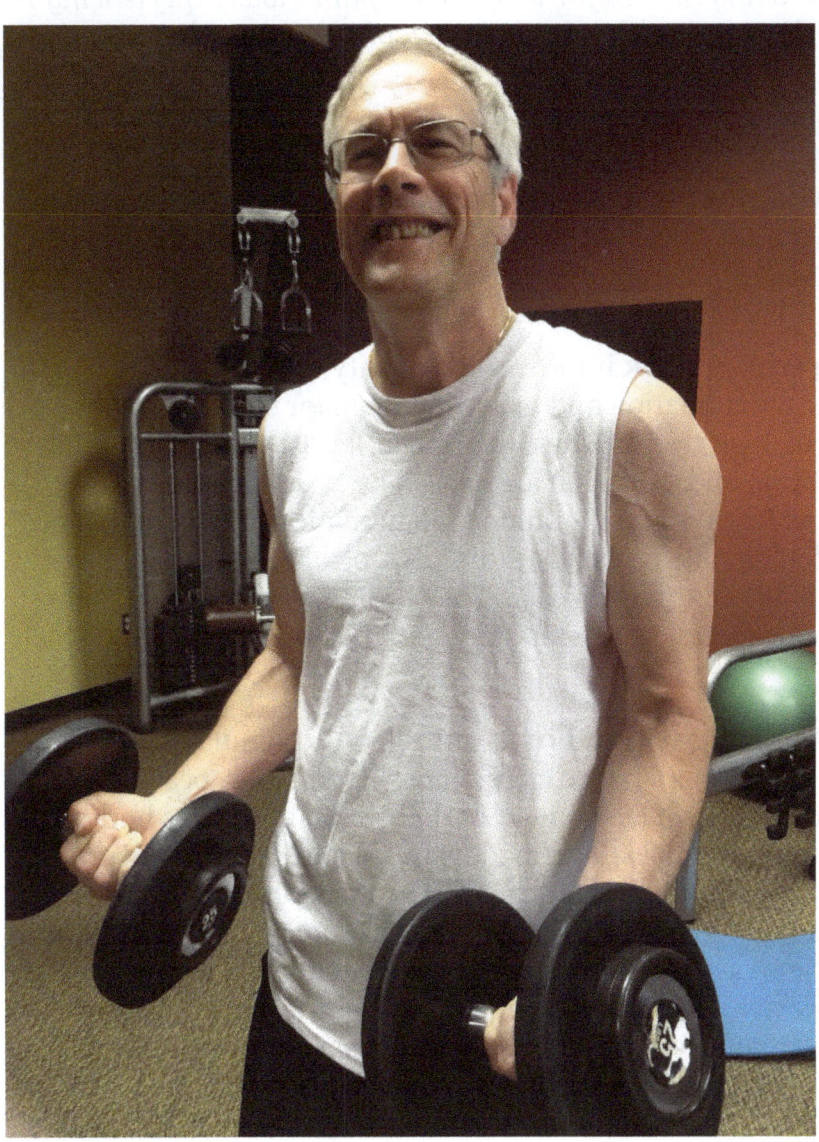

John Gilmour, Age 57

In April of 2013 I weighed 255 lbs and had several health issues. I was a Type 2 diabetic with hypertension, high cholesterol, and sleep apnea. My job as a Senior Operations Manager could be demanding and highly stressful. Looking toward retirement, I realized I needed to make changes in my life in order to enjoy retirement. After making the decision to get my health back, I joined the gym and was scheduled to meet with Ronnie Rowland to discuss training and nutrition. Ronnie explained his Functional Diet, Basic Functional Training, and the need for Functional Testosterone Replacement Therapy. He set me up with a three-day workout plan and my physician put me on testosterone therapy. I wasn't always good at sticking to the diet, but stayed close. I kept a food journal for the first two months, and it made a big difference in understanding what I was eating. My weight started to drop after the first week and continued down at a steady rate of around 2 pounds each week. After a few months of workouts I asked Ronnie to redo my training to a four-day workout plan. For my Functional Cardio I ride my bicycle 2-3 times a week. The results of my lifestyle change have been dramatic! Within 2 months of starting Functional Training with a Fork, I was able to stop taking Micardis for my high blood pressure. Then after 6 months, I was taken off of the Metformin that was treating my Diabetes. At this point, my weight was down to about 215 and I had more muscle tone and vascularity than ever before. A year and a half later, my weight had stabilized at 200 and I no longer needed to sleep with a CPAP machine. Finally, after two years, my cholesterol was low enough that I was able to stop taking Simcor for it. The knee pain I was experiencing is practically nonexistent. Now that my health is back, I am looking forward to enjoying my upcoming retirement!

Functional Alert: If you have any of the following: high blood sugar, high cholesterol, and high blood pressure, ask your doctor about **Functional Training with a Fork**!

Functional Training with a Fork improves the quality of your blood, which helps prevent chronic systemic inflammation and oxidation (a major source of high blood pressure, high cholesterol, high triglycerides, high sugar levels, and heavy metal poisoning). Systemic inflammation and oxidation are caused by excess amounts of pro-inflammatory cytokines and free radicals! Systemic inflammation and oxidation are the root cause of all life-threatening illnesses such as diabetes, stroke, aneurysm, heart attack, cancer, Alzheimers, and autoimmune disease. They promote aging by damaging the function of blood cells, blood vessels, organs, tissues, and the immune system, which leads to systemic dysfunction.

Without **Functional Training with a Fork**, your blood accumulates Dysfunctional Toxins, such as undigested food, excess lipids, blood sugar, pesticides, heavy metals, decayed cells from free radical damage, and fibrin that prevents both toxic waste from being removed and oxygenated blood from reaching cells, tissues, and organs. These Dysfunctional Toxins will interfere with normal joint and immune function, making you feel tired and increasing everyday aches and pains. Whether you are an athlete, young person, or an aging adult, healthy oxygenated blood is the key to having good health and longevity. Having good circulation is critical to good health because oxygenated blood allows your body to repair itself. It even helps white blood cells fight infection in the body. Along with food, blood is the fuel your body needs to function properly!

Functional Training with a Fork will optimize your:

- Self-confidence.
- Sexual function for enhanced intimacy.
- Mood to combat stress, anger, anxiety, and depression.
- Cognitive function for better learning, memory, communication, and reaction time.
- Relationships all across the board.
- Systemic function for deterring all diseases and enhancing longevity.
- Joint function and comfort.
- Production of cytokines and free radicals.
- Blood viscosity (thinner blood) and clotting factors.
- Red blood cell count for improved delivery of oxygen to the body's tissues.
- Inflammatory responses for better delivery of white blood cells to repair inflamed tissues and to fight off infection caused by a bacterium, virus, or fungus.
- GI tract function.
- Cholesterol levels.
- Blood sugar and insulin levels.
- Lung and respiratory health for improved oxygen intake and carbon dioxide release.
- Cardiovascular health.
- Overall appearance and lean muscle mass-to-body-fat ratio.
- Longevity.
- Immune System.

We have written this book to give you an opportunity to change your life. The basic concepts of body-fat loss, muscle tone, and better health and functionality are straightforward and they will fit together like a giant puzzle after you finish reading this book!

Our Children

We also need to focus on our children's health and well-being. Overweight adults are not the only ones who face a wide range of social, physiological, and psychological challenges. Overweight children find it more difficult to make friends and are often regarded as lazy. They are more likely to have a low self-esteem that can last a lifetime. Overweight kids also face a host of medical problems at an earlier age. Some struggle finding employment as overweight adults because they are viewed as a medical liability.

Many adults fail to realize that skinny kids with a fast metabolism are also doing damage internally by eating a lot of unhealthy foods. Doctors are treating more young people for high blood pressure, diabetes, and ADHD/ADD. When we were young we played in the neighborhoods all day and food was the last thing on our minds. We rarely went back for seconds because we wanted to get back outside as soon as possible to play with our friends. Frequent bouts of intense exercise help children stay less stressed. When you're stressed, you forget things! Experts say that a lack of exercise and/or a poor diet makes certain brain conditions worse, such as ADHD.[4] For a few children with ADHD, Functional Exercise and a Functional Diet can actually be a replacement for prescription drugs, but, for most, it's complementary.

Acute bouts of stress cause a temporary increase in blood pressure. Stress triggers the release of adrenaline and cortisol. Abnormally elevated levels of adrenaline (epinephrine) cause the heart to beat faster and the blood vessels to constrict, resulting in a temporary increase in blood pressure.[5] If stress becomes chronic, it puts kids at risk for chronic high blood pressure because their rapid heartbeats and restricted blood vessels are never able to recover.[6] Without exercise a kid's body will secrete higher levels of cortisol in response to stress. This causes them to lose muscle tone and eat more foods higher in carbohydrates and fats than kids who exercise properly and secrete less cortisol. Too much cortisol can also suppress the immune system by preventing the reproduction of t-cells![7,8]

Most of today's kids have replaced activity with video games, and they often snack on junk food throughout the day. It's a vicious cycle that must be broken. Both parents and the school system have the ability to offer students foods that are healthy, appealing, tasty, and filling (no one wants to eat a piece of baked, dried, under-seasoned chicken) instead of junk food such as pizza. Teaching kids to eat healthy while they are young will lay the proper foundation for life-long healthy-eating habits.

Our Schools

Teaching the Functional Diet is necessary in the schools. We believe our school systems are currently making a huge mistake by not making it mandatory for students to take classes on what constitutes proper nutrition from elementary through high school.

Educating and reinforcing our children about the importance of proper nutrition is one way we as a society can cut health care costs to a very noticeable degree in the future!

Our children need parents and teachers who truly care about their health, well-being, and cognitive abilities so they can excel academically. We believe controversy regarding what constitutes proper nutrition needs to be worked out among parents and teachers. We have seen first-hand the damage that can be done to children. During his sophomore year in high school, our son, Austin, gained 20 pounds of body fat from eating the fattening foods they prepared in his culinary arts class. Once we found out how he was gaining the weight, we put him back on the Functional Diet and he lost all the weight.

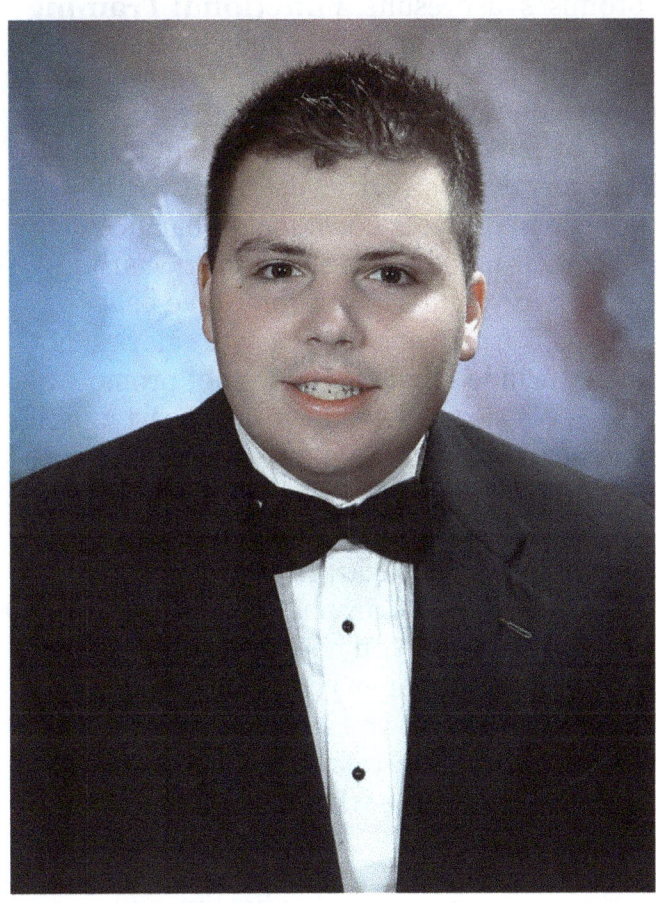

Austin Rowland

After losing the weight, my thinking was much clearer. I was happier, looked better, and had more energy and self-confidence. I never want to allow myself to become overweight again!

Too many carbs coming from any source—especially processed white flour, wheat, grains, and starches—are linked to chronic inflammation, chronic oxidation, and weight gain. The same goes for eating too many fat sources, especially trans fats and saturated fats. Therefore, we believe it's wrong when carbs and fats make up the base of the food being served in our school systems. Protein and fibrous, plant-based foods should be the base of the Functional Diet.

The Fitness and Weight-Loss Industry

Due to massive changes in diet and activity levels over recent years, about two-thirds of our U.S. population is now overweight and many are unhealthy.[9] Some of the other one-third still have health problems due to inactivity and poor food choices. From 2003 to 2013 (only 10 years) the global population of obese people rose from 1 billion to 2 billion.[10] The yearly revenue of the U.S. weight-loss industry is approximately 20 billion dollars.[11] A large percentage of this money comes from people looking for a quick fix or an easy way out that doesn't exist! We believe that a lot of people spend their hard-earned money on bogus weight-loss supplements, fad diets, and colon cleanses, and on dysfunctional exercise equipment and workout routines. These are all marketed toward people who have the same hope: the belief in quick fixes to get rid of their depression and disgust from allowing themselves to become overweight. For many people, the psychological cost of having to permanently give up their fattening diets and sedentary lifestyles seems too great. So they keep trying all these whacky fad diets and exercise programs that don't bring lasting results. Never forget that nothing good can come from a diet or exercise program that promises fast results. **Functional Training with a Fork** teaches you the best way to lose body fat gradually and keep it off forever!

Physicians have jumped on the money-making wagon by selling people so-called natural fat-burning supplements and by putting people on no-weight training, 500-calorie-per-day diets and by prescribing a very expensive drug called HCG. The HCG diet causes a loss in muscle tone and bone, and disrupts hormonal imbalances. Dieters are set up for long-term failure because their metabolism shuts down, causing depression, reduced mental clarity, agitation, lethargy, and a lower libido. We believe that the weight loss experienced while using HCG is from consuming fewer calories, not the HCG itself. In fact, 24 clinical studies have concluded that HCG does not promote body-fat loss or cause a decrease in appetite![12, 13] We also believe the loss of heart muscle from a 500-calorie-per-day diet contributes to heart problems and a Dysfunctional Immune System. Our experience in working with people who have tried the HCG diet has shown that the reduction in appetite some experience at first is not from injecting HCG, but changing over to a high protein diet and avoiding sugar. In addition, some people are being prescribed potentially harmful stimulants or amphetamines along with the HCG to reduce their appetite even further. We can show you how to succeed where doctors and big drug companies usually fail. The lifestyle change you will experience by using **Functional Training with a Fork** is going to get you away from all the gimmicks and non-truth by showing you once and for all how to lose body fat and keep it off without feeling deprived. In fact, **Functional Training with a Fork** fixes many of the underlying problems in today's society!

Fortunately, more people are turning their attention to staying heathy, and as a result, the fitness industry is booming. Unfortunately, dysfunction is running rampant there. Our gyms have spent billions of dollars on effective muscle-building equipment. We think it's sad that about 75% of gym members don't know they are using exercise equipment improperly. It's even sadder when people pay money and get hurt while trying to do something good for their bodies.

Innovators of the 7 Types of Functional Training

Choosing the right personal trainer is very important! As personal trainers we should all have a good attitude and try to work together so we can all be on the same page. Some kind-hearted, talented people fail as personal trainers because they don't have a strong work ethic or they get poor information and stick with it. Some let their egos or past teachings get in the way. The fact is, exercise and nutrition can be complicated—especially with all the misleading information going around. Personal trainers, more than ever, need to understand how the human body works so we can evaluate new exercises and nutritional philosophies being thrown at us.

Our experiences illustrate both the bright and the dark side of the industry. The bright side serves to help everyone. The dark side harms not just individuals, but personal trainers and the gyms where they work! It concerns us when people start out with the best of intentions and the will to change their bodies, yet end in disappointment and feelings of inadequacy.

The average person or personal trainer who learns how to properly apply the seven different types of Functional Training discussed in this book will be able to progress forward with great confidence, knowing they are using the right type of Functional Training for their unique situation. The intimidating exercise maze that prevents many people from joining a gym will be erased with **Functional Training with a Fork**. Likewise, personal trainers will have a reference manual for teaching. We see no value in performing exercises, routines, and diets that can't be maintained long-term as a healthy lifestyle (e.g., CrossFit® and the Ketosis diet). The biggest complaint we hear from clients about their past experiences with personal trainers is that they felt they weren't getting results. We believe that proper nutrition, intense weight training, and some cardio are—and always have been—the foundation for getting fit. If, for example, a female client tells us she wants to lose fat on her abs and tone up overall (especially her upper arms and legs), the most effective and safest method we have found involves the Functional Diet (about 70% of her regimen), Basic Functional Training or Advanced Functional Training (about 20%), and Functional Cardio (about 10%). If she can't do it using these methods, then nothing exotic is going to do it for her! Proper nutrition, intense weight training, and some cardio have always been the foundation for getting fit. We see people spending hours in the gym doing various forms of cardio and practically useless exercises, with very little to show for it.

Obtaining the best results requires using common sense, hard work, and consistency, and sticking to the basics. We believe when you make something too complicated or hard, people don't want to follow it. What you eat is by far the most important thing when it comes to losing body fat; cardio training helps some, but not nearly as much as most people think. Functional Training, when combined with a Functional Diet, is the most effective means for reducing body fat and building muscle tone. We believe the best cardio is Functional Cardio that improves the cardiovascular system. You shouldn't approach cardio as a means of losing weight at all costs, but rather as a way to improve your heart's efficiency. Losing weight isn't the same as losing body fat. You can lose weight while actually increasing body-fat levels!

Take a long hard look at all the people you see now who are 35 years and older. A lot of them walk with a limp from bad knees, lower backs, and hips. Their shoulders are often in bad condition and many have some form of chronic pain. Approximately half of these injuries are related to overuse through improper exercising or to some form of injury that occurred outside the gym. The other half are caused from a lack of Functional Training to build muscle tone and support connective tissues.

It's not fun having chronic joint pain throughout your entire body. It hinders your ability to function during everyday activities. The great news is that improving your ability to function during daily activities can be done safely by performing the same exercises and training methods used for muscle toning and body-fat loss!

High-risk doesn't equal high-reward when it comes to exercise. High-risk exercise equals low-reward. Unfortunately, we have seen a lot of people come into the gym and take the old "get into shape or die trying" attitude. They go full steam ahead with the mindset that if they get injured, they will get over it. They don't consider the more extreme scenario that has them struggling to walk from their bedroom to their bathroom without having to take a break, trying to live on disability payments, becoming dependent on painkillers, and possibly never stepping foot in a gym again. It's crucial to get proper instructions on how to use weight-lifting equipment and learn the proper techniques. Your body is too valuable to take advice from someone without a credible education and experienced background. Roughly a million Americans from 1990 to 2007 were injured when they joined a gym to lose weight and improve their functional abilities and muscle tone.[14] Almost 460,000 people were sent to the hospital in 2012 alone for injuries and approximately 32,000 were hospitalized or dead upon arrival to the hospital![15] Today, the number of injuries has increased because of the recent CrossFit® fad. It's the fastest growing fad that is teaching others how to exercise improperly. We believe CrossFit® is leading to increased rates of unemployment, disability claims, and health care cost! On the other hand, proper Functional Training leads to increased rates of employment, fewer disability claims, and lower health care costs.

Authors' Note: *This book teaches you how to get built for function!*

CHAPTER 1

The Functional Diet

In today's society people are finally starting to become more concerned about their looks and health. They don't just want toned muscles; they want to be healthy, functional, energetic, sexual, and live a long life. The Functional Diet is the single most important component for improving your ability to function in everyday activities. Controlling both the quality and quantity of food you put in your mouth every day will be the #1 deciding factor in how much body fat you have to lug around and how well your organs function. The more body fat you have, the more you will weigh and the slower you will move. You will also lose flexibility and balance and experience joint pain. You will start having memory loss, depression, and sexual problems. Internal organs won't function optimally, causing a vast array of medical conditions. Weight causes more stress on your joints and heart during daily activities, which dramatically increases your chances of becoming injured and having a heart attack. It becomes a chore to do simple things such as standing, walking, and going up and down stairs. You will snore and have breathing problems. Being over-weight causes early signs of degeneration in the lower back, knees, hips, feet, and ankles. Obesity is strongly linked to various life-threatening diseases such as heart disease, diabetes, and cancer.

Functional Alert: It will be easier to follow a Functional Diet once you become educated about what you are putting in your mouth with a fork!

The Functional Diet will determine approximately 70% of your body-fat loss success. Functional Training makes up roughly 20% and Functional Cardio is about 10%. Functional Hormone Replacement will also play a significant role when females approach menopause and males approach andropause.

There is a lot to be said for common sense, and if you don't begin with the proper foundation, you have already set yourself up for failure. For instance, belly fat can't be targeted with specific exercises, no matter how hard you try. Flat abdominals are mostly made in the kitchen, not in the gym! Meaning your diet is what makes them defined. You can build the abs and make them stick out farther, but you can't spot reduce. Fat loss occurs throughout your entire body as you begin to lose inches, and people lose faster in some areas than others due to their genetic makeup. Every time you lose body fat, it will always come off in a specific order. For some of you, it may come off your legs first and abs last. Or maybe it will come off your abs first and legs last.

Functional Alert: The abdominal muscles are considered a small muscle group. This means you won't burn many calories while training them regardless of the intensity applied!

Learn Your Genetic Limitations

Losing body fat can be a totally different experience for men than it is for women. For example, a male who is an endomorph (has a slow metabolism) can lose body fat easier than a female who is an endomorph because he has higher testosterone levels. Maintaining six-pack abs year round isn't a realistic goal if you don't have the genetics to sustain it without feeling miserable. A certain degree of body fat is acceptable. Some people find they have to starve themselves to death and feel miserable to maintain such a condition. This is unhealthy and not sustainable. Some of the models you see in infomercials and magazines are genetically gifted. They can easily maintain abs year round while others can't. The ones who aren't genetically gifted have to starve themselves to get to that point and are able to maintain that condition for only a few days. They show up to photo shoots for magazines dehydrated, weak, and dizzy! It's unfortunate how most magazine covers have created unrealistic expectations for what fit people should look like. Some people can't maintain that look by eating a Functional Diet and working out. It's important to learn your genetic limitations so you can find your functional "sweet spot"—the place where you feel good and have a lot of energy, while remaining relatively lean for your body type. The key to losing body fat and good health is finding that spot and maintaining it as a lifestyle, not yo-yoing up and down in weight.

Functional Alert: When you follow the Functional Diet properly, you shouldn't feel as if you are on a diet. The Functional Diet works where others often fail because it involves consuming more non-starchy vegetables (Free Foods), and lean protein in order to crowd out excess processed sugars and unhealthy fats in your diet. It also allows you to adjust both calories and macronutrient ratios in accordance with your exercise program and body type or genetics. This brings forth permanent body-fat loss so you can be proud of your body and stay on it as a lifestyle!

Some people have tried to complicate things by looking for an easy way out that doesn't exist. They have done the exact same thing with exercise and it doesn't work! Your goal should be to consume just enough carbs and fats to supply your body with fuel and then just a little extra for reserves. The rest of your calories should come from protein and fibrous plant-based Free Foods. Some examples of non-starchy carbs (Free Foods) are spinach, lettuce, broccoli, peppers, green beans, Brussels sprouts, zucchini, greens, cabbage, and celery.

While using the Functional Diet, our clients feel full longer and don't get that mid-day crash. They have cut back on both carbs and fats, replacing them with Free Foods, lean proteins, and more water. They have also decreased their sugar/insulin spikes not only by reducing carbs and fats, but keeping carbs and fats separated in most meals to the best of their ability. For the majority of our clients, their body-fat levels dropped, causing their blood sugar, blood pressure, triglycerides, and cholesterol to reach good levels. Many no longer need to take medication to control these conditions. Simply put: The Functional Diet allows everyone to stay satisfied and energetic while meeting their calorie requirements. They feel better, have more energy, look better, and lab results from their doctors show they're healthier!

Functional Alert: America wouldn't need to spend so much money on health care plans to cover all these medical issues if they would eat right, keep their hormone levels healthy, and exercise properly!

We know perfectly well that people can lose weight by just counting calories. Many have done that but, in the process, lost a lot of muscle tone! Developing more muscle tone means you can actually consume more carbs without turning them into triglycerides and being stored as body fat. When you have less body fat, it also means you have less space for Dysfunctional Toxins (anything that damages the cells, tissues, and organs that activate the immune system) to find refuge, so they can be more readily eliminated.

The Functional Food Spectrum

The Functional Food Spectrum is a scale showing how foods are ranked in terms of the amount of protein, fiber, probiotics, prebiotics, nutrients, phytonutrients, carotenoids, antioxidants, sugar, and the types of carbs and fats in food; how much the food is processed; whether fish is farm-raised or wild-caught; and whether produce and meats are U.S. organic or non-organic. Also, it shows if they are from the U.S. or other countries.

It's of the utmost importance to eat foods ranked on the higher end of the Functional Food Spectrum. They are extremely important for improving your looks and overall health! These foods are high in protein, fiber, probiotics, prebiotics, unsaturated fats, nutrients, phytonutrients, carotenoids, and antioxidants. They are low in refined sugar, saturated fats, trans fats, heavy metals, antibiotics, and high-risk synthetic pesticides. Consume as many unprocessed foods as you can, as well as meats free of antibiotics and hormones and wild-caught fish on the bottom of the food chain that contain fewer heavy metals (such as mercury). All foods should come from the United States.

You need to significantly reduce your intake of foods ranked on the lower end of the Functional Food Spectrum. These foods are low in protein, fiber, probiotics, prebiotics, unsaturated fats, nutrients, phytonutrients, carotenoids, and antioxidants. They are high in sugar, saturated fats, and trans fats; they are highly processed; and they contain antibiotics, hormones, larger amounts of heavy metals, and larger amounts of high-risk synthetic pesticides. Farm-raised fish containing antibiotics are on the lower end of the spectrum, along with wild-caught fish on the top of the food chain, which have a higher heavy-metal content (e.g., albacore tuna). All foods coming from different countries (e.g., China) are on the lower end of the Functional Food Spectrum. Shopping on the outside aisles of the grocery store usually offers foods higher on the Functional Food Spectrum, whereas foods on the inside isles are generally ranked lower on the Spectrum.

Functional Alert: Foods on the lower end of the Functional Food Spectrum cause the body to release more pro-inflammatory cytokines and free radicals. This means your body has to deal with more inflammation and oxidation. Foods on the upper end of the Functional Food Spectrum cause your body to release fewer pro-inflammatory cytokines and free radicals. This results in less inflammation and oxidation!

We are concerned for many people because their lifestyles are comparable to a slow death by poison. There are multitudes of various Dysfunctional Toxins listed on food labels that are causing health problems. However, it may come as a surprise to many of you that a highly processed pack of crackers might contain fewer Dysfunctional Toxins than a piece of fruit! Some apples have been found to contain very high amounts of high-risk pesticides (Dysfunctional Toxins). The pesticides might be more damaging for your particular body chemistry than the chemicals and preservatives (both Dysfunctional Toxins) that are found in crackers. However, the apple contains nutrients, antioxidants, carotenoids, phytonutrients, and usable fiber that the crackers don't! This makes the apple less damaging to the body because the fiber will eliminate a lot of the Dysfunctional Toxins through your digestive system before they get stored in the blood stream and fat cells, while the nutrients, antioxidants, carotenoids, and phytonutrients will minimize damage to your cells and immune system.[1,2]

On the other hand, if all you eat is a pack of crackers, the lack of fiber will allow almost every dysfunctional toxin contained in the crackers to be stored in your blood stream and fat cells and will harm your immune system. Furthermore, the crackers are practically void of nutritional value (nutrients, antioxidants, carotenoids, and phytonutrients), which accelerates cell damage. This lack of fiber and proper nutrition causes chronic inflammation and oxidation, which blocks the ability of your digestive tract, fat cells, organs, and arteries to properly communicate to the immune system. Your body requires some inflammation and oxidation to be healthy because it provokes the immune system to dispatch white blood cells to repair the body. However, if excess amounts of white blood cells are released due to chronic inflammation, they begin destroying the inside of your body.[3]

When we go shopping, we buy liquid egg whites, organic chicken and turkey, wild-caught salmon, 94-96% organic lean hamburger, organic potatoes, non-GMO Smart Balance® Omega peanut butter a registered trademark of Boulder Brands, PB2 Powdered Peanut Butter, CARBmaster® yogurt, and organic Ezekiel® breads found in the freezer section. Our shopping list also includes both conventional and organic fruits and vegetables (we don't have the money to buy all organic), lemon juice, and caffeinated organic coffee grown in the United States. We never buy juice or milk because they're loaded with sugar. Our condiments are organic mustard, and various spices.

We consume a lot of Free Foods that have a high nutritional value, stay away from sugar and highly processed foods, as much as possible, and limit artificial sweeteners. The only artificial sweeteners we usually get from food/drinks are in Powerade Zero™ and CARBmaster® yogurt. The only cereals we eat are non-GMO original Cheerios® and organic oats which are low in sugar. We limit saturated fats, avoid trans fats, and stay away from oils (except spraying a little no-stick coconut oil on a pan for cooking purposes) because they are high in calories due to their fat content. Instead of using highly processed, fattening salad dressings, we sprinkle on a tiny amount of organic cheese and/or crushed organic nuts. On occasion, we mix organic mustard and a tiny amount of artificial sweetener in a little water to make a low-calorie honey mustard salad dressing.

Exercise Is Not Enough

You can't out-train a diet that is too high in calories for your metabolism. As personal trainers, we find that the majority of the time our clients stop losing body fat, the problem is their diets. Ninety percent of the time those same clients mistakenly think they are undertraining with cardio. As personal trainers, we can help a morbidly obese person who weighs 300 pounds get below 200 pounds, but we can't help a morbidity obese 300-pound person who is stuck in their ways. If there is anything we have learned in gyms over our many years as personal trainers, it's that people are often dishonest about what types of foods and how much they are eating. They fear we will think badly of them. We rarely call them out on it because we understand that it's a process. For some people, it takes longer to figure out what and how much they can eat in order to lose body fat and sustain it as a lifestyle. It doesn't take much of the wrong types of foods to have negative consequences. Most people are not going to reach their weight-loss goals having two cheat days per week. In fact, it only takes eating 500 more calories per day for everyone to gain a pound per week.[1] In the first week, they end up gaining one pound of body fat. Twenty weeks later they have gained 20 pounds! Genetics influence whether or not we tend to gain or lose body fat more rapidly than others, but so do our activity levels, hormones, and the foods we consume. Increasing body fat or losing body fat is dependent on a number of factors, which include resting metabolic rate, active metabolic rate, hormones, caloric intake, the types of foods consumed, the times of day certain foods are consumed, the types of foods combined in each meal, macronutrient ratios, amount of exercise, and the amount of muscle tone we possess.

Functional Alert: When people eat lunch at a fast-food restaurant, they usually eat anywhere from 1,500-2,000 calories in one sitting. That's enough calories for the entire day for someone with a slow metabolism!

There are plenty of diets that try to show you how to stay healthy through portion control only. These diets may sound good on paper, but fall way short of being effective when applied in real life. This is because you are eating foods on the lower end of the Functional Food Spectrum. You must consume foods ranked on the higher end of the Functional Food Spectrum in order to control hunger and make your body as toxic free as possible.

In normal cells, two types of metabolisms are going on at all times, but normal health requires that an aerobic (good) metabolism dominates. A good way of knowing that your body has shifted toward an anaerobic (bad) metabolism is if you often crave junk food! Refined sugar is the fuel source of anaerobic metabolism and it's a significant risk factors for developing cancer, heart disease, diabetes, etc.[2] Once body-fat levels are reduced and muscle tissue is increased through regular exercise, less blood sugar/insulin will be secreted in relation to food consumption and more Dysfunctional Toxins will be eliminated from the body, thus making it easier for your aerobic metabolism to dominate.

Macronutrients

The Functional Diet works where others sometimes fail because its customized macronutrient meal composition, along with the adequate protein and fiber intake, keeps people full and increases their metabolisms!

It's very important to consume a high-protein diet: approximately 40% of your daily caloric intake. Those who fail to do so will lose some muscle tone, their metabolism will slow down, and they will struggle more with body-fat loss because they are often hungry. A high-protein/high-fiber diet is a requirement for everyone looking to keep their body-fat levels down, improve muscle tone, and enhance overall functionality. We have learned that a low-protein, higher-carb, and higher-fat diet leads to overeating, body-fat gain, less muscle tone, and chronic inflammation and oxidation.

Protein, carbohydrates, and fats are macronutrients. The macronutrient ratios we recommend for those trying to lose body fat and be healthy are approximately 40% protein, 30%-40% carbohydrates, and 20%-30% fats. What constitutes too many carbs and fats varies from person to person depending on genetics, insulin sensitivity, hormones, how many carbs and fats are burned during exercise, and how much muscle one has to store glycogen before the leftover gets stored as body fat. As people get older, they often find themselves more sensitive to carbs, especially women. What we have learned as personal trainers throughout the years is that if you have good insulin sensitivity, low insulin secretion, and a fast metabolism, you will usually do better on a higher-carb (40%), lower-fat (20%) diet. On the other hand, if you have poor insulin sensitivity, high insulin secretion, or a slower metabolism, you will usually do better on a lower-carb (30%), higher-fat (30%) diet. (People who have poor insulin sensitivity and high insulin secretions experience weight gain, lethargy, and increased appetite from eating more carbs than fats.) Insulin sensitivity determines how you would set up a Functional Diet to prevent chronic inflammation and oxidation in accordance with your metabolism. We recommend a baseline Functional Diet consisting of 40% protein, 30% carbs, and 30% fats for starters in order to see where you stand.

Functional Alert: You may love carbs, but the question is: Do they like you?

People who are overweight and have become insulin resistant often do better reducing carbs until they reach their target weight goal. Their bodies simply can't metabolize carbohydrates efficiently until they lose body fat. Once they become sensitive to insulin again through losing body fat and adding muscle tone, they sometimes find they can gradually change over to a higher carb, lower-fat diet and keep the weight off and function just fine. Some of our clients find that they must stay on lower carbs and higher fats permanently in order to remain functional and keep their weight down because they are so carb sensitive.

Functional Alert: Fats also cause your blood sugar and insulin levels to increase, but not to the extent of carbs!

The body needs a certain amount of glucose to maintain regular function! Carbs are what provide the body with glucose. When one is objective about the science of lipids (cholesterol and triglycerides) and how they are metabolized in the body, high-fat diets can be just as dangerous as high-carb diets. When you consume more calories from carbs and/or fats than your body uses for fuel, they get stored as body fat (triglycerides) and your health suffers!

It's a myth that going into ketosis (consuming 40 grams of carbs or less per day) automatically causes your body to use its own fat for fuel. This is only true if calories are reduced. We've seen plenty of people gain weight in ketosis because they ate too many calories. Furthermore, the ketosis diet is a fad diet that's not sustainable as a lifestyle. Removing all carbohydrates from your diet will put you on the fast track to dehydration and constipation. It's not uncommon for people to lose 5-8 pounds of water weight during their first week. It will make you feel lousy and deprived. Cutting all carbs significantly lowers serotonin levels, which often causes depression. It's also notorious for causing bad body odor in the form of sweat and bad breath! You need to consume enough carbs to prevent going into ketosis or going in and out of ketosis. Reducing your carb intake too much causes your body to try to go in and out of ketosis. This causes extreme sugar/insulin imbalances, which cause the release of excessive amounts of pro-inflammatory cytokines and free radicals. Even if you stay in ketosis, high levels of ketones and/or a lack of antioxidants (neglecting to eat fruits and vegetables) make the blood acidic, which can damage the immune system.

Functional Alert: Females should not go below 90 carbs per day and males should not go below 110. This will ensure you stay away from ketosis and have the energy needed to function properly!

When it comes to body-fat gain and your overall health, there is no escaping your diet! Excessive amounts of carbs or fats are bad for your health and will ruin your body composition (the body's relative amount of fat-to-muscle in the body). The proper balance of each is what you need to feel good, look better, and live a longer and healthier life.

It's up to you as an individual to decide which approach is best for your body type. Even if the perfect macronutrient ratios of food are consumed, you will still gain body fat and do harm to your overall health if your daily caloric intake is too high! One of the most common things yo-yo dieters say when they are not losing body fat is, I feel I am not eating enough calories to lose body fat because it's making my metabolism slow down. That is like someone who is trying to gain weight saying, I feel like eating too many calories is preventing me from gaining weight because it's speeding up my metabolism! The point we are trying to make is, we have worked with numerous new clients who were yo-yo dieters. They would eat very little for a couple of days, then turn around and gorge. This type of yo-yo dieting causes your metabolism to become slower because it resets your basal metabolic rate (the number of calories your body burns while at rest, working out, or sleeping).[1] It also causes muscle loss and a lack of energy needed for continued exercise.

Functional Alert: You can't work out effectively on a diet that is very low in both carbs and fats. You need a certain amount of carbs and fats in order to have energy for exercising!

As long as you keep yourself in a caloric deficit, you will lose body fat regardless of whether you take the higher-carb route or the higher-fat route. However, many of you will be able to maintain one route as a lifestyle change much easier than others due to your genetic makeup and activity level. Some of you will stay hungry and lose strength taking the higher-carb approach, whereas others will feel more satisfied and energetic. On the other hand, some will stay hungry and lose strength while taking the higher-fat approach, whereas others will feel more satisfied and energetic.

Functional Alert: Choose the macronutrient ratios that allow your body to function to the fullest extent possible!

The amount of calories you need to consume is determined by your basic metabolic rate. Stay within your macronutrient guidelines as closely as you can, even though you may not always be 100% accurate. Some days you will have more carbs and other days more fats. Sometimes you might undershoot or overshoot protein by a few grams. As long as you are consistently staying close to your macronutrient guidelines, you will reach your mark! When you consume different types of foods for your meals containing a similar macronutrient breakdown, it's still going to work as long as these foods are on the higher end of the Functional Food Spectrum! Once you figure out how to lose body fat and create meals that fit within your macronutrient guidelines, you will never need another meal plan again. You will no longer be confined to eating the same foods day in and day out, unless you are one of those people that actually prefer eating the same foods every day. We have found that some people enjoy their diet to be varied to some degree, while most like sticking to the same foods because it's easier for them to track. Personally, we find that we are creatures of habit and mostly eat the same food every day. However, we are constantly changing the flavor by adding different spices and low-calorie sauces.

A 2,000 calorie baseline Functional Diet is a good starting point for many who are exercising consistently while trying to lose body fat without feeling sluggish or deprived. Let's say you are shooting for a daily caloric intake of around 2,000 calories on Sunday, Monday, Tuesday, Wednesday, Thursday, and Friday with macronutrients composed of 40% protein, 30% carbs and 30% fats. The best way to lose body fat on a 2,000 calories per day Functional Diet is to combine this with Functional Training and Functional Cardio. Males should never go below 1,500 calories per day to lose body fat and females should never go below 1,200 because weakness, muscle loss, and hunger will occur, setting you up for Functional Diet failure. You need to track calories through macronutrient requirements.

Authors' Note: *The options are many and your diet doesn't have to be perfect to obtain good results. However, the closer you get to perfection, the better results you will obtain.*

Sample Baseline Functional Diet

Sample Baseline Functional Diet for Males and Females	
2,000 Calories, 5 Meals Per Day, 6 days per week	
Sunday, Monday, Tuesday, Wednesday, Thursday, and Friday	
Meal 1	(Breakfast) 40 grams of protein, 60 grams of carbs, and 0 grams of fat. Two cups of organic caffeinated coffee. **NOTE:** Fats are not needed for breakfast!
Meal 2	40 grams of protein, 20 grams of carbs, and 0 grams of fat. Consume plenty of Free Foods in this meal.

Meal 3	(Pre-workout/late afternoon meal) 40 grams of protein, 60 grams of carbs, and 40 grams of fats. You'll need fats in this meal for an energy boost before workouts and to prevent energy crashes during daily activities! This is the best time to take vitamin and mineral supplements because the extra dietary fat enhances the absorption rate. Consume Free Foods as needed.
Meal 4	40 grams of protein, 0 carbs, and 0 grams of fat. Make sure to eat plenty of Free Foods, such as a big salad, along with your protein source. **NOTE:** Add 25 grams of fat to this meal if you don't eat fats in meal #5! Consume 5-15 grams of psyllium husk fiber or organic flax seed along with a minimum of 8 ounces of fluid before eating dinner.
Meal 5	(Dessert) 40 grams of protein, 12 grams of carbs, and 25 grams of fat. This meal should be consumed 1-3 hours after meal #4.
Total Calories and Macronutrients	
1 gram of protein = 4 calories, 1 gram of carbs = 4 calories, and 1 gram of fat = 9 calories.	
Total daily proteins	200 grams = 800 calories (approximately 40% of daily caloric intake)
Total daily carbs	152 grams = 608 calories (approximately 30% of daily caloric intake)
Total daily fats	65 grams = 585 calories (approximately 30% of daily caloric intake)

Total daily calories	1,993 (approximately 2,000 calories)
Total daily fiber intake	30 grams
Cheat Day	
Saturday (Large Calorie Increase one day per week)	
Saturday is a much-less restrictive diet. You increase your calories and have the foods you desire beginning at dinner and lasting until you go to bed. For example:	
100 grams of proteins	400 calories
400 grams of carbohydrates	1,600 calories
130 grams of fats	1,170 calories
400 + 1,600 + 1,170 = 3,170 calories on cheat day	

Functional Alert: Counting macronutrient ratios enables you to stay within a certain calorie range while keeping your carbs, fats, and proteins where they need to be for your particular body type!

Ronnie's Functional Diet Plan

I basically consume the same food every day. My Functional Diet is composed of approximately 40% protein, 40% carbs, and 20% fats. I have a pretty good response to insulin and can consume more carbs. However, my body functions horribly on fast burning (refined) carbs containing flour, such as waffles, bagels, biscuits, pancakes, and most breads. I eat flourless organic bread that has to stay refrigerated. My body doesn't do well with most breakfast cereals, fruit juices, milk, dried fruits, pasta, macaroni and cheese, and many processed foods that rapidly break down to sugar. They cause me to feel tired and very hungry. Too many fats, especially saturated fats from red meat and cheese, make me gain body fat and don't provide me with as much energy as slow-burning carbohydrates composed of natural sugar. If I lower dietary fats too much, I always feel hungry!

I consume five meals daily. My meals consist of protein and carbs during the first three meals and then I cut out carbs during my last two meals and replace them with fats. I find fats to be very satisfying at night, but carbs make me hungry! I still eat Free Foods such as salads, green beans, etc., throughout the day. I have learned it's very important to add fats to meals three (pre-workout meal or 3:00 p.m. on non-training days) and five in order to remain fully functional. I never eat carbs without protein because it will stimulate my appetite! I consume protein and fiber at every meal to obtain a variety of amino acids and prebiotics. I drink two to three CARBmaster® yogurts/liquid egg white shakes daily to obtain adequate amounts of protein and probiotics. My fiber intake is around 35 grams per day. I consume 10-15 grams of psyllium husk (prebiotics) in 8 ounces of Powerade Zero™ before dinner. My sodium intake is around 2,000 mgs per day. I consume roughly 2,500 calories per day: 1,000 calories from 250 grams of protein, 1,000 calories from 250 grams of carbs, and 500 calories from 55 grams of fat. On my once-a-week cheat day, my calories are around 4,500. I tend to both carb- and fat-load on my cheat day. All my meals stay the same as on non-cheat days except for my dinner and nighttime snack. I find that cheating in the early part of the day leads to overeating, body-fat gain, and excessive fatigue.

Kathy's Functional Diet Plan

I basically consume the same food every day. My Functional Diet is composed of approximately 40% protein, 30% carbs, and 30% fats. I gain too much body fat consuming a lot of carbs because I don't have a very good response to insulin. It doesn't matter whether the carbs come from natural sugar or refined sugar; they both increase my appetite and cause my belly to swell. However, the refined carbs are much worse! I have more energy and less bloating, stay fuller longer, and gain less body fat by eating a little more dietary fats and a little less carbs. The key for me is to eat only a very small amount of fruit and starchy carbs. Primary emphasis is placed on non-starchy carbs (Free Foods), assorted fats, and lean protein!

I consume five meals daily. I take in a variety of fats (unsaturated and saturated) three times per day. However, approximately three-fourths of my fats come from peanut butter, cashews, almonds, and mixed nuts. The other fourth comes from cheese (saturated fat). I add fats to meals three (pre-workout meal or at 3:00 p.m. on non-training days), four, and five. I have carbs during meal one (breakfast) and during meal three (pre-workout or at 3:00 p.m. on non-training days). I have learned that it's very important to add some carbs to meal three to remain fully functional. I only consume carbs during breakfast and pre-workout! I never eat carbs without protein because they stimulate my appetite. I always consume enough carbs to keep me from going in and out of ketosis. This prevents excessive blood sugar/insulin imbalances and the release of excessive amounts of pro-inflammatory cytokines and free radicals. I still eat Free Foods such as salads, green beans, etc., throughout the day. I consume protein and fiber at every meal to obtain a variety of amino acids and prebiotics. I drink two to three CARBmaster® yogurt/liquid egg white shakes daily to obtain adequate amounts of protein and probiotics. My fiber intake is around 35 grams per day. I consume 10-15 grams of psyllium husk (prebiotics) in 8 ounces of Powerade Zero™ before dinner. My sodium intake is around 2,000 mgs per day. I consume roughly 1,800 calories per day: 720 calories from 180 grams of protein, 540 calories from 60 grams of fats, and 540 calories from 135 grams of carbs. On my once-a-week cheat day, my calories are around 3,800. I tend to both carb- and fat-load on my cheat day. All my meals stay the same as on non-cheat days except for my dinner and nighttime snack. I find that cheating in the early part of the day leads to overeating, body-fat gain, and excessive fatigue.

Functional Alert: Our Functional Diets have helped our immune systems significantly, guarding against colds, infections, viruses, and various types of flu. Our immune systems could not have done this prior to starting the diets. According to recent data released in a joint study by Gallup and Healthways, sick days cost the U.S. economy $84 billion each year.[2] Except in Washington, DC, and San Francisco, employers are not required by law to provide paid sick days for employees. Therefore, approximately 70% of workers typically go to work when they are sick with the stomach flu or other contagious diseases.[3] Clearly this means it's time to start doing some immune system building using **Functional Training with a Fork**!

Dessert

Our last meal of the day is considered our dessert. We usually eat it 1 to 2 hours after our dinner. Some people think eating before going to bed will cause them to gain weight, but just the opposite is true when you incorporate a carb curfew! If you avoid eating before going to bed, it causes you to feel deprived. It's a classic example of why people give up and binge on junk food late at night! Unfortunately, the vast majority of people think the most effective way to lose weight is by not eating anything late at night before going to bed. Not eating after dinner creates a problem for many people. They suffer hunger pangs throughout the night and eat a huge breakfast the following day, which makes them tired and affects their daily performance. Eating the proper macronutrients/food late at night is a key factor in remaining on a Functional Diet! It's what you eat at night that makes you gain weight, not eating at night. If you eat a lot of junk food high in carbs and/or fats before going to bed, you are going to pack on the pounds.

The following nighttime dessert helps us get rid of any cravings we may have for sweets. It also completes our daily nutritional requirements and helps us get a good night's sleep. We add 1-2 CARBmaster® yogurts into a plastic cup. Then we add 6 oz of non-cooked liquid egg whites, and 1 level tablespoon of Non-GMO Smart Balance®

peanut butter and/or PB2 peanut butter powder, and stir before eating with a spoon. We prefer CARBmaster® yogurt because it's lower in carbs/sugar and taste better than the other yogurt we currently have access to.

You can also make this dessert using 2 scoops of low-carb/low-cholesterol whey protein powder in water, along with Non-GMO natural peanut butter or PB2 peanut butter powder. More than 90% of the fat is removed from the peanut. PB2 can be ordered off the Internet or found in local grocery stores. It makes a great choice for those who struggle to control their intake of peanut butter or need to avoid fats during the last meal of the day. We avoid fats (peanut butter) during our last meal (dessert) if the fat limits have been reached during dinner (meal #4).

If we are still hungry, we have our choice of Free Foods such as microwavable green vegetables or something crunchy we can eat with our hands (such as celery or carrots). We have learned that mindless eating with one's hands leads to weight gain. By changing the types of foods you eat with your hands, you lower your caloric intake and lose weight. This allows you to turn a bad habit into a good habit!

Authors' Note: *Note that 8 ounces (one cup) of liquid egg whites contain 25 grams of protein. Liquid egg whites are pasteurized in liquid form, not raw egg whites separated from whole eggs that can cause salmonella. Liquid egg whites mix well with your favorite protein powders, yogurts, smoothies, drinks, or food with or without cooking and are 100% absorbable by the body. They contain no fat or cholesterol, unlike meat, and can be cooked or drunk. This makes them the purest, healthiest, and most versatile form of protein known to man! Liquid egg whites are odorless, virtually tasteless, and are extremely convenient for people on a busy schedule. They taste like a cold melted milkshake when combined with CARBmaster® yogurt that is made from whey protein concentrate! We recommend starting out gradually until your stomach adjusts to the extra protein coming from the egg whites.*

Some of our clients prefer to strain their liquid egg whites while pouring them on top of their yogurt before mixing. A stainless steel mesh wire strainer with a handle works great. Do not use a blender to mix up the liquid egg whites and yogurt because it will make them taste bitter! A large number of Americans have high cholesterol, which increases your risk for heart attack and stroke. Make smart decisions at mealtime by incorporating liquid egg whites into your daily diet to help lower your cholesterol, body-fat levels, and excess fluid trapped in the tissues of the body. Liquid egg whites (cooked or drunk) are healthier to consume on a frequent basis than all meats. Liquid egg whites don't contain cholesterol, but whole eggs contain a substantial amount.

Many of our dedicated clients have accomplished amazing body-fat loss transformations by drinking liquid egg whites mixed with one CARBmaster® yogurt (Kroger's grocery store brand that contain only 60 calories per container) or other brands of yogurt that are very low in sugar and calories, for 2-4 of their daily meals. The beauty of pasteurized liquid egg whites and yogurt is that they can be conveniently mixed in a shaker and packed in a cooler.

Protein

Protein should make up the base of all your meals (e.g. skinless chicken breast, fish, lean beef, and liquid egg whites). It helps stabilize blood-sugar levels and it helps counterbalance the effects carbs/sugar have on the pleasure center of the brain (the part of the brain that tells you, I want more food) by stimulating the reward center of the brain (the part of the brain that tells you, I've had enough food)! In order to remain on a Functional Diet, you must consume enough protein in each meal to keep you full and to maintain stable blood-sugar levels. Most Americans do just the opposite! They consume mostly carbs and/or fats in a meal, causing sugar levels to skyrocket, which promotes hunger!

The body also has more difficulty turning protein and fibrous Free Foods into body fat than carbs and fats. You need to consume plenty of protein in every meal throughout the entire day, but not so much that you begin to gain body fat or can't lose weight. Consuming too much of anything—even protein that increases your metabolism approximately three times more than carbs or fats—can cause you to gain body fat. The proper amounts of protein help keep you full so you can avoid the more fattening foods composed of carbs and fats. Dietary protein not only builds stronger bones and muscles, it also builds stronger tendons and ligaments, especially when incorporated with Functional Training.

Functional Alert: Consistent intake of protein on a daily basis reduces your appetite by signaling the reward system in the brain.[5] This reward system consist of a group of neural structures that strengthen future behavior!

Protein usually takes longer to leave your stomach than carbs and this keeps you fuller for longer periods of time. Protein also causes the body to secrete a hormone called leptin, which tells our brains that our stomachs are full. However, if you have very high body-fat levels, you are more than likely leptin-resistant. Once you get your body-fat levels down, you will no longer be resistant to the hormone, and the protein you consume will cause your body to secrete the proper amounts of leptin to help control your appetite. The protein-based foods we consume, especially liquid egg whites, contain an essential amino acid called tryptophan that leads to serotonin production. Serotonin is a hormone and neurotransmitter that is vital for regulating mood, appetite, and GI tract function.[6] Approximately 90% of serotonin is found in the GI tract.[7] A deficiency of serotonin from not consuming enough protein can lead to irritable bowel syndrome, depression, and anxiety as well as a tendency to eat more high-carbohydrate foods.

When most people hear the word protein, they mistakenly think of it only as a muscle-toning agent instead of understanding that its nature's primary appetite suppressant. In order to beat hunger and have energy throughout the day, you have to stay well-hydrated and eat enough lean protein and fiber in every meal. When you consume the right food, you burn a good amount of calories in the digestion process. The burning of calories through digestion is referred to as the thermic effect of food. All calories are not the same! This is because for every 100 calories of protein consumed, approximately 30 calories will be burned through digestion, which increases your metabolism. In contrast, for every 100 calories of carbs or fats consumed, only about 10 calories will be burned through digestion. Therefore, consuming more calories from protein than fats and carbs leaves less body fat for Dysfunctional Toxins to take refuge in or cause chronic inflammation and oxidation!

Allow us to illustrate:

Thermic Effect of Food	
Protein	30% metabolic boost
Carbohydrates	10% metabolic boost
Fats	10% metabolic boost

Daily calorie burn during digestion of 2,000 calories	
2000 calories coming from protein alone	600 calories burned during digestion
2,000 calories coming from carbohydrates alone	only 200 calories burned during digestion
2,000 calories coming from fat alone	only 200 calories burned during digestion

You burn 3 times more calories during the digestion of protein than carbs or fats.[8] In the estimates above, 600 calories are being burned during digestion from protein, 200 from carbs, and 200 from fats. In addition, a higher thermogenic effect is observed after a meal composed of whole foods containing fiber, than after an equivalent calorie meal composed of highly processed foods containing no fiber. Consuming more protein and fiber improves metabolic function and decreases appetite! This leaves fewer calories to cause obesity, diabetes, heart disease, cancer, etc., because more calories are being burned when food is being digested. In addition, you will consume fewer calories by replacing a modest amount of carbs and fats with protein. The accumulative effect of combining a high-protein, high-fiber diet has obvious benefits for anyone who is trying to control their body-fat levels and improve their functional health. It's hard to stay full when you cut calories from carbs and/or fats, if you don't replace an adequate amount of those calories with lean protein. In fact, the lack of consuming enough lean protein in each meal in order to satisfy the reward center of the brain to stay full is often the primary reasons for a failed body- fat loss program!

If you are one of those people who can't stomach a diet composed of 40% protein or you are involved in a lot of endurance-type exercises, then you may have no choice but to reduce protein just a little and make up the extra calories with carbs and/or fats. No one, including bodybuilders, needs to take in more than 300 grams of protein per day spread out over 6 meals, at 50 grams per meal, regardless of their body weight, how fast their metabolism might be, or how many calories they burn through exercise. At that point, you would need to add more carbs and/or fats to fulfill your daily energy requirements.

Functional Alert: A crock pot makes lean meat (protein) tender!

Healthy Carbs and Fats

You need to consume enough carbs derived from natural sugar and healthy fats to fuel your body. In order to train with the needed intensity to get results, feel good, and have proper brain function, you need some carbs and fats! Protein stimulates the "reward" center of the brain and makes you feel satisfied. Carbohydrates stimulate the "pleasure" center of the brain and makes you want more! Therefore, carbohydrates should never be consumed without adequate amounts of protein to counterbalance the appetite stimulating effects that blood sugar has on the brain! Small to moderate amounts of fats, on the other hand, can be consumed without protein or with Free Foods. This is because fats alone won't cause sugar levels to soar as carbs will when consumed alone.

Free Foods List:

Broccoli	Celery	Artichokes	Garlic
Green beans	Cucumbers	Mushrooms	Ginger
Asparagus	Lettuce	Eggplant	Scallions
Cauliflower	Okra	Turnips	Dill Pickles
Brussels sprouts	Green peppers	Sauerkraut	Chili peppers
Spinach	Zucchini	Radishes	Tomatoes
Greens	Squash	Chives	
Cabbage	Onions	Alfalfa sprouts	

Authors' Note: *These are some of the Free Foods available that don't count toward daily total calories or carbohydrates. They have no appreciable effect on blood-sugar levels and caloric intake. These are the only kind of carbs that can be consumed without the presence of adequate protein. The vegetables on this list are mostly composed of fiber and vital nutrients.*

If you skip breakfast, you are going in the wrong direction! After fasting all night, your body has become depleted of blood sugar and amino acids. If your breakfast doesn't include carbs and protein, you will lose muscle, experience fatigue, and binge eat later on in the day. Over time, this slows down your metabolism. Most breakfast cereals are carbs with refined sugar on them! If you get up in the morning and eat a bowl of cereal with milk (both mostly carbs and sugar), you will be starving an hour or two later due to the rapid rise and fall of your blood sugar. It's a desperate feeling! In addition, the lack of protein and excess carbs/sugar causes leptin levels to remain too low, which tells your brain that you are still hungry for food. Leptin is a hunger hormone produced by the fat cells in your body. Leptin levels go up when you gain body fat. Likewise, they go down when you begin losing body fat. This often leads to increased hunger at the beginning of a body-fat loss program. However, a high-protein, lower-carb/sugar diet helps counterbalance this effect. Consuming egg whites (protein) and oats (fibrous carb) for breakfast instead of foods such as sugary cereals, bagels, pancakes, juices, and milk will prevent you from going hungry and cause you to lose body fat! In order to prevent leptin resistance, you need to consume plenty of fiber and lean protein for breakfast and lay off the refined sugar. Leptin resistance occurs when your leptin is excessively high. The receptors that leptin bind to stop functioning properly and fat cells keep signaling the brain that the body is hungry! [9] If you have a lot of body fat, especially in the midsection, it's a sign that you are leptin resistant! A higher-protein, lower-carb diet makes it easier for leptin to reach the brain so that you feel satisfied eating fewer calories.[10] This helps reduce leptin resistance and your metabolism increases.[11] Researchers have shown that testosterone therapy also helps prevent leptin resistance.[12]

Functional Alert: Over time **Functional Training with a Fork** eliminates leptin resistance. This makes it much easier to remain on a Functional Diet!

Refined Sugar and Artificial Sweeteners

Refined Sugar is a highly destructive Dysfunctional Toxin. It's even more destructive than saturated fat! Refined sugar is rarely listed as an ingredient. Instead, it usually shows up as high-fructose corn syrup, dextrose, honey, maltose, maple sugar, molasses, evaporated cane sugar, agave nectar, and fruit juice concentrate. Artificial sweeteners are also considered Dysfunctional Toxins. We believe some are worse than others. The artificial sweeteners that cause the most negative effects on gut bacteria are obviously the worst and, we believe, put the largest damper on body-fat loss. If you experience stomach upset, headaches, or dizziness from a particular artificial sweetener, your body is letting you know it's harming the good bacteria in your gut! It's important to understand that lowering good bacteria in the gut slows down the metabolism to some degree.[1]

Functional Alert: Consuming plenty of probiotics and prebiotics help counterbalance the effects artificial sweeteners have on the gut!

Artificial sweeteners don't contain calories or spike blood sugar and/or insulin levels to any appreciable degree.[2] Therefore, you are much better off using them in small amounts to replace real sugar. However, using none at all is best, especially if you get a bad reaction such as a headache or stomachache. It's important to note that we don't experience headaches or upset stomachs using tiny amounts of most artificial sweeteners, but we have with large amounts! That's our body sending us signals to let us know what's right and wrong. Many people, including us, also get headaches and/or stomachaches from refined sugar. It appears artificial sweeteners and all refined sugars have some degree of negative effects on gut bacteria![3,4] But unlike refined sugar, artificial sweeteners don't increase your appetite if consumed in small amounts.[5,6] We don't know the long-term consequences of using artificial sweeteners, but we do with refined sugar!

Functional Alert: The consumption of refined sugar has been associated with a significant reduction in leptin levels. It also stimulates the pleasure center of the brain.[7]

This means refined sugar will make your appetite soar!

We believe refined sugar is much worse than artificial sweeteners for causing life-threatening medical conditions such as diabetes, heart disease, cancer, and obesity. Artificial sweeteners do lower good bacteria in the GI tract, but they must be consumed in very large amounts to be as lethal as refined sugar.[8] It's best to keep sugar consumption to an absolute minimum and consume artificial sweeteners in small amounts to optimize your health.[9] It's hard to believe there are highly educated people who still consume beverages such as sweetened tea, colas, fruit juices, and sports drinks full of sugar on a daily basis. Many are unaware that fruit juice isn't the same as intact fruit and usually has as much sugar as classic sodas. Beware of food labels that claim fruit juices and smoothies have a lower sugar content than soda. If they do, it's usually not by much!

Functional Alert: People who drink beverages containing sugar consume more calories on those days than on the days they don't have sugary drinks.[10] Sugar adds to their daily caloric intake and stimulates their appetites. Some people are getting all of the calories they need in a day from drinking sugary drinks alone. In addition, some people drink diet drinks so they can eat more junk food. That just doesn't work for losing body fat!

All carbs eventually turn into sugar, including those from fruits (e.g., apples) and many vegetables (e.g., sweet potatoes). However, consuming slow-burning fibrous carbs (plant-based foods) creates fewer sugar/insulin spikes; slows down the digestion rate of food, keeping you full longer; provides more energy and essential nutrients; and doesn't stimulate your appetite like faster-burning carbs (refined carbs) that produce more insulin. A lower-insulin-producing diet containing foods high in fiber lowers the risk of most life-threatening diseases and of becoming obese.[11]

Functional Alert: Refined sugar appears to be just as addictive as recreational drugs!

Refined carbs such as pure sugar are considered unhealthy because they are lacking in nutrients and there is no fiber to slow down the rate of digestion, thus causing a spike in blood sugar/insulin followed by a crash. The rapid drop in blood sugar stimulates your appetite, making you hungrier and more fatigued. This means if you consume food containing a very small amount of sugar, you need some form of protein and fibrous food in order to slow down the absorption rate and help deter the release of blood sugar/insulin. For example, if you are going to have a bowl of non-GMO Cheerios™, instead of adding milk—which contains more carbs, sugar, and very little protein—add liquid egg whites mixed with CARBmaster® yogurt or protein powder mixed in water.[21] You can add something (e.g., blueberries) to enhance the overall nutritional value.

Sugar Alcohols

Sugar alcohols are contained in diet foods such as protein bars. They do contain calories and do spike insulin levels. Each gram of sugar alcohol can turn into as much as 2.4 calories per gram compared to 4 calories per gram of sugar.[1] When counting carbohydrates from protein bars made with sugar alcohols, subtract half of the grams of sugar alcohol listed on the food label. If the protein bar says it contains a total of 20 carbohydrates on the nutritional label (10 coming from sugar and 10 coming from sugar alcohol), we recommend counting this as 15 carbs toward your daily macros. Sugar alcohols may cause gastrointestinal (GI) distress, so eat with caution.

Alcohol

Alcoholic beverages would be considered a carbohydrate equaling 7 calories per gram. For those who have a daily drink, it goes toward your daily macronutrients. It's best to avoid drinking a lot of alcohol before going to bed—it increases triglyceride levels and slows down your metabolism. The effects are even worse when a lot of alcohol is mixed with dietary fats.[1,2] Furthermore, when your body gets finished metabolizing the alcohol, it disrupts your deep-sleep cycle, which decreases growth hormone output.[3,4]

Functional Alert: Alcoholic beverages will boost daily caloric intake, blood sugar, and insulin. They can also stimulate your appetite. One drink consists of one 4 oz of wine, 12 oz beer, or 1 oz of liquor. Excess alcohol is defined as having more than one drink per day. Excess alcohol causes an increase in pro-inflammatory cytokines and free radicals!

Mixing Carbs and Fats

Avoid mixing a substantial amount of carbs and fats in the same meal, except before your evening workouts or late afternoon meals on non-workout days and in your weekly cheat meal. It's much easier to eat fewer calories if you don't combine significant amounts of carbs and fats in the same meal because the carbs stimulate your appetite, causing you to eat more fats, which are high in calories.

Functional Alert: The Functional Diet keeps your energy level stable throughout the day! There are no highs and lows that are experienced on diet plans that allow you to eat moderate amounts of sugar, eat carbs alone, or combine a considerable amount of carbs and fats in each meal!

Natural sugar (e.g., bananas) increase one's appetite and causes a spike in blood sugar/insulin. However, a banana would create a much smaller blood sugar/insulin spike than refined sugar because it contains some fiber and its chemical makeup is different. Take note that non-starchy carbs on our Free Foods List don't cause blood sugar or insulin spikes! These foods don't contain any appreciable calories and are okay to combine with fats. A good example is a big salad with one tablespoon of extra virgin olive oil used as dressing. Add some extra-lean meat and you have a healthy meal that will keep you full. In other words, you can eat an extra-lean steak and salad for dinner, but you need to avoid having a baked potato. Likewise, you can have a baked piece of fish, a potato, and a salad for lunch, but don't add any fats such as olive oil or butter to the fish or potato, or any type of dressings or oils containing fats to the salad. However, you should mix some carbs and fats around 3 p.m. before evening workouts and on non-training days to remain energetic.

Functional Alert: Keeping carbs and fats separated lowers blood sugar and insulin spikes. This lowers the body's production of pro-inflammatory cytokines and free radicals, thus lowering inflammation and oxidation in the body![1]

The single largest factor that has contributed to the obesity epidemic in America is gorging on a mixture of carbs and fats during dinner and/or before going to bed! This often causes chronic heartburn and acid reflux. A lot of people who fall into that category tend to skip breakfast because their GI tract was under assault the night before. Stop consuming any measurable amounts of carbs before going to bed to help prevent body-fat gain. It's best to stick to fats, protein, and Free Foods that don't provoke an insulin response late in the day, regardless of whether your body responds better to carbs or fats. Moreover, consuming a lot of carbs before going to bed will cause a spike in serotonin levels.[2] You want serotonin to be at its lowest levels during deep sleep and highest when fully awake during the daytime. This helps prevent bouts of falling asleep and waking up throughout the night. It also helps keep you happier during waking hours.

Functional Alert: What are you bringing to the dinner table that could be sabotaging your body-fat loss efforts?

Pre-Workout Meal

While it's fine to consume slow-burning carbs and protein after a workout completed earlier in the day, the most important time to be fully fueled is before workouts. How you arrange carbs and fats allows you to choose what your insulin spikes do in terms of what is getting bigger: your muscle cells or fat cells. Your body does best with just protein and carbs before an early morning workout in order to jump-start protein synthesis (building muscle tone). However, as the day lingers, energy levels will plummet, and you'll do better consuming fats along with your carbs and protein before an evening workout in order to jump-start protein synthesis. The prolonged insulin secretion from combining carbs and fats in the same meal helps store protein (amino acids) in muscle cells.[3] A pre-workout meal in the late-afternoon composed of protein, carbs, and fats allows you to double dip: You reap the benefits of elevated blood amino acids and insulin during and after your training session. This elevation of amino acids and insulin will help reduce the muscle-eating hormone cortisol following an intense training session.[4] It also prevents you from having to take in carbs post-workout! Adding protein, carbs, and fats prior to your evening training sessions primes the pump and encourages muscle tone, better muscle contractions, and more vascularity, and provides you with sustained energy so you can train with greater intensity through the entire workout.

Functional Alert: Never work out on an empty stomach and always give your food time to digest. If you plan to work out and it has been more than three hours since you last ate, it's time to fuel up. If you neglect to eat protein, carbs, and fats before working out in the evening, you can expect to run out of energy fast and possibly pass out from low blood-sugar levels. Fats are difficult to digest for breakfast and can actually interfere with a workout performed earlier in the day. You don't require fats, in addition to carbs and protein, prior to workouts performed earlier in the day because energy reserves will be much higher. As the day progresses, your dietary fats will begin to deplete and they will need to be restored. Fatigue from a lack of fuel or improper fuel before an intense workout is one of the reasons why people cut their workouts short!

Timing Carbs

The most important time to consume carbs is breakfast and late afternoon/evening pre-workouts, when they will more readily be used for fuel. Eating an appreciable amount of carbs 2-3 hours before going to bed, even if it's during late evening post-workouts, prevents a lot of people from losing body fat. We believe that consuming a lot of fast-burning carbs (e.g., maltodextrin or refined sugars) post-workout is a big mistake! First of all, this causes hypoglycemia, resulting in a huge spike in blood sugar followed by a rapid drop.[1] People feel lethargic instead of energized. Second, taking in refined sugars post-workout can cause irritable bowel syndrome. The refined sugars increase bacteria's ability to form biofilms that stick to the intestinal epithelial cells, which cause stomach distress.[2] Anytime you overindulge in carbs, some of the extra sugar will escape into the colon and will feed the bad bacteria in your GI tract, which will build up Dysfunctional Toxins in your colon. Not only do these Dysfunctional Toxins cause many medical conditions, they are partly to blame for obese people having distended stomachs.[3]

Functional Alert: Consuming fast-acting carbs within an hour after exercise is not needed to fuel muscle tone. In fact, many so-called recovery protein shakes often contain lots of refined sugar that will sabotage your body-fat loss efforts. A high sugar snack or so-called recovery drink (containing high sugar) after working out will stop some of the benefits of exercise- induced growth hormone and damage your endothelium (inner lining of arteries)!

Timing Fats

The most important time to consume fats is before workouts, in the evening, and/or before going to bed. Fats provide a sustained release of energy to ensure you don't run out of fuel while working out. They also take a long time to digest, which helps prevent insomnia and waking up in the middle of the night hungry. Fats deter muscle breakdown by preventing amino acids from being burned for fuel while sleeping. Consuming fats before going to bed also allows the body to release more growth hormone while asleep than carbs.

Growth hormone burns body fat, builds muscle tone, and makes you appear more youthful. This hormone is released multiple times while you are asleep.[1] Protein and fats don't blunt the release of growth hormone when ingested before going to bed.[2] However, carbs do decrease growth hormone output when consumed in substantial amounts 2-3 hours before going to bed.[3] Consuming a lot of carbs before going to bed keeps blood-sugar levels elevated as your body begins to release growth hormone while asleep. This interferes with your cells' ability to uptake blood sugar and get it out of the blood stream. The leftover blood sugar turns to body fat and some remains in the blood stream. The extra blood sugar and insulin that is secreted while sleeping often causes you to feel sleepy and sluggish the following day. When your blood sugar is high at night, your kidneys try to get rid of it by urinating, and you end up going to the bathroom all night long.[4] Consequently, the following day you are tired and end up eating more to try to get energy. When people switch from carbs to fats before going to bed, while consuming the same amount of calories, they lose more body fat because they experience less hunger, sleep better, increase growth hormone output, and have more energy the following day!

Functional Alert: If at any time you get ravenous hunger pangs or start feeling shaky throughout the day, it's a sign you are low on carbs and/or fats. In order to stabilize your blood-sugar levels, eat the macronutrient or macronutrients you are lacking and some protein!

Consuming a little bit of dietary fat goes a long way in keeping you full and providing you with the energy needed to function. Fats contain 9 calories per gram. Alcohol contains 7 calories per gram. Protein and carbs contain only 4 calories per gram.[5] When looking at healthy fat sources such as extra virgin olive oil or natural peanut butter, the label reads 1 tablespoons as one serving for extra virgin olive oil and 2 tablespoons as one serving for peanut butter. If you have ever actually measured this out, it's not a lot in quantity, but it's a lot of calories. It's very easy to get more than you think! Unfortunately, many people add a lot of fattening dressings or oils to their salads, and they end up having as many calories as hamburgers and fries from a local fast-food restaurant. Never order a salad at a restaurant without asking them to put the dressing on the side. Then use a very tiny amount, if any at all. In cases like this, we believe a lot of people know how to eat right, but just refuse to do it or think they can't do it. The reason they often think they can't is because they have not allowed enough time for their hunger hormones (leptin[6], ghrelin[7], insulin[8], cortisol[9], serotonin[10], dopamine[11], and testosterone[12,13]) to stabilize so they no longer crave those types of foods.

The Best to Worst Fats

It's important to be aware of the types of fat you are consuming from food. Unsaturated fats, omega-3s, omega-6s, saturated fats, and trans fats affect the body in different ways. The following is a list of the best to worst fats.

1. Monounsaturated fats and omega-3s tie for first place.
2. Omega-6s
3. Saturated fats
4. Trans fats[14,15]

Foods containing monounsaturated fats
- Macadamia nut oil (safest monounsaturated fat spray oil for cooking)[16]
- Extra virgin olive oil (second safest monounsaturated fat spray oil for cooking

due to its high antioxidant content, which helps prevent oxidation)[17,18]
- Avocados
- Olives
- Nuts (also very high in omega-6s)
- Peanut butter

Foods containing omega-3 fats (polyunsaturated fats)
- Fish (wild caught salmon is our #1 pick)
- Macadamia nut oil
- Flax seed
- Macadamia nuts (contains the least amount of omega-6s of all nuts)[19]
- Cashews and almonds (contains a moderate amount of omega-6s)
- Walnuts (contains a high amount of omega-6s)
- Grass-fed beef (also contains saturated fats)

Foods containing omega-6 fats (polyunsaturated fats)
- Nuts
- Corn oil
- Soybean oil
- Sunflower oil
- Safflower oil
- Cotton seed oil[20]

We recommend avoiding all omega-6 spray oils for cooking, except macadamia nut oil and olive oil, due to their ability to easily oxidize under high-heat conditions.[21] In addition, GMO cooking oils such as corn, canola, and soybean are potentially toxic without being exposed to heat.

Foods containing saturated fats
- Coconut oil is the safest cooking spray oil under high-heat conditions (even safer than macadamia nut oil and olive oil) because it does not oxidize.[22,23]
- High-fat cuts of meat
- Coconut and palm oil
- Cheese
- Butter
- Lard
- Whole-fat dairy products (ice cream, milk, and cream)
- Chicken skin

Foods containing trans fats
- ☐ Fried foods: French fries, chicken, fish, tortilla chips, etc.
- ☐ Commercially-baked pastries, doughnuts, cookies, muffins, cakes, pizza dough, etc.
- ☐ Packaged snack foods: crackers, candy bars, chips, etc.
- ☐ Stick margarine and vegetable shortening
- ☐ Most fast food[24]

Replacing saturated fats and omega-6 fats with monounsaturated fats and omega-3 fats can help lower inflammation and oxidation throughout the body. This promotes healthy functioning of your metabolic, endocrine, cardiovascular, and immune systems. Another major benefit is improved brain function! We advise consuming more omega-3s and monounsaturated fats to lower inflammation and oxidation; limiting omega-6s to lower inflammation and oxidation; keeping saturated fat consumption very low to aid in preventing insulin resistance and increasing LDL cholesterol levels; and avoiding all trans fats to deter chronic inflammation and oxidation.[25-31]

There is no ideal ratio of omega-3 and omega-6 intake because there isn't enough evidence to determine where the line should exactly be drawn. All we know is that omega-6s create more inflammation and oxidation than omega-3s.

Functional Alert: Eating fried or baked food cooked in hydrogenated oils or omega-6 oils is linked to health-threatening conditions. Using oil repeatedly or making it smoke will make it oxidize sooner. Think about this the next time you are tempted to eat fried food at a restaurant!

It's wise to replace some omega-6s with omega-3s (e.g., salmon) and monounsaturated fats (e.g., peanut butter). Omega-6s are found in seeds and nuts and in the oils extracted from them. The omega-3 to omega-6 ratios of cooking oils vary greatly. Some of them contain mostly omega 6s. For example, corn, soybean, sunflower, safflower, and cottonseed oil contain the most omega-6s, and are almost completely lacking in omega-3s. Unfortunately, these five oils are most commonly used in highly processed food because omega-6s won't turn rancid like omega-3s do. Omega-6s are used to extend the shelf life of unhealthy processed food and they are inexpensive with high profit margins. Another thing to consider is how easily omega-3 supplements such as fish oil can rapidly turn rancid on the shelf. Once they turn rancid and become excessively oxidized, they can damage your body at a cellular level. For example, taking fish oil supplements was shown to cause prostate cancer in a study performed by Fred Hutchinson Cancer Research Center in Seattle, Washington.[32] Therefore, we believe taking fish oil supplements should be avoided until they figure out a way to prevent the oil from turning rancid and oxidizing. In addition, the fish oil would need to be obtained from wild-caught fish on the bottom of the food chain in the cleanest waters available (e.g., the Pacific Northwest) to prevent excess mercury exposure. The key to getting healthy omega-3s is eating more real food such as wild-caught fish on the bottom of the food chain caught in the most unpolluted water.[33-36]

Functional Alert: We believe it's very dangerous to consume fish oil containing fish coming from China!

Basic Concepts of Losing Body Fat

The basic concepts of losing body fat are simple to understand. While your body is at rest, it burns on average about 50% carbs and 50% fats for fuel.[1] The average overall resting metabolic rate during sleep is the same as your resting metabolic rate during the day.[2,3] Walking around performing daily activities without getting your heart rate elevated also burns approximately 50% carbs and 50% fats. When you are exercising intensely, your body switches over to burning approximately 70% carbs and only 30% fats for fuel.[4,5]

Functional Alert: It takes longer during intense workouts for a female's body to change over to using carbohydrates as the dominant energy source. This is one of several reasons that many females function better consuming fewer carbs than males![6]

Formulas that calculate your needed daily caloric intake are a mere estimation due to countless variables such as age, body-fat percentages, weight, lean muscle mass, activity level, and individual differences in our bodies. Its mere guesswork and nothing else! Caloric totals are often not accurate on restaurant menus and contain more calories than listed.[7] This is one of several reasons to avoid restaurants if you are trying to lose weight!

It's very important to realize that deviating from your diet by only 250-500 calories per day is all it can take to stall your long-term body-fat loss goals, thus making portion control of the utmost importance. You must get on the right plan and stick to it. Males should never go below 1,500 calories per day to lose body fat and females should never go below 1,200. Everyone's body type is different, and your metabolic rate changes as you begin to add muscle tone and increase energy expenditure through exercise.

Functional Alert: If you have a slower metabolism, then you will have to eat less food than someone with a faster metabolism. Those who desire to gain weight simply need to gradually eat larger quantities of healthy food. Loading up on junk food to gain weight is very unhealthy and so is eating junk food to lose weight!

Everyone should eat the maximum amount of calories for their body type that allows them to lose weight at the appropriate rate. Those of you with a slow metabolism may need fewer overall calories than the 2,000 calorie per day sample baseline Functional Diet we have provided to get body-fat levels where they need to be. Others will need to increase calories beyond the sample baseline Functional Diet. Once you hit a plateau and are unable to lose any more inches, then you will want to reduce calories by 250-500 per day while keeping protein at approximately 40% of your total daily caloric intake. This constitutes 1,750 to 3,500 calories a week reduction from diet alone, allowing you to lose around one pound of body weight per week. By cutting 500 calories a day, you may find you lose around 2 pounds a week when training hard with weights and adding in some cardio. This rate of weight loss is considered reasonable and healthy.

Strive to lose one to two pounds per week on the Functional Diet until you reach your body-fat loss goal. The more body fat you have, the longer it will take to get it off. At first, it may be tempting to cut out over 500 calories per day, but a realistic and lasting weight change happens gradually. Some can expect to lose as much as 5 pounds during their first week of a Functional Diet because reducing carbs decreases water weight.

Even if your body fat is at a dangerous level, give yourself enough time to lose weight and don't think you need to drop another 500 calories every week just because you are not losing weight in a linear fashion. Healthy body-fat loss occurs in increments over time! If you don't drop weight after 4 weeks, then you can reduce calories by another 250-500 per day if you are consistent with your Functional Exercise program. If you automatically start your weight-loss goals by consuming only 1,000 calories per day, you are going in the wrong direction! There is a problem with decreasing calories too abruptly, especially while exercising vigorously. Once you reach the point where calories get too low, you will have nowhere to go. You will begin to feel weak and lose muscle tone and strength, and the weight comes off slower because your body's metabolism slows down due to the drastic decrease in calories and muscle loss.

Losing body fat requires patience! Being stuck at a weight-loss plateau for weeks eventually happens to everyone who tries to lose weight, even though they are eating and exercising properly. Don't get discouraged and revert back to your bad eating habits. The body fat will eventually come off if you stay on track! If you stall for a month or longer, you need to exercise more and/or reduce calories. Using the same approach that worked at first will maintain your body-fat loss, but it may not lead to more body-fat loss. However, if you are new to weight training, you will still be losing body fat, even though the scale doesn't show it, because you will be building muscle. If you have been working out for a long time prior to going on the diet, then you will not build additional muscle while losing body fat. Your goal would be to maintain as much muscle as possible while reducing body fat gradually.

Success requires that you learn from mistakes along the way rather than losing hope and giving up. Failure is not uncommon when trying to do the right thing! If you are not getting results over time and feel as though you are doing the proper things, then either you aren't on the right diet or you are not following the proper work-out program to meet your individual needs. One of the most important factors in losing body fat is learning how to recognize why you failed, and then making the necessary adjustments to correct the problem.

Body-fat loss will still occur over time when following a super-low-calorie diet, but you will feel miserable and be highly prone to relapsing. This form of lifestyle isn't sustainable! This is why we highly recommend you stay away from fad diets that promote yo-yoing in weight and cause poor health. No one lasts long on starvation diets and they always end with a period of binge eating. You must not treat body-fat loss as a race in order to be successful. No one is successful over the long haul following fad diets! Experience has taught us that a lifestyle change is a gradual process for most. If you try to do everything at once, you can fall off the wagon.

Functional Alert: Don't punish yourself for being overweight by going on a starvation diet. It doesn't work!

You must begin your lifestyle change by stop eating at restaurants. That's step #1! The only time you should allow yourself to eat at a restaurant is during your designated once-a-week cheat day. Even healthier-sounding restaurant menu items usually sneak in extra calories by adding butter, oils, sugar, and MSG (appetite enhancer).[8] They also serve large portions because the obese and gluttonous people who keep restaurants in business want a lot of food. If you can't accomplish step #1, the chance is high that you won't be able to make it to step #2. Step #2 involves consuming more non-starchy vegetables (Free Foods), fruits, healthy fats, and lean protein in order to crowd out excess refined sugars and unhealthy fats in your diet. This allows you to focus on delicious food that should be part of any Functional Diet plan. Step #3 comes later, once you have adjusted to step #2. In step #3, you reduce calories by 250-500 per day if needed, while keeping macronutrient ratios in balance. It's very important that you follow these steps in precise order to avoid Functional Diet failure!

Functional Alert: Losing body fat requires replacing bad habits with good habits!

We understand that proper nutrition is by far the hardest part for people to stick to upfront; however, once you begin to see results and understand the relationship between diet and disease, it becomes an enjoyable lifestyle. Many people are confused about what constitutes a Functional Diet. In order to lose body fat and keep it off, you must also select the food you eat based on what it's doing to the inside of your body, not just how it's going to make you look. The Functional Diet is not a fad diet, but a sustainable lifestyle change. With a Functional Diet, it becomes easier to reduce your consumption of bad food because you know such food causes destruction to the body both internally and externally. When you begin to add in more food ranked high on the Functional Food Spectrum, it eventually crowds out the food on the lower end. Over time, this brings about a permanent lifestyle change. The Functional Diet works where others sometimes fail because you are adding Free Food and protein and lowering carbs and fats. The problem with most diets is that they have you taking away too much food at the beginning instead of adding the right kind of foods. This is the single biggest mistake one can make when making a permanent lifestyle change! People learn that they can no longer eat as much of the bad food once they start adding in the good food. On the Functional Diet you should not worry about counting caloric intake until your body adjusts to the added healthy food. Then you can gradually lower your calories if needed in order to lose body fat. Using an apps on your phone is a valuable tool for helping you stay on course. Once a weight-loss goal is reached, it's all about maintaining that weight from that point forward.

Everyone's body type is different and your metabolic rate changes as you begin to add muscle tone and increase energy expenditure through exercise. If you have a Functional Personal Trainer, he or she will make any needed adjustments to the baseline Functional Diet provided as you progress (for example, caloric and macronutrient increases or decreases). When people are overweight, they often struggle to control food cravings. Skipping meals can actually have a negative impact on long-term healthy weight management. In order to keep your metabolism speeding along, you need 4 to 6 smaller meals throughout the day. Calorie consumption shouldn't be the main focus in losing body fat. It's important to balance out the food you eat so there is less refined produce, plenty of fiber from raw food, and lean protein.

Losing body fat requires more than just counting calories. One of the problems with placing emphasis on calorie counting is that it focuses too much on the quantity of food rather than the quality. If you just think in terms of overall calories and replace protein with more carbs and fats, you will begin to get hungry and sluggish, lose muscle tone, get a soft appearance, slow down your metabolism, and put your body into fat-storing mode. Over the long-term, people notice they get too hungry to continue with a lower-calorie diet unless they are taking in the necessary lean protein and generous amounts of fiber. The end result is a failed body-fat loss program!

All males and females have something they want to change about their physique. We think it's the number one factor motivating us to continue pushing ourselves in the gym. We have noticed that more people are becoming fixated with their bodies. In today's society people are finally starting to be more concerned about their health. They don't just want the toned muscles, they want to be healthy, functioning, and energetic and live a long life filled with quality.

When it comes to exercising and eating healthy, there is no point in negativity. You just have to look forward and do the best you can. Functional Training and a Functional Diet go hand in hand. Functional Training is one of the best motivators for helping you stay on a Functional Diet. When people stop exercising, their healthy eating habits usually fall by the wayside. Lifting weights can get boring and repetitive and cardio is far worse, which is why some people quit. We urge you not to give up! Instead, hire a Functional Personal Trainer and ask them to change your Functional Training regimen with something new and different. It must stay inside the realm of what's outlined in this book (e.g., changing from straight sets to single-drop sets).

We are aware that genetics play a role in how everyone looks after they have done everything right, diet- and training-wise. However, from what we have seen as personal trainers, on the whole it's mostly lifestyle! If most thin adults had been brought up eating more with less activity, they would be overweight. Your genetics determine how much muscle you will be able to maintain while in a calorie deficit. Individuals who are genetically blessed will lose less muscle while dieting down. Some people have problems getting rid of fat and they lose muscle when they drop their calories too low. This has to do with something called a "partitioning effect" (where calories go when you eat more or where calories come from when you eat less).[9]

Genetically-gifted individuals (the lucky ones) have a much better partitioning effect than people with poor genetics. If you have great genetics, you will be able to store more calories in muscle cells and fewer in fat cells when you are in a calorie surplus. You will also use more calories from fat cells and less from muscle tissue when you are in a calorie deficit or performing cardio. You can expect to stay leaner and gain muscle tone easier than the average person. The beauty of the Functional Diet is that you can customize it to fit your own individual needs. We all have our strengths and weaknesses and are very special in our own unique way. It's important to be realistic and not waste your time comparing yourself to others. God has a purpose for each and every one of us. It's up to you to seek it out!

Most people fall somewhere in the middle when it comes to genetics. You can slow down a fast metabolism and you can speed up a slow one. Diet is the most important factor, weight training is second, and cardio is last. Everyone's metabolism begins to slow down around the age of thirty. If you have inherited a slow metabolism then you know what happens if you slack off your diet, weight training, and cardio. You start losing muscle and gaining body fat again! The great news is that your body chemistry will change over time as you acquire more muscle tone and eat a Functional Diet. Eating a Functional Diet, combined with Functional Training and Functional Cardio, greatly improves insulin sensitivity, your resting metabolism, and your active metabolism. This makes it easier to maintain a steady weight once you lose body fat and build some muscle tone.

Functional Alert: Since everyone has different metabolisms, workout routines, and food preferences, nutritional and exercise advice has to be specifically targeted for each individual!

Food Preparations

If you are serious about living a functional lifestyle, you must make food preparation a top priority! Prepare your meals in advance. Time management plays a key role in staying healthy and fit. Poor time-management skills leads to procrastination, which can lead to irresponsibility. Irresponsible food preparations is the #1 enemy in losing body fat and remaining unhealthy.

Food preparation is where the official work begins. Responsible people will consume the right food. This is what we refer to as doing the actual work. Once the week has been completed, you will feel satisfaction and reward yourself with a cheat day. Irresponsible people are not against preparing their meals in advance. However, when the actual moment arrives to begin food preparations, they can't see any instant gratification and this prevents them from following through with the task. In other words, they neglect to take small steps and become organized in order to achieve long-term goals. Food preparations is the easy part. If you find yourself struggling to do the easy part when life tests you, then simply look around and see all the wonderful things life has given you. This prevents you from making excuses and allows you to continue with food preparations.

When it comes to incorporating a permanent lifestyle change, we believe it's important for each individual to acquire the right mind-set! You do this by making your mind believe food preparation and exercising are just a regular daily routine such as going to work. In other words, they're not an option, but rather something you do every day without having the big over-reaching goal in mind. If you neglect to learn how to become a responsible person, you will be going in circles for the rest of your life!

Functional Alert: Many of you will need to hire a Functional Personal Trainer to motivate and hold you accountable for food preparations, weight-loss goals, and Functional Training. Being in the gym around other people exercising helps you stay focused on your goals. It's positive reinforcement!

In most cases, changing your lifestyle will involve not just yourself, but your family as well. Getting them on board may not be easy at first. Compromise is crucial for getting any stubborn family members to change their dietary habits. It's extremely important to listen to what your family members have to say to prevent them from getting angry and turning the whole ordeal into an argument. You must listen to their points of view and be able to verbalize it back to them. A tip for helping them give up their bad lifestyle habits is to have them think they are not giving up anything. Instead, make them believe you are the one making most of the sacrifices. For example, a reluctant spouse may say he's not going to eat healthy because he doesn't have time to prepare his meals. Tell him you will prepare his food. He will believe you are the one making most of the sacrifice, but in reality you are already preparing your own meals, and making some additional food is really no sacrifice for you. Now you will have both reached a point of compromise!

Functional Alert: Never allow yourself to be influenced by people who are unwilling to work at improving their health and looks. You must learn self-discipline so you can avoid picking up other people's bad habits!

Food preparation isn't instantly gratifying, but the long-term benefits are amazing! All too often, people over-extend themselves by getting involved in too many activities or become workaholics in search of instant gratification. This prevents them from consistently preparing their meals in advance. Having the wrong priorities causes unhappiness and early death. The more irresponsible you become, the worse you feel about yourself, and the more you fail. Defeating irresponsibility requires gaining control over your life. A lot of what makes you happy or sad is your level of satisfaction and self-worth. The way you decide to spend your free time will significantly determine your success in living a functional lifestyle. We schedule our weekly food preparation and workouts just like we would schedule a doctor's appointment. Some of you may find the need to get up 30 minutes earlier to prepare food for the day if you fail to prepare it at night. If your schedule is extremely busy like ours, you may find the need to prepare meals twice a week (e.g., Sundays and Wednesdays). In these particular cases, we recommended cooking a lot of lean meat at one time and storing it in large plastic containers.

Functional Alert: If you have time to watch TV, get on Facebook, the Internet, or text your friends every day for instant gratification, then you have time to prepare your meals in advance! In order to be responsible, you have to use your time wisely. The time taken waiting in line for food at restaurants could be the time spent preparing your healthy food. We prepare a couple of days' worth of food in the time it takes to visit one restaurant and we also save a lot of money!

Too much instant gratification leads to feelings of guilt and anxiety because you are always chronically procrastinating and nothing gets done, which causes a Dysfunctional Heart. Constantly seeking out instant gratification is often a sign of having ADD/ADHD or chronic depression. On the other hand, a life without any instant gratification is boring. In regard to food, your designated once-a-week cheat day is your instant gratification! We have found that the best way to prevent falling off the lifestyle change wagon, is to schedule a guilt-free pleasure time by incorporating a once-a-week cheat day. The cheat day is not there to discourage you, but to inspire you. It shows you how far you have come and how fattening food no longer control you!

Have one designated cheat day. Once-a-week cheat days are composed of extra carbohydrates, fats, and calories above your normal calorie intake. The extra calories come from an extended cheat meal. We define a cheat day as consuming the same food you normally eat, but you consume more calories by having an extended cheat meal later in the day. This extended cheat meal starts at dinner and lasts until you go to bed. The extended cheat meal can be anything you want (e.g., pizza, popcorn, and ice cream). This means you can go eat at your favorite restaurant for dinner once a week and come back and snack on popcorn and/or ice cream until you go to bed. Most people prefer to have their once-a-week cheat day on Saturday. As your lifestyle change continues, you'll find out that your stomach will shrink and you won't be able to eat as much as you used to during cheat days. We have found it's best to stay on your normal diet until dinner time. This will prevent you from over doing it earlier in the day. Caloric intake should be considerably higher on this day in order to enhance your metabolism. The once-a-week cheat day will prevent you from hitting a body-fat loss barrier, and it gives you something to look forward to every week such as visiting your favorite restaurant. We've noticed that everyone's metabolism begins to slow down after six days of eating fewer calories and requires a cheat day once a week. The extra food on your cheat day significantly enhances your ability to lose weight. We would like to point out that any additional water weight you gain isn't going to be body fat, assuming you don't go ridiculously overboard. If water weight is gained, it will leave in 1-2 days depending on your metabolism and activity level. Some find they wake up the next morning lighter due to their fat burning and anabolic hormones gaining momentum.[10-13] Over time, you will learn not to overdo the calories during your extended cheat meal. If you do, you can expect to feel very sluggish the following day. When the cheat day is over, you will not want to experience that bloated, ugh feeling until the next cheat day rolls around. It's very important that you get back to your normal eating habits the following day. Two extended cheat meals per week will cause you to gain body fat. You should skip your designated once a week cheat day, if you didn't stick to your diet the other 6 days of the week!

Functional Alert: Your designated weekly weigh-in should always be on your cheat day morning before breakfast. This will give you an accurate reading on how much weight you lost for the week or your true weight. Having a sensible once-a-week extended cheat meal is not yo-yo dieting because any weight gained is only a little short-lived water retention, not body fat!

In order to be successful on a long-term basis, you have to learn to be responsible while still rewarding yourself with some instant gratification. This is also important for maintaining a Functional Heart. You can still procrastinate to some degree and be responsible as long as you get the task at hand completed, which, in this case, is preparing your food in advance. The big picture is having some patience and taking smaller steps. Otherwise, you will feel overwhelmed and staying on a Functional Diet may seem impossible. It's all about perception! We all handle things better in smaller steps coupled with organization.

Functional Alert: Don't become a workaholic to avoid meaningful work!

Visualization

Visualization is needed to succeed with food preparation. Your mind (logical thinking) and heart (emotional thinking) control your actions. A lot of people know in their minds they need to lose weight, but their hearts are not into it. In life, your heart has the final say so, and if your heart is not into it, you won't succeed in whatever you do. To get into shape, you must visualize the outcome you want for your body by eating the right kinds of food. This persuades the mind (how you see and perceive things) to coincide with the heart (controls the actions you do intentionally) so the two are going in the same direction!

We believe confessing your visualization with your mouth and having a change of heart toward healthy food preparations is very important! We will use the Bible as an example to explain why it's so important. In Romans, Chapter 10, the Bible speaks of the gospel (death, burial, and resurrection of Jesus Christ). It goes on to say that everyone who believes with their heart that Christ died for their sins and was raised again on the third day shall be saved. Now please pay close attention to Romans, Chapter 10, verses 8-10 (KJV):

> *"But what saith it? The word is nigh thee, even in thy mouth, and in thy heart: that is, the word of faith, which we preach; That if thou shalt confess with thy mouth the Lord Jesus, and shalt believe in thine heart that God hath raised him from the dead, thou shalt be saved. For with the heart man believeth unto righteousness; and with the mouth confession is made unto salvation."*

Notice that the Bible states in verse 10 that confession is made unto salvation. This does not mean that a person is saved by his mouth confession, but rather, the mouth testifies readily of receiving Christ for our sins by believing from the heart. In other words, in order to be saved or born again on a spiritual level, you must come to the place where you believe with all your heart that the work Jesus performed on the cross is your only hope to be freed from the bondage of sin. Believing the gospel or calling on His name brings you into a personal relationship with God. This same concept holds true for the Functional Diet. Many people try to approach a Functional Diet from a logical point of view (head knowledge) instead of putting their hearts or emotions into it. This results in book knowledge, but not the change of heart that's required to be truly dedicated to a Functional Diet.

We recommend that you meditate on the following to change your actions:

Visualize from your heart what is putting a barrier between you and healthy food preparation and how you are going to overcome that barrier. Now confess it with your mouth to testify you are readily receiving it. *Congratulations! You are ready for a Functional Diet!*

As you are mentally visualizing from the heart, we would like you to verbalize what you are seeing in order to make things clearer in your mind. As you verbalize your step-by-step plan, you will notice each step becomes clearer and much simpler to organize and understand. This gets rid of negative visualization (e.g., you don't have time) and replaces it with positive visualization (e.g., you figure out a way to make time).

Having a Dysfunctional Heart means you are not able to get things done. It can control you by making you think negative thoughts such as, I might as well skip food preparations and workouts since we are all going to die eventually anyway! You can't let mentally challenging barriers at work, home, etc., get in your way. The longer you allow yourself to become controlled by external factors, the more valuable time you have wasted. You owe it to yourself to spend time on your health, because you are worth it!

Functional Alert: Life can be tough at times, but with heart, you will definitely achieve success. Getting your heart right enables you to eat right year round (spring, summer, fall, and winter)!

Functional Heart

The Functional Diet requires having a Functional Heart. Logical thinking is attributed to your mind, but emotional thinking is when your heart takes first priority over your mind. A Functional Heart is defined as reaching a logical conclusion about what is right and what is wrong and then following through with action.

A very important thing we have learned while working with the public is that most people have been through a great deal of pain in their lives. This is why it's important to not judge other people and to show compassion. You would be surprised to find out that a lot of people became overweight due to a single stressful event that occurred in their lives. You can almost draw a line through their lives. Once there was this happy person who spent time with the people they loved most in life. Everything was sheltered, protected, and comfortable. Their face had this light, but then one day something happened and they took a hard corner and the light went out. They ended up all alone! It could be a lot of things, such as the death of a loved one, loss of employment, an ugly divorce, a chronic medical condition, an accident leaving them disabled, etc. Some mourn their losses and never let them go. This is often a sign of having PTSD. These same people usually think their weight-loss failures are solely from a lack of will power, but they are wrong! They are also caused by hormonal imbalances and by depression from not being able to let go of emotional baggage and move on with their lives. The bottom line is, they use food for comfort during times of what they perceive as emotional stress or they use food as a reward for what they perceive as good behavior (or a time of celebration).

Functional Alert: The heart is the battleground. Loving self and others helps overcome loneliness!

Perceived stress deceives us by making us think we can find comfort in food. This is how compulsive overeating or gluttony begins. It's all downhill from there! When under stress, we fail to respond appropriately to perceived threats. Stress causes our bodies to overproduce cortisol and other stress hormones, causing a disturbance in bodily functions. This puts us at a much higher risk for developing mental, health, and weight problems.

Having a Functional Heart and implementing the other principles found in **Functional Training with a Fork** are the best ways to cope with stress in your life. The key to stopping the destructive pattern of overeating is to replace stress with a Functional Heart. People who have intense feelings of deprivation when they try to give up gluttony have yet to find a Functional Heart. The heart is what makes your brain tell you what to eat. If you don't heal the root cause, you can't expect to win the battle against food. Everyone battles food on a daily basis, and it's one battle you can't afford to lose!

Functional Alert: The #1 thing that gets people into trouble emotionally and "paves the way" to obesity is allowing perceived stress in their lives to control them, instead of having a positive sense of power to produce a desired result!

Binge eating is an attempt to escape painful self-awareness brought forth by negative emotions. It's comparable to using alcohol to alter consciousness in order to cope with the situation at hand. This is why drunkenness and gluttony are both considered sins. The relationship between our health and lifestyle choices is very complex and it not only affects our self-image, but our sex life, dating, marriage, other family members, friends, co-workers and job performance.

Most of our clients eventually admit that when they are under a lot of stress, healthy-eating habits are more difficult to maintain. They eat to try and fill a perceived emotional void while causing another emotional void: weight gain! Many choose fast food and making poor choices while eating in restaurants instead of preparing their meals in advance and/or taking their food along with them in a cooler when they are away from home. They don't take time out for themselves, not realizing that this is actually hindering their ability to be better caregivers to their families! They live stressed-out lifestyles that takes years off their lives. Living a lifestyle under chronic stress shows up both physically and emotionally.

Some of you are in a bad place and you're trying to get out! That is only going to happen when you stop dwelling on the past and learn how to forgive yourself and others. Some people become pathologically stuck in the past instead of moving on with their lives. This kind of anger and resentment often causes people to see the negative in every situation instead of the positive. You need to tell yourself, I am moving on with my life instead of holding hate and anger in my heart. The next step involves training yourself not to worry about things you can't change. This means you have to come to the realization that the vast majority of your concerns are not realistic. You must also stop making excuses about eating the wrong kinds of food or too much food, and exercise regularly to help reduce emotional stress. This requires making a permanent lifestyle change by creating goals that are super easy and that you really want, instead of worrying about whether or not you can successfully achieve them.

Many of you reading this book have failed at body-fat loss in the past thinking it was all from a lack of discipline. We want you to know it's not only a lack of discipline, but also a lack of knowledge about what food and portion sizes you should be eating, as well as the emotional baggage you are holding onto, that has built up unresolved emotional issues. At this point, it becomes your responsibility to figure out your priorities in life so you can build new memories—good memories! Getting your priorities in order requires responsibility and strength, but you can't obtain these things until you get character! You build character when you stand on the foundation of what is right and what is wrong. You keep your promises and always do what you say! Your character is what separates you from the next person.

Functional Alert: Having poor character brings forth a lot of unwanted stress in your life which increases inflammation and oxidation inside the body. Living a life of good character decreases inflammation and oxidation!

It's important to hang out with people who have good character and the same purpose in life. They will make you feel like family. When you feel wanted you'll have more self-confidence to achieve your body-fat loss goals. We've seen self-confidence help people succeed time and time again in our careers as personal trainers. By following the principles outlined in **Functional Training with a Fork** you can get where you need to be in life instead of being a dreamer who won't take real steps to make a reality of their vision!

Sometimes you'll need to go against the norm in order to do what is right. When you display good character you are being the person you were made to be and everything that surrounds who you really are. Character is based on your actions! People who lack character say one thing, but they don't perform the action they promised. All too often, people fail at making a lifestyle change because they don't perform the action they promised themselves. In essence, they pretend to be making a lifestyle change for the purpose of gaining acceptance. If you know and love yourself, you will find it easy to be true to yourself. This is a requirement for making a functional lifestyle change! If you don't display good character, other people will get hurt and you will hurt yourself.

Functional Alert: Don't allow financial difficulties to prevent you from being a person of great character. Having character cost $0.00. Money doesn't define your self-worth, character does!

Although all of us are genetically different, our behavior is largely influenced by how we see others. Some of you reading this book are allowing other people to prevent you from changing over to a functional lifestyle. You have steered away from two very important rules in life: Don't waste your time blindly following others and don't waste your time judging others; use that time and effort to focus on making yourself happy! Being more accepting of other people doesn't mean agreeing with them on every topic, approving of all their actions, or abandoning your own rights. But understanding other people better helps you not to judge them or walk in step with them. If you will begin to listen to your heart, you'll find strength and the chains of emotional baggage will break free. This results in you becoming your own best friend and it produces the type of character that causes you to do the same productive things every day because your heart is now functioning properly. *Congratulations! Now you are ready to remain on a Functional Diet!*

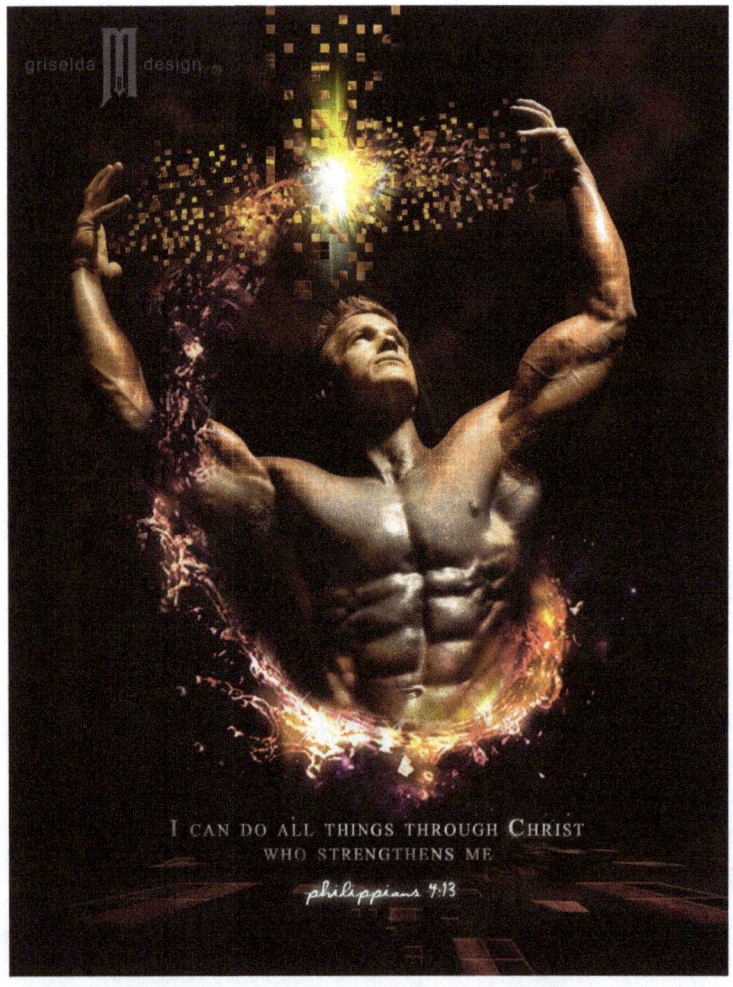

Photographer: jasonellisphotography.com
Graphic Designer: griseldaMdesign.com

Functional Alert: Hate produces the opposite effect of love. Hate produces bad character, which causes people to become unpredictable and nonproductive. Love produces good character, which causes people to be predictable and productive. You'll need good character to remain on a Functional Diet!

James Ellis

Good action requires love. Loving God, myself, and others helped motivate me to win the WBFF Fitness Model World Championship in 2011. I no longer compete, but continue following a Functional Diet as a lifestyle. If you will devote yourself to developing your love walk in these three areas (loving God, self, and others) doors will open for you that have not opened in the past!

You must train yourself not to overeat when you are upset! If you believe deep down that you are worthless and nobody loves you, then how do you expect to remain on a Functional Diet? You can't! Losing body fat requires accepting and loving yourself so the anger, depression, and low confidence can leave. We want you to know your life does matter and no one is perfect!

Functional Alert: Your sense of self-perception plays a huge role in whether you will begin and continue with a Functional Exercise and Functional Diet program!

As fitness professionals, we know that in order to lose weight and keep it off, you must fix your perception issues and become responsible. We do our best to try and understand each individual's situation because we all have stress to contend with on a daily basis. Life isn't perfect, so you have to learn how to distinguish between true tragedies and the hassles of everyday life. If you obsess over everyday hassles, you will eat more food and damage your immune system. When you allow hassles to overwhelm you, life will turn out to be much less than it could be and your stress levels will soar out of control. You must learn to let the small things go.

Functional Alert: The hassles of life are always going to be there!

It's impossible to avoid all situations and people that generate stress. However, you need to try and avoid people who often push your fight-and-flight reactions until you learn better coping skills. If they say things to put you down, just try to ignore them and understand that they are the ones with problems. Sometimes you will meet a person who is impossible to deal with, and it's best to avoid them as much as possible.

Functional Alert: Respect yourself by having the courage to walk away from any relationship that is dysfunctional!

We've met a lot of obese people who felt as if their lives didn't matter and that they may never matter again. We can promise you it doesn't have to be that way! It takes more than Functional Training and eating a Functional Diet to fix these kinds of problems. You also have to invest some of your time, money, and love in other people. By doing this you will help someone else in need and increase your own feelings of self-worth. We all have gone through pain and loneliness in our lives. It's what made us who we are today. You need to love yourself, so you can love others and become a functional member of society. Functional Love is impossible if you hesitate on the side lines. In order to have Functional Love, you have to persist in loving others as time moves forward.

Functional Alert: When you begin to love yourself (not to be confused with being in love with yourself) it becomes contagious. This means by loving yourself you actually help others learn to love themselves!

As we have seen, dysfunctional eating is caused by a lack of responsibility and stress generated from negative emotions. There is a third factor that plays an important part: hunger hormones linked to stress. Putting an end to obesity and poor eating habits requires fixing both our psychological functions and our physiological functions. The mind and heart control our psychological functions and our hormones control our physiological functions. The mind, heart, and hormones of people who can't control their food intake have a hard time distinguishing what is a real threat and what isn't. So, they often end up on high alert, which causes their bodies to secrete hormones that make them hungry. The most destructive of these hormones is cortisol! It binds to the hypothalamus in the brain, provoking a person to eat food high in carbs and fats.[14] High cortisol elevates blood sugar/insulin, which causes hunger pangs.[15] Cortisol also reduces leptin levels, which is a hormone needed at healthy levels to lower one's appetite.[16] Cortisol also lowers testosterone.[17] The hormone testosterone blunts your appetite by reducing your perceived stress levels and increasing insulin sensitivity.[18] When the stomach is empty, the hunger hormone ghrelin is secreted causing you to feel hungry. When the stomach is stretched, the secretion of ghrelin stops, causing you to feel full.[19] Ghrelin is also secreted in larger amounts due to stress, making your brain think your stomach is empty even though it's full.[20]

Functional Alert: When your body releases excess cortisol, it lowers your metabolism and you gain weight!

Laughter, like exercise and sex, causes the body to release dopamine while simultaneously lowering the stress hormone cortisol. This lowers your appetite for food. Laughing also helps control your appetite by getting your mind off of food cravings. It also improves the function of your immune system, helps relieve chronic pain, increases sex drive, and boosts your energy and mood.[21, 22] If you pay close attention, the happiest people are the ones who are drawn toward people who make them laugh. People react much more positively when you are kind, gentle, patient, honest, respectful, humble, and have a great sense of humor. Why is this so important? It increases your social connections with others by allowing you to finally trust yourself and give others the trust they have earned. This sense of security keeps perceived stress levels down because it allows you to share and laugh with one another. Social connections play a huge role in helping people heal from trauma and reducing appetite!

Functional Alert: Laughing reduces inflammation and oxidation inside the body. It gives us peace and joy which enable us to see the bright side of life despite all the negativity we have to endure!

Training yourself to laugh more is accomplished by changing your mind-set, surrounding yourself with people who are more optimistic than pessimistic, and not overworking yourself. Instead of dwelling on negative things, be grateful for the positive things you have been given in life so new doors can open. Whatever you focus on is where your energy and thoughts go. Pleasant experiences with others have a long-term effect in creating happiness whereas materialism is a happiness that is short-lived. True happiness comes from a state of mind.

You also have to change your mind-set and believe you are being treated fairly even though conditions may have not changed or your surroundings may not be as good as you wish. Constantly worrying about things you can't change or getting involved in unnecessary drama causes a Dysfunctional Heart. This keeps you stressed out because you are always anticipating undesirable outcomes!

Functional Alert: Drama can be addictive because certain chemicals in the brain are produced from the adrenaline rush. When you get in touch with your heart, you will feel more connected to the important things in life. This allows drama to disappear. The worst kind of drama is caused by one's self. You can make just one mistake and feel as though the whole world is crushing you! Everyone makes mistakes. Forgive yourself and try not to make the same ones. Less drama in your life reduces inflammation and free radical damage going on inside the body and it reduces your appetite for food!

We have never seen anyone depressed or angry because they stopped eating food on the lower end of the Functional Food Spectrum, but we have seen plenty of people depressed and angry from being overweight. When you are mentally depressed, you become physically suppressed! This makes it more difficult to follow through with healthy food preparations and Functional Exercise. Emotions affect your physical body as much as your body affects your feelings. Some claim they eat from depression, but it's actually unresolved anger. Anger leads to anxiety and anxiety leads to depression. Are you angry? Do you work or associate with angry people? Anger is the strongest and most devastating emotion for both your mental and physical health![23, 24] Being around angry people can bring you down with them. It often becomes a vicious, three-way cycle (anger-anxiety-depression)! All three emotions are often masked upfront by overeating because the body releases serotonin and dopamine levels when large volumes of carbs and fats are consumed.

Functional Alert: It's not uncommon for a person to face his or her worst times alone. It's often during this time that keeping your body-fat levels down becomes a real challenge. This can be the perfect time to join a gym and hire a Functional Personal Trainer to keep you motivated!

Extended Access to Fattening Food

We have learned throughout the years that obese people have an extended access to foods that are high in sugar and fat. When presented with a choice between high-calorie food that have more taste and low-calorie food that are comparatively bland, obese people choose the fattening food! They end up consuming 2-3 times as many calories and that's why they can't lose the weight. They get used to eating fattening food high in calories and their taste buds can no longer detect the flavor in blander food that are low in calories. We promise you that after you have been on a Functional Diet and stop eating fattening food, the blander food begins to taste great when you get hungry. In other words, blander food becomes the new norm for your brain!

Functional Alert: After approximately one year of being on a Functional Diet, you'll develop an intolerance to unhealthy food and their food-poisoning-like effects. You'll feel so much better on a Functional Diet you'll never want to stop. In addition, if you can make it through the holidays the first year without gaining weight, it will be much easier to have self-control in the years that follow!

Please pay close attention to what we are about to say: The only way the vast majority of you are going to be able to lose body fat and/or eat healthier is by removing the temptation of high-fat, high-carb foods in your home. It's mostly the people with easy access to fattening food who have the desire to overconsume them. If you cut off your access to fattening foods and begin eating blander, low-calorie food, you will eventually like the way they taste!

On the flip side, eating food that is too bland can get boring fast. For example, a plain, baked chicken breast isn't appealing for most because it lacks flavor. In order to stay on the right path without feeling deprived, most people have to add low-calorie spices and sauces to their food to get a variety of flavor! Spices, sauces, and even a little artificial sweetener can make highly-bland food taste great. Be cautious not to go overboard with sauces if they contain a measurable amount of calories. You can find plenty of healthy cooking recipes in various books and on the Internet.

It takes around 3-6 months to re-train your taste buds so you stop craving the wrong types of food. Cravings for comfort food are in your brain, not your body. Bad habits are in your mind because you have trained yourself to eat the wrong food. It's a learned behavior! You must learn to balance your macronutrient needs and re-train yourself to make healthier choices. It's the same as breaking a drug habit such as smoking. Once you quit smoking, you don't want to be around cigarette smoke. Likewise, once you stop eating food full of fats, carbs, and salt, you avoid being around places where this is served. Excess of anything can become an addiction and this is particularly true with fattening food high in carbs, fats, and salt.

In order to break bad eating habits, you have to learn to eat what your body needs, not what your mind wants! We have heard people complain that they get tired of eating the same food all the time during their sugar withdrawal phase. We have learned that when you get hungry enough, a sweet potato will taste like a piece of chocolate cake! You can train your mind to enjoy eating mostly the same healthy food all the time. Visualize what you want to look like and feel like before you put the food into your mouth. Is this food choice going to make me fat and sluggish or is it going to make me lean and energetic? The choice is yours!

You must learn to read food labels. All packaged food comes with a nutritional label. We are surprised to find the number of people who don't have a clue about what they are eating because they neglect to read food labels or search the Internet to find the macronutrients for each type of food they consume. This information is necessary to help you stay on track with your daily targets, while avoiding poor food choices.

Many people don't realize that food such as conventional yogurt, juice, and milk are full of sugar. Flavored milk (e.g., chocolate milk) has tons of added sugar. Many think peanut butter, cheese, and nuts are protein sources, but they are mostly fat sources. Some think the carbs in fruit and beans won't make them fat. Others overindulge in calorie-dense food such as olive oil or peanut butter since it is touted as healthy. There is no way you can expect to eat healthier and lose weight if you don't take the time to learn what you are putting into your mouth! It's essential to pay very close attention to food labels and the macronutrients of all food in order to lose body fat. If you want to be successful at counting calories indirectly through macronutrients, you must acquire this skill. You should know how to find a food's macronutrient content, caloric content, and its serving size. Most people consume too many fats, too many carbs and added sugar, and combine too many fats and carbs in multiple meals. They also neglect to consume enough protein and fiber in their diets!

Functional Alert: Too many fats (e.g., cheese, olive oil, or peanut butter) will make you just as fat as too many carbs (e.g., potatoes, pasta, and fruit)!

Another tool for losing body fat is to keep a food diary in order to give yourself a clear picture of your current diet. In this way, you can evaluate the changes needed to be successful. Recording what you eat in a food journal lets you see what you are taking in so you can make any needed adjustments to your diet if you aren't making progress. Some people like to use diet-tracking apps (e.g., MyFitnessPal) on their phones or computers until they figure out what they need to eat in order to lose body fat. The apps work great because they make this task easier. After you build your food database with the food that you eat, you can log in all of them in a very short period of time. These apps do the math and have a huge database to search caloric and macronutrient content for each food. They summarize the information for you, making it easy to track and record food requirements. You'll be able to record everything that you've eaten over the past year. This makes the apps great monitors for how much food you have been eating. Prior to apps, many didn't realize how many excess calories they were consuming. Apps help prevent people from overeating and help them identify where the problem areas occur. Once you start tracking your food intake, you start making smarter choices.

Functional Alert: Using an app on your phone can be much simpler than writing your food list down in a food journal!

Stop Overeating

You must train yourself to stop overeating. The end of obesity and type-2 diabetes starts with you! Learn how to put the proper portion of food on your plate and avoid going back for seconds. It takes your brain at least 20 minutes to register that your body has had enough food. If you wait to stop eating until your brain tells you that you are completely full, then it's too late and you will have already overeaten. You have to learn to eat the proper food until you are satisfied, not until you are completely full.

Functional Alert: If you are still hungry after eating, drink around 12 ounces of some form of sugar-free beverage and the hunger pangs will usually leave. Many find sugar-free organic coffee to be a great appetite suppressant!

Many obese people eat until they feel extremely bloated and then turn right around and do it again about four hours later. Their depression, appearance, and overall functionality often become a living nightmare! They have to be near food everywhere they go. In restaurants, it's very common for them to eat appetizers and desserts in addition to their main course meal, which is already exceeding their caloric intake for the day. Some even top it off with a bottle of wine. Overkill is putting it mildly! They eat not for health, but rather to get their money's worth. They often eat family members' leftovers. As a result of overeating, they not only gain more body fat, but they also develop body odor and bad breath. This comes from a lack of fluids and consuming junk food on the lower end of the Functional Food Spectrum, instead of food on the higher end.

Functional Alert: It's not uncommon in today's society for an obese person to justify their weight problem because they see morbidly obese people in worse shape than they are. In addition, they see a lot of people with similar body-fat levels. In other words, they become desensitized to obesity and eventually become comfortable because they blend in with the crowd. They don't see obesity as a big problem and begin to accept it as the norm. Don't buy into the idea that being obese is normal!

It will be very difficult for the majority of you to know when to stop eating if you are eating a bunch of food ranked on the lower end of the Functional Food Spectrum. These kinds of food don't fill you up and actually increase your appetite. In other words, the more carbs and fats you take in, the more you crave! These foods, which are lacking in fiber and lean protein, include fast food, pizza, pasta, ice cream, cookies, cakes, doughnuts, biscuits, rolls, French fries, chips, etc.

Food full of carbs (sugar) and fat temporarily increase dopamine levels in the brain comparable to drugs like nicotine. Carbs and fats work in the same way as nicotine. When you become addicted to nicotine you get a huge feeling of relief after you smoke a cigarette. The same goes for food high in carbs and fats. As time passes, your brain tells your body you need more of the drug or food to be satisfied. Eventually, both drug addicts and food addicts reach a point where they need their "fix" more frequently or in larger quantities to feel normal. People who have learned to eat healthy and stop eating before they are completely full are the ones who never become overweight in the first place and have to experience food withdrawals. Likewise, those who have never smoked cigarettes are the ones who never have to suffer from nicotine withdrawals.[25, 26]

Functional Alert: Food withdrawal symptoms range from mild to extreme. They can last anywhere from several days to several months. Food rehabilitation programs begin with a plan for handling withdrawal symptoms. The best way to get over these symptoms is working with a Functional Personal Trainer!

If you are eating food on the lower end of the Functional Food Spectrum that are high in calories and increase your appetite, then how do you expect to be able to control your appetite? You can't! Once you put on a lot of weight, it can take a very long time to get rid of it because your hormones get out of balance, making your metabolism slow down and your hunger skyrocket. It can be compared to starting a new prescription drug that slows down your metabolism and makes you crave bad food. You begin to gain weight even though your activity levels haven't changed. The take-home message is never allow yourself to become overweight, unless you want to suffer through some nasty withdrawals when you decide enough is enough!

Functional Alert: Some people are eating a lot of unhealthy fattening foods and/or taking recreational drugs to get more dopamine and mellow out. What they fail to realize is that dopamine is more readily available in Functional Exercise and even Functional Sex for many!

Shrinking Your Stomach

Expect to be a little hungry and irritable upon beginning a Functional Diet to shrink your stomach. This is normal because you have overeaten and stretched your stomach. Stay on track and it will eventually leave and you will feel energized and start seeing transformations. If you are often feeling as though you are starving, you will need to increase your total caloric intake from food on the upper end of the Functional Food Spectrum! You need to wean yourself off a food journal as soon as you are ready so you don't become unhealthily dependent on it.

Functional Alert: Always emphasize eating smaller portion sizes because regardless of how many calories you consume in a particular meal, you will be hungry again in about 3-4 hours. For example, if you eat a huge lunch loaded with calories on the lower end of the Functional Food Spectrum, you will still be hungry 3-4 hours later. Eating fewer, more filling foods on the higher end of the Functional Food Spectrum enables you to control your appetite until the 3-4 hour time frame of needing to eat again rolls around. This keeps your body-fat levels down and your energy levels up. Furthermore, overconsuming Free Foods doesn't usually make you fat directly, but it can indirectly, by stretching out your stomach and increasing your appetite for non-Free Foods!

Proper macronutrient ratios and timing will enhance your metabolism and allow you to remain full and energetic. Consume 4-6 small meals/snacks daily to shrink the size of your stomach. Eating smaller meals throughout the day will shrink it comparable to gastric by-pass surgery. Your stomach will shrink considerably after 3-6 months of consuming smaller meals more frequently. In return, you will eat less food without going hungry. What you are going to find out is that you don't need nearly as much food as you think in order to remain satisfied. Overeating is simply a bad habit you have to stop. People don't become overweight because they are hungry, but rather because they get into a bad habit of overeating! Then they feel miserable every time they overeat. How many times have you overeaten out of habit, only to regret it later?

Functional Alert: Always eat before you go shopping and have a grocery list so you won't be tempted to buy the wrong foods. Use medium-sized plates and small bowls to cut down on portion sizes. Never keep junk food in your house or you will be tempted to eat it. Don't eat before a meal and never go back for seconds!

You need to stay satisfied and this requires eating small meals more frequently in order to avoid making bad choices, such as foods containing refined sugar, starches, and bad fats. These are the cheapest calories without a lot of preparation. These kinds of food will also make you fat, while lean proteins and green leafy vegetables don't!

Large meals slow down your metabolism by making you become inactive, which results in burning fewer calories. Your body can only use so many calories for fuel in one meal. The excess calories that are not used for fuel are turned into triglycerides and stored as body fat. Furthermore, your body releases more blood sugar causing excess inflammation and oxidation, and more wear and tear on the immune system. When you overeat, you stretch out your stomach and it makes you hungrier even sooner. Now, it's going to take more food to satisfy your appetite; and the more you eat, the fatter you get and the fatter you get, the more you eat!

Functional Alert: If you feel guilty and get angry with yourself after overeating, then you can stop! If you don't have those feelings, then you will never stop because you perceive this form of behavior as acceptable. If you can't stop on your own, hiring a Functional Personal Trainer would be a wise decision!

Yo-Yo Dieting

We believe that a lifestyle of constantly bringing the wrong types of foods into your home is comparable to slowly poisoning your family members. It completely changes people and their lives. People can make up all the excuses they want to support that kind of lifestyle, but it's a very poor decision. God has blessed us with food that is delicious and nutritious. All sin is sin in the eyes of God and gluttony is one of them! There are consequences for all sin. For example, if you eat a lot of junk food and/or allow yourself to become overweight, chances are great that you will have health issues, relationship issues, and mental issues, which will take years off your life. We are not saying that gluttony makes you a bad person because we all sin to some degree every day. What we are saying is, food will destroy your life just like anything else that is done in excess.

The overindulgence in food is the biggest challenge you will face when trying to lose weight. Losing body fat is something you have to want to do for yourself in order to be successful. To do this, you must come up with a game plan for food preparation in order to avoid yo-yo dieting! If you prepare your food in advance and always have access to it, you will have no choice, but to eat the right food in the proper portions. If you don't prepare your food in advance and take it with you wherever you go, then you will eat whatever is available. This almost always ends in poor food selections on the lower end of the Functional Food Spectrum, resulting in weight gain and/or health problems. Food preparation becomes easy once you get into a routine!

Find ways to keep yourself busy so you won't always be thinking about food. To prevent yo-yo dieting, you will want to eat at scheduled times to the best of your ability and not skip meals. Yo-yo dieting also occurs because you are not eating enough protein and fiber in each meal to remain full. When you eat, it's important to eat the proper macronutrient ratios during specific times of the day to control the hunger hormones leptin, ghrelin, insulin, dopamine, cortisol, and testosterone.

Functional Alert: Most people overeat because they've been taught to eat a diet that promotes hunger!

If you are not serious about sticking to a Functional Diet and Functional Training program, then you can't expect to lose the weight and keep it off. Success requires a lifestyle change. Wishful thinking never brings forth lasting results. It only causes you to get caught up in a miserable circle of losing a few pounds and gaining it all back!

Functional Alert: Don't allow yourself to become hungry. Hunger leads to gorging, causing you to get off your Functional Diet!

Take Responsibility

Take responsibility by making positive changes. Staying busy helps prevent you from overeating. Sitting around the house bored all the time watching television can make one think about food. If you allow yourself to become distracted while eating, it often leads to consuming more food. Working out helps people get away from excess food, drugs, etc. Hanging with peers at work who eat fattening food for lunch or bring in junk food, such as doughnuts, is a huge problem in today's society! If you can't control the urge to eat these foods, then you are better off eating alone, while letting your co-workers and friends know you are on a Functional Diet. We can assure you that you are not missing out by eating lunch alone or avoiding social events, if that is what it takes to remain healthy and fit. The lure of excessive alcohol, food, and sugary drinks is making people overweight and unhealthy.

No one can make you overweight unless you allow it to happen. Don't blame your spouse, family members, and friends for not being able to control what you eat and drink. There comes a point in life where you have to grow up and take responsibility for your own actions! The world is full of temptations. It's up to you to make the right choices. If you choose to eat junk food because your friends and family members make you feel guilty for not doing so, then you are only hurting yourself. You are also setting a bad example for your family and friends. In order to become healthy and fit, you have to become fixated on being healthy and fit.

Functional Alert: If you are overweight, it's time to put down the fork and stop overeating. No one is forcing that fork into your mouth!

When someone refuses to change over to a healthy lifestyle, it's hard not to treat it like a war between good and evil. The fight against gluttony and laziness often becomes a spiritual warfare! In the grand scheme of things, every person has a duty to take care of themselves and others. It's very common for people to let their upbringing and pride get in the way, causing them to behave in an irresponsible manner. Obesity and/or eating junk food is often fueled by excess pride which leads to negative emotions. Some people remain obese or sick because they don't want others telling them what they should and shouldn't be eating. People with this type of mentality often boast about eating unhealthy fattening food and how great they taste. What many people fail to realize is that excess pride isn't only linked to disliking what others have to say, it's also linked to staying uneducated about certain topics because they already think they know it all!

The best solution for overcoming excess pride is to learn to think for yourself instead of blindly following the crowd. The things you have been subjected to as a child often distort your ability to discern between what is right and wrong. Until you learn to think for yourself, you will remain in a state of pride. Pride often leads to a lifestyle of chronic complaining and chaos because deep down you don't like the person you have become. This prevents a lot of people from changing to a functional lifestyle. They always find excuses as to why they are unable to make the needed changes, yet are unaware that the negative emotions generated from pride is what's hindering them. You would be surprised to find out how many people we have successfully trained who eventually tell us that their original refusal to change their lifestyle was due to their excess pride. In other words, they simply refused to do it!

We all have some degree of pride because we are still in the flesh. We have found the best way to get rid of excessive pride is to humble ourselves. This will help you attack body-fat loss and exercise with confidence and humility instead of arrogance. Practicing humility is much more difficult when you surround yourself with close-minded people. Practicing humility opens up your heart to the voice of reason. This makes you teachable and smarter. Humility helps you to evaluate your personal traits without feeling embarrassed.

Functional Alert: We have seen people lose the function of their internal organs over pride. A diet too high in calories and/or junk food causes their organs to work overtime!

Food Pushers

Food pushers are the equivalent to flies buzzing in your ear. It doesn't take long to get off track if you listen to other people who are eating the wrong kinds of food. Food pushers can be your best friends, co-workers, family members, an insecure spouse, a workout partner, people in need of praise for their cooking abilities, etc. You just have to put the "smack down" on them without thinking twice. When an overbearing host tries to force junk food on you explain to them in a polite manner that you are watching your diet. You have the right to eat what you want, so don't let others push food on you. Sincere people will understand.

Some food pushers will intentionally try to sabotage your diet hoping you will fail. They know they are not dedicated to a lifestyle change and deep down they are envious that you have made a lifestyle change and they have not! If you watch closely, these same people always seem to make your social gatherings a special occasion. They say things like, Oh, come on and have a piece of this cake. It's a special occasion! They are trying to get you to change your mind—but don't give in! They probably see you as being fixated on food, when in reality they are the ones with the problem. We often ask both skinny and obese people this question, "Would you push alcohol on a family member or friend who is a recovering alcoholic?" The answer should be no! Well, the same answer should apply to food addictions. If you are going to eat food that is fattening, please don't push it on someone who needs to lose body fat or improve their health.

The fact is, some people are not envious of your new body and lifestyle. Simply put, they don't want to convert to a healthy lifestyle because they have not been convinced of its importance. In these situations, they need more help attaining the same goals and lifestyle changes you have made. Invite them to the gym with you and offer them some good-tasting, healthy food to get them on the right track.

Functional Alert: It makes things much easier when friends and family members work together as a team to improve their eating habits. Are you guilty of enabling a family member or friend to remain obese by bringing them fattening food or taking them out to a restaurant?

Communication is paramount if you want good relationships! It's highly important to remind others you are making a lifestyle change to enhance your overall functionality and looks and to feel good about yourself. Let them know that you want to spend many years of quality time with them and how much you would appreciate their support!

It's not only adults that are being affected. We have seen the wrong kind of guidance and rewards being handed out to and by all age groups. Junk food shouldn't be looked at as a love gift or as a way to gain acceptance from others. The only things to be gained are body fat and disease! Fortunately, **Functional Training with a Fork** is waking up some people and they are making changes.

We have seen some ugly divorces where kids get put in the middle and are used as pawns. We think it's ignorant when divorced couples use their kids to drive their ex-spouses crazy instead of finding ways to work as a team to do what is in the best interest of their kids. It's wrong to use your kids to get revenge, because you are not just hurting your ex-spouse, you are destroying your kids from the inside out! An ugly divorce can cause emotional eating disorders in children that last into adulthood. In addition, grandparents and ex-spouses often try to use food to make the child/children feel better about the situation. Sometimes, ex-spouses no longer care and just let them eat whatever they want. Sadly, this happens every day to children all across America.

Functional Alert: Routine, structure, and the proper guidance are vital to a child's life! They must be taught how to control themselves emotionally in order to overcome being easily frustrated and always desiring instant gratification. The collapse of family structure in America is negatively affecting the ability of our current generation and future generations to function in a variety of circumstances!

Even well-meaning parents and grandparents are hurting children with junk food! It gets extremely frustrating when you see parents, grandparents, etc., who love kids, yet are bad influences on them. It's not uncommon for them to offer kids seconds and desserts during a meal. One of the worst mistakes that parents and grandparents can make is filling a child's plate with a ton of food and telling them they must eat it all before they can have a dessert. These poor kids reluctantly eat more calories than their bodies need just so they can get a sugary dessert at the end, which does further harm. This type of family dysfunction is inconceivable and unacceptable! It teaches kids to mimic what is being taught. In other words, instead of learning self-control, they learn how to eat out of control. Furthermore, a lot of people simply don't want to take the time to prepare a healthy meal; instead, they run their kids through a local fast-food restaurant. Many of them don't know the difference between healthy food and unhealthy food. Greasy burgers, salty fries, and milk shakes overflowing with fat and sugar become the norm. The time to make a change is now in order to spare the health of our children and break this dysfunctional cycle!

Functional Alert: Don't overfeed or starve your kids! Feed them healthy, tasty food, in the proper portion sizes for their metabolism. This will keep them healthy and energetic, and prevent obesity!

Dysfunctional fundraising is running rampant in America! The hypocrisy of selling and buying junk food to save lives utterly astounds us. If you want to donate to organizations, just write a check directly. Avoid labeled junk food containing trans fats, refined sugar, and other suspected cancer-causing ingredients.

On a personal note, what kind of message are organizations sending to our kids when they sell junk food, such as cookies, to raise funds? We say, find different ways to make money! We see parents getting angry about the banning of junk food in schools, when they should be getting mad at junk food manufacturers and concerned about what the junk food is actually doing to their kids' looks, health, and academic performances. One of the worst frustrations a parent can endure is not knowing what's wrong with their child and then not being able to do anything about it. However, in these particular cases, we know the problem and it can be fixed.

Functional Alert: In 2010, the food and drink business spent over $40 billion lobbying congress against regulations. Some of the regulations they lobbied against would have decreased the marketing of junk food to our children.[27, 28] We believe it's wrong for the food industry to use bribery such as cartoon characters and free giveaways to entice kids and adults into buying junk food. It's setting our kids up for future obesity, health problems, and early death!

Many people are allowing the food industry to control themselves and their kids. Never underestimate the persuasiveness of advertising because it changes people's attitudes! Did you know that more than 95% of food ads on television are promoting junk food, such as sweetened cereals and beverages, prepackaged snack food, fast food, canned food, and frozen meals?[29] Research has confirmed that there is a strong association between the increased marketing of junk food to children and the rates of childhood obesity.[30] It's easy to see why childhood diabetes is on the rise! Junk food is so inexpensive that poorer kids often end up consuming more calories than the wealthier ones. Healthy food costs more because you get what you pay for.

Functional Alert: Ask yourself this question: As a parent, how much am I really protecting my kids if I keep them away from second-hand smoke, yet allow them to eat junk food such as fast-food?

We know parents love their kids and grandparents love their grandkids. However, offering them cheap junk food is doing them a great disservice because they will learn to associate those kinds of food with loving nurture and have a hard time breaking that cycle as they move into adulthood. Kids need to be taught by adults how to have a good attitude toward healthier food choices. Ask yourself this question: Do I love my child/children enough to stop feeding them in a way that will take years off their life?

Functional Alert: Attitude is everything when it comes to making the proper food choices in childhood and adulthood. What's preventing you and your kids from making good food choices?

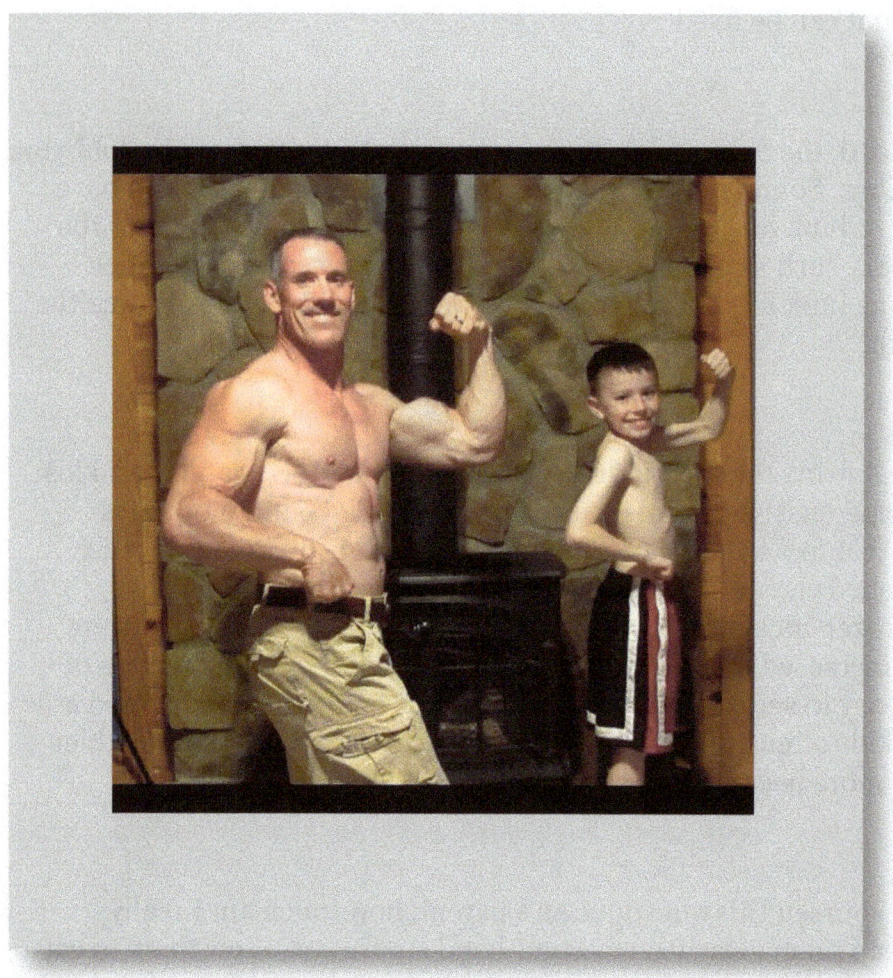

Jimmy Corbett and his son, Jace Corbett

I take my role as the man of the family very seriously. I do my best to be a good provider, protector, leader, and teacher of my family. I follow the principles found in **Functional Training with a Fork**. *I believe the principles found in this book are necessary to be a good person and live a full and meaningful life. A lot of people go to gyms and work out very hard, yet never lose body fat. Why? It's because they look past the necessity of a Functional Diet! A key point to keep in mind about what the authors are saying is that we must teach our kids by example. Simply telling our children what to do is not very effective. Our children mostly learn by observing what we eat, the way we choose to exercise, and how we treat others and God. They won't always do everything we do, but it's the best way to teach them honesty, responsibility, and coping skills. I feel the breakdown of today's American family is a major problem and* **Functional Training with a Fork** *is putting people back on the right path!*

Take Command

Take command of your own health. Being on a sustainable Functional Diet doesn't mean you are making a big sacrifice! It just means becoming more aware of what you are eating and being smarter about it. You will know you are going in the right direction when you become more sensitive to the things you eat. When you know the food is unhealthy and/or you are eating too much, you turn away quickly! Restaurants you used to like to visit won't appeal to you anymore. You will spend time searching for healthy food instead of fattening food. Your diet becomes more structured and your workouts more intense. You begin to rejoice in your new lifestyle instead of looking at it as a burden. Barriers are viewed not as a dead-end, but as an opportunity to make yourself better. Working out at the gym with others will be more inspiring because of the group mentality.

Functional Alert: The best way to predict success is to create it!

It's up to you as an individual to gauge your health by monitoring your cholesterol, triglycerides, blood pressure, general overall well-being, libido, sleep patterns, satiety (fullness), hydration, digestive system, and levels of blood sugar, pain, energy, and body fat. There is usually a measurable difference between carbs and fats in relation to how each one affects your body. The difference can sometimes be seen short-term through laboratory tests that are non-invasive. Over the long-term, more invasive diagnostic tests can be your guide. You will need to figure out whether it's the carbs or the fats that stimulate your appetite the most, causing you to gain body fat. Then you can lean more toward the one you can control. For some of you, your weakness will be carbs, (e.g., cereals, pastas, potatoes, or breads). For others, it will be fats (e.g., cheese, nuts, peanut butter, or oils). Once you stop the food that you crave and have a hard time controlling, the cravings will lessen!

Carbs, fats, and salt activate the brain's pleasure center. The big picture boils down to your brain chemistry, and the best way to avoid eating the wrong food is to stop bringing them into your home. It's also imperative that you stop going to restaurants where you will be tempted. Most people who struggle to lose weight can't eat out at restaurants more than once a week and keep the weight off. If more people would accept this reality, we would have less of an obesity problem today! Some people would rather eat what they want, when they want, and be fat and miserable, and not live as long, than to eat in moderation and exercise regularly. One of the main joys in their lives is eating fattening food and socializing at restaurants. They use food as a sedative instead of exercise, proper nutrition, and sexual intercourse to deal with their stress. As a result, their hunger controlling hormones and weight gain begin to spiral out of control!

If you are obese, you are allowing the large food companies to control you! Food companies have manipulated food to make it taste better so you eat more and keep buying their products. The tobacco company did the same thing by adding more nicotine to cigarettes! They knew they would keep people addicted to their products. The biggest sin of the food industry is putting profits before others' health. The calorie-dense food with a long shelf life (e.g., chips, cookies, crackers, cakes, ice cream, pasta, pizza, macaroni and cheese, etc.) that seem to taste the most fulfilling upfront will actually leave you the most unfulfilled—it's a short-lived pleasure that does great harm to the body. Anything with a long shelf life makes a profit for the company producing it, but "it's going to cost you in more ways than one."

Functional Alert: Food companies have added hidden sugars and chemicals, such as MSG, to keep you addicted to their products! [31]

Major food companies seem to be labeling things so that you will imagine what's in them rather than know what's inside. Many of the food labels at the grocery store are deceptive. For example, marketers try to entice you to buy sugar-laden cereal by stating that it's full of vitamins, minerals, and fiber, and low in fat with no added sugar. Some labels on cereal boxes claim to have fruit, but it's not usually real fruit. In fact, most of the fruit fillers in highly processed food are actually Dysfunctional Toxins that can be made to look like fruit. One of these is the chemical propylene glycol—it's found in antifreeze and used to winterize RVs to keep their pipes from freezing.[32]

Manufactures often use a food additive in processed food to enhance flavor. This food additive is called MSG (monosodium glutamate, also known as sodium glutamate) and it's in just about everything (e.g., most fast food, restaurant food, and processed food). MSG is a chemical given to labs rats to drastically increase their appetite so they will gain weight.[33] It's used on rats because, under normal circumstances, they won't overeat and gain weight. MSG causes the rats' blood sugar and insulin to skyrocket. Food manufacturers are aware that many consumers would prefer not to have MSG in their food. In order to hide the name on food labels, it's often disguised under another name—Hydrolyzed Vegetable Protein.[34]

Functional Alert: Have you ever noticed how small the print is on food labels? Even a person with good eyesight can barely read them!

Another example of hidden Dysfunctional Toxins in your food is **high-fructose corn syrup**. Food manufacturers use it because it's cheap to produce and sweeter than regular sugar. High-fructose corn syrup comes from GMO corn and it's highly addictive and fattening.[35, 36] It's the single largest calorie source in many Americans diets![37] The next time you consume sugar, monitor yourself. You'll feel happy for a very brief time, and then begin to feel extremely hungry and tired. Many people are not eating real food, but rather food-like products with added sugar and hydrogenated oils. Sugar and fat are addictive, like recreational drugs. When you violate your body it comes back to violate you. High nutrition and low calories are the key to remaining healthy and losing body fat, not low nutrition and high calories. Even when you are on a high-calorie diet low in nutrition, you begin starving on a cellular level because your body gets low on essential nutrients.

Functional Alert: Fat-free labels on food products usually means they're loaded with sugar! No sugar added doesn't usually mean sugar free!

Support Groups

Some of you may find the need to join a support group. While losing body fat is a very individual process, having additional group support, in addition to a Functional Personal Trainer or the gym, can help your short- and long-term success. Food addiction is like any other addiction. Some can walk away easily while others cannot. Some people need additional reinforcement from a group to keep them accountable or they will fail at losing body fat. We have seen people lose weight by regularly attending a weight-loss support group and even eating unhealthy prepackaged food. Unfortunately, once they reached their goals, they stopped going to meetings and slowly put the weight back on. They lost their drive because they no longer worried about what others in the group would think about them if they gained weight during the week. However, the biggest problem was that they never learned how to shop and prepare their own meals. In other words, they were never eating a Functional Diet!

The group meetings aren't for everyone. If you don't enjoy group meetings or don't have time to attend, you can use the Internet. An Internet search will help you find weight-loss blogging message boards. There are also Facebook groups for weight-loss support. If the idea of joining a support group appeals to you, look for a group whose weight-loss goals match the principles found in this book. You should stay away from groups that push eating unhealthy prepackaged food, diet pills, HCG (a hormone produced by a portion of the placenta) shots, and rapid weight loss.[38] The Functional Diet requires that you shop and prepare your own healthy food. This prepares you to keep the weight off if you ever decide to exit the support group.

Quitters

Don't be a quitter! When you quit you can lose everything. We have a news flash for you: Life isn't always easy! You're going to have to work hard for everything you get, just like everyone else. For years, we have seen people complain about how bad their lives were, but they've never done anything to make them better. Losing body fat isn't magic! You can't just whine and complain about it and expect things to change. The sad thing is, most obese people try to find excuses to justify their bad eating habits. If someone waits too long to change their lifestyle and is already suffering from a terminal illness or the end of an intimate relationship, they're going to look back and become extremely disappointed that they didn't try harder.

Functional Alert: Whatever it is you want to do with your looks and health, start today, don't delay. Make a plan and start now!

In today's society, a lot of people waste precious years of their lives fantasizing about losing body fat, toning up, improving overall functionality, and gaining the respect of others. It takes a long time (and a lot of negative experiences) before they realize that the real reason they never accomplished their goals is that they really didn't want them badly enough in the first place. They love the thought of having these things, but don't love the work involved to get them. Therefore, they fail repeatedly! Now we have a question for you: Do you really want to lose weight, build muscle tone, improve your overall functionality, and gain the respect of others, or do you want to be one of those people who make excuses and whine about not reaching their goals because they don't enjoy the work required to get there? Everyone has to make sacrifices for the things they want most in life. People who have to make some sacrifices to obtain their goals appreciate them more. People who have everything handed to them are often unhappy in life because they didn't do anything special to deserve it. Living a functional lifestyle requires challenge, learning, and adaptation. The best life has to offer usually comes when you have to overcome adversity. You don't have to do anything in life perfectly. All you have to do is show up, perform, learn what works, and move forward.

The exciting part about accomplishing a goal is that if you really want it, you won't feel deprived. For example, parents who are willing to take on more responsibilities to ensure that their kids are well taken care of, don't feel deprived because they enjoy making sacrifices for them. In fact, parents feel blessed to have the opportunity because their kids bring joy into their lives! On the other hand, a parent who resents having kids would feel deprived. The same scenario applies to those who want to lose weight. A person who really wants to lose weight won't feel deprived when they walk past a friend at work who is eating a doughnut or piece of cake because they love what eating healthy does for them. A person who doesn't really want to lose body fat will feel deprived because they are unwilling to make a sacrifice to look and feel better. The only time a dedicated person feels deprived is when they aren't trying to reach or maintain their goals. Trying to reach new goals makes life more exciting! We have met a lot of people who are stuck in the past. They are always talking about how great their bodies use to look in high school. Now that high school is over, it's time to decide what you want your body to look like for the rest of your life and how long you want to live in good health. We ask that you take this incredible opportunity to change your lifestyle with Functional Training with a Fork so you don't have regrets later in life.

Functional Alert: Don't pass up happiness by clinging to things that make you unhappy and bring forth a false sense of security!

The longer you eat the wrong kinds of food, the harder it is for you to stop! The good news is that when you do decide to eat healthier food, you will become a stronger person and it becomes easier to maintain healthy eating habits. Each time you reach a new level in body-fat loss and improved functionality, you will view it as a milestone. If you quit, then you are not giving it everything you have. We are not asking you to step onto a stage at a local physique competition. What we are teaching is that quitters have nothing to gain but additional body fat because they have stopped trying!

Functional Alert: Struggle always precedes greatness. Some of us have to struggle more than others to get there. If you expect anything less than greatness from yourself, then you have set your standards too low!

We are all creatures of habit! When we successfully change bad habits into good habits, the good habits remain with us for a lifetime. Body-fat loss is not something you deserve; it's something you need. People who stay in shape have to work at it. We didn't get in shape overnight. We have had to work within reasonable limits on a persistent basis. Body-fat loss is not something that can be given to you or purchased. Just thinking about losing body fat in your head is not going to get you anywhere. That's only the beginning! You have to pursue body-fat loss with consistency. Then you can help others with their weight problem.

Some of you reading this book are overweight because you suffer from food addiction. You eat fattening food to the point of feeling bloated and sluggish. You keep telling yourself, I'm going to stop! However, you continue down the path of destruction.

You feel miserable, you look bad, and you are ashamed and disgusted with yourself. Where's the fun in that? Being overweight and self-conscious go hand in hand. If you are obese, you probably see yourself as being the center of attention. You are embarrassed when people watch you eat. You are embarrassed when your clothes are tight. You wear long pants to cover your legs and over-sized shirts to try to hide your belly. When you feel embarrassed all the time, it destroys your self-confidence and makes you give up hope. Even though you aren't working out and following a Functional Diet, you are still constantly thinking about them. Your mind is distracted, you feel guilty, and it's preventing you from feeling good about yourself and your life. Let's face it: It's urgent that you commit to making a lifestyle change today so you don't keep putting it off as you have so many times in the past!

Functional Alert: Being unable or reluctant to make decisions is linked to a lack of hope and self-confidence. We ask that you find your hope and self-confidence today and make a decision to start **Functional Training with a Fork**. We know you want to be set free, so don't start thinking of excuses. It's time to face reality and change your lifestyle—you deserve to be happy!

CHAPTER 2

Functional Training

The fitness industry has always been about Functional Training. Functional Training makes you look more attractive to others and feel good about yourself. In today's fitness world, the term "Functional Training" is being misused just like the term "Core Training!" What some are referring to as Functional Training is actually Dysfunctional Training (e.g., most of the exercises performed in CrossFit®). Likewise, what some are referring to as Core Training (e.g., some of the exercises being taught in mat Pilates) is actually weakening the core!

The basic idea of Functional Training is to perform repetitions of exercises that mimic movement of daily activities to build muscle tone, strength, and enhance overall functionality without becoming injured in the process. Functional Training is very important because it helps you perform your daily activities more easily without getting injured. This means any type of training that safely helps you perform better and builds muscle tone and strength is considered Functional Training! For example, squats mimic getting in and out of a chair. Functional Training gently stretches the muscles as it strengthens the muscles through resistance exercise. This alleviates tightness in muscles and prevents them from becoming stiff. Functional Training, combined with Functional Hormone Replacement, is the #1 way to prevent bone fractures and osteoporosis, not taking bone-building drugs that often have side effects. The truth is, there are pros and cons for each type of Functional Training, and the most important component comes down to safety for the individual. Every Functional Training method produces results, some more than others. You have to find the method of Functional Training that works best for you.

Functional Alert: Improving functionality becomes craziness when you stray from basic exercises. The best way to get functional is to perform basic weight-training movements. Don't fool yourself into thinking wacky exercises that put you in an awkward position and/or make you feel uncoordinated is Functional Training!

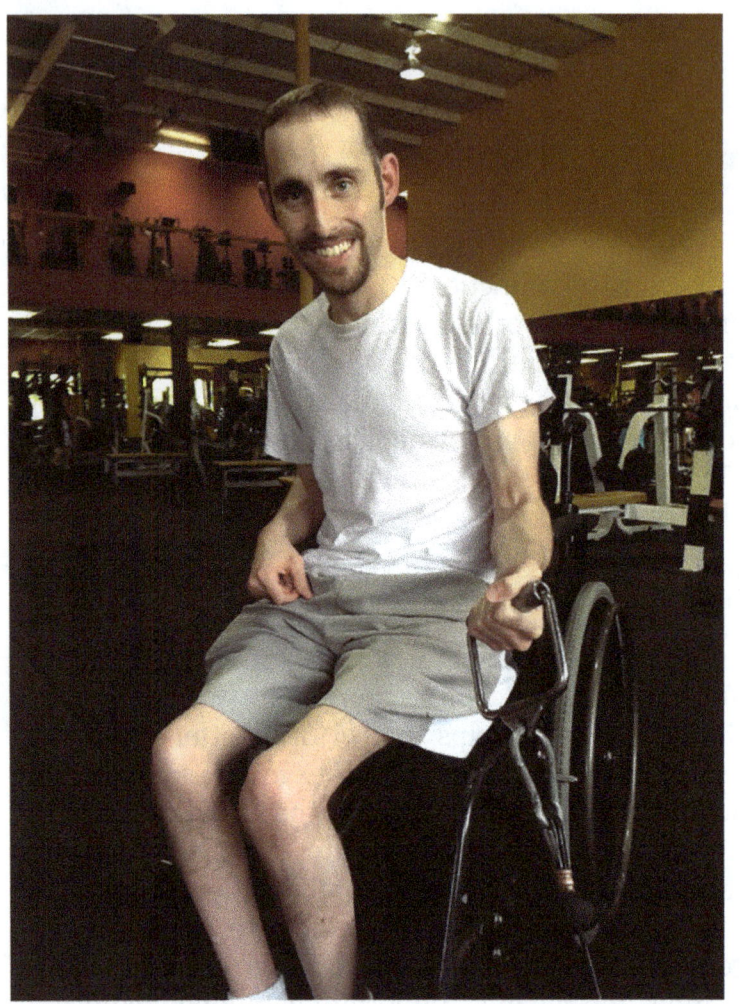

Joshua Van Buren

I'm thirty years old and work in Enterprise Information Technology as a desktop engineer. I was born two and a half months premature in a complicated delivery via C-section. As a result of this, I have a variant of cerebral palsy called spastic diplegia, which mainly affects my lower body and causes me to need a wheelchair. To deal with the extreme tightness in my hamstrings I underwent hamstring-release surgery at the age of twelve in 1997. As a result of this surgery I developed CRPS (complex regional pain syndrome) due to nerve damage. This healed for the most part, but left me with some lingering issues in my feet and toes.

I began weight training once a week at the age of sixteen, and now I use Basic Functional Training for my upper body and Rehabilitative Functional Training for my lower body four or five days a week. Functional Training, combined with a well-balanced diet, has improved my health and quality of life. I have been able to maintain a positive attitude, healthy immune system, and a good body weight and to remain mobile, minimize joint damage from continuous sitting, and stay strong enough to do everything I need to do in daily life!

Sculpting your physique and building muscle tone is approximately 20% Functional Diet and about 80% Functional Training. When people lose weight without incorporating the proper type of Functional Training, they lack shape, have a soft appearance, and develop saggy skin. If you want to remain functionally active as you age and have muscle tone, then Functional Training is for you! Functional Training greatly enhances your functional ability and social participation. There are seven options of Functional Training being offered by Functional Personal Trainers worldwide: Slingshot Functional Training, Basic Functional Training, Advanced Functional Training, Highly Advanced Functional Training, Group Functional Training, Rehabilitative Functional

Training, and Post-Catastrophic Functional Training. You will lose a lot more body fat by focusing on a Functional Diet and Functional Training rather than on of a Functional Diet and Functional Cardio. You can lose body fat with any type of Functional Training if your diet is good, but some forms of Functional Training are far more effective than others in terms of building muscle tone and burning calories.

You will gain more muscle tone by implementing, Slingshot Functional Training (SFT), Basic Functional Training (BFT), or Advanced Functional Training (AFT), than following any other method of Functional Training. Everyone reading this book can participate in some form of boot camp training using only body-weight exercises to the point you are pouring sweat and nauseated, and feel very sore for the next several days. Will you gain as much muscle tone as you would using SFT, BFT, or AFT? The answer is no because nothing has changed in terms of lifting more weight to cause a substantial increase in muscle tone! That isn't to say that training with more frequency, intensity, and volume are not a part of the equation, but lifting more weight lays the foundation for building maximum muscle tone, strength, and improving functionality. Furthermore, just because a muscle gets sore after a training session doesn't mean additional muscle tone will occur. Some people get sore in certain body parts while others don't. You don't have to get a muscle sore to make it get toned. Just because a particular muscle group gets sore after a training session doesn't mean you will experience an increase in muscle tone. Extreme muscle soreness in the days following a workout is usually caused by your muscles having done something they aren't used to doing (e.g., a new exercise) or not working out on a consistent basis!

Functional Alert: Many of the people you see on infomercials who claim they built their body using this form or that form of boot camp-style training often leave out the part where they are also lifting weights on the side and eating a clean diet. Some of them also have a lot more type-2 muscle fibers than the general population!

Unfortunately, the wrong kind of exercise can do you more harm than not exercising at all because it severely disrupts normal alignment throughout the body, causing further wear and tear on bodily structures. Many who have exercised improperly are now dealing with chronic injuries that changed their lives forever! CrossFit® is the fastest growing fad, and we strongly believe they are teaching others how to exercise improperly.[1]

Functional Alert: The best way to prevent injury is knowing how to prevent it in the first place!

The great news is that improving your ability to function during daily activities can safely be done performing the same exercises and training methods used for muscle toning and body-fat loss. Functional Training is the best way to prevent muscle imbalances and overuse injuries. As personal trainers, the exercises we provide for our clients and the order in which they are performed can mean the difference between being injury-free and being disabled. The ideal training program is to use free weights, machines, cables, and bodyweight exercises if health permits. As personal trainers, we find that free weights are harder on some of our clients' joints versus the machines or bodyweight exercises and vice versa.

We have learned we must train our clients in a way that provides body-fat loss, muscle toning, and improved functionality in a timely manner. These types of workouts are manageable both time-wise and energy-wise for most people. It's nothing short of remarkable that such modest investments in Functional Training can produce such profound physical outcomes.

Functional Alert: A Functional Personal Trainer will demonstrate the proper use of gym equipment and explain what muscles are being worked!

Connective tissue (tendons, ligaments, and fasciae) and joint pain can result from not being in the correct position for your particular body on any exercise. The movements that work best for you don't always work for someone else. You must pay careful attention to how your connective tissues and joints feel on various exercises.

The contraction of muscles maintains body posture and joint stability. Your muscles work in much the same way as shock absorbers on a motocross bike. They cushion the joints, take stress off of connective tissue, and help maintain proper alignment, which helps the body to function properly. If muscles get weak, they become ineffective shock absorbers, resulting in damaged muscles, tendons, ligaments, fasciae, cartilage, and discs.

Muscle imbalances and injuries are likely to occur due to obesity and/or weakness in either the agonist muscle (initiates a specific movement) or the antagonist muscle (controls movement). In order for muscles to accomplish their daily functions, they must work in harmony. A functional limitation results in the loss of ability to perform athletically or do everyday activities. Muscle tone, strength, and functionality wither away fast if you're not working out on a consistent basic, and they wither away even faster as a person ages!

FUNCTIONAL TRAINING

Functional Alert: You cannot expect your muscles to protect your disc, tendons, ligaments, and cartilage if you are carrying around a lot of extra body fat. Building muscle protects whereas building fat destroys!

Improving muscle control through strengthening the muscles and enhancing neuromuscular coordination minimizes trauma. Coordination is directed by your brain, but is affected by muscle or bone loss and changes in the joints, tendons, ligaments, and discs. These changes affect your posture and gait, which lead to weakness, slower movement, and loss in balance. Weakness in larger muscle groups results in instability in the ligaments and tendons, causing increased compression forces on cartilage and disc throughout the entire body and wear and tear over time.

Certain types of balance training can make up a very small portion of Rehabilitative Functional Training and Highly Advanced Functional Training. However, weight-lifting exercises for the legs, especially compound movements, are a lot more effective at improving the kind of balance needed to lower the risk of falls than exercises such as the stork swim or the tree pose used in yoga classes. This is because weight training dramatically strengthens the stabilizing muscles that are used to continually shift your body weight during daily activities and sports. There is little transfer from balancing exercises to improve balance in daily activities.

Functional Alert: Muscle imbalances create a domino effect. For example, a weak lower back and glutes causes tight hamstrings because your pelvis tilts forward. The tightness of the hamstrings, originating from the lower back/glutes, increases compressive forces all the way down to the ankle!

As you can see, everything must remain in proper alignment or balance in order to run smoothly. The body is in a constant state of change. An exercise that feels perfectly fine now may cause you to experience debilitating joint pain several months down the road. A Functional Personal Trainer is of great value during these situations. These trainers have the ability to troubleshoot the problem by finding a substitute exercise that works the muscles in a similar fashion or by changing your body position to make the exercise fit your biomechanics.

Functional Alert: Proper Functional Training causes the synovial joints to secrete synovial fluid.[2] This fluid performs the functions of making it easier for cartilage and bone to move past each other and it cushions the joints. The continual release of synovial fluid over time helps maintain joint health!

Improperly training the muscles also results in damaged muscles, tendons, ligaments, fasciae, cartilage, and discs. A good example is CrossFit®. The most common injuries sustained in CrossFit® are of the spine and shoulders.[3] Other injuries include the elbows, wrist, feet, ankles, hips, and knees. The result is increased cost of health care and, for some, lost wages and living in chronic pain, all of which can have detrimental effects on family life.[4] Hypermobility in the joints from stretched out ligaments and tendons reduces proprioception (sensory receptors commonly found in muscles, tendons, and joints that give your brain feedback about the movements and position of the body). An unstable joint means that tendons and/or ligaments have been stretched/injured and allow the joint to move around too much. The extra movement slowly injures the cartilage in the joint and causes degenerative disc disease. This causes weak muscles and reduces stamina, having an adverse effect on gait and posture, and causing chronic pain.

Signs of joint instability include soreness or swelling after activity. However, by keeping muscles, tendons, ligaments, fasciae, and bones strong through proper Functional Training, you help prevent wear and tear on the discs of the spine and cartilage in the joints. In other words, proper exercise helps keep everything in line where it should be so nothing wears out before its appointed time, thus allowing you to remain functional.

Functionally Fit

Functional Training helps your body function more efficiently on all levels. It's very unfortunate that many people's sedentary lifestyles results in unfavorable outcomes in terms of disease and disability. Functional Training:

- ☐ Significantly lowers production of pro-inflammatory cytokines and free radicals when actively training the muscles and while your body is at rest.[1-4]

- ☐ Changes the chemistry of your brain.[5]

- ☐ Helps you remain on a Functional Diet.[6]

- ☐ Causes your heart to pump blood and deliver oxygen to working muscles and all major organs, such as the brain. The cells in your brain start functioning at a higher level, making you feel more alert during Functional Training and more focused after you finish. Over time, you will experience a lower resting heart rate and your brain will function more efficiently.[7]

- ☐ Helps with your digestion after a meal.[8]

- ☐ Plays a dramatic role in helping you cope with the stress you face in everyday life. It's even more effective for managing stress than cardio. Stress often becomes

FUNCTIONAL TRAINING

unmanageable, causing a Dysfunctional Immune System.[9]

- [ ] Helps you control anger, anxiety, and depression.[10]

- [ ] Gently stretches your muscles under a load during training, providing them with a deep myofascial release or massage. Not only does this help alleviate stress and muscle tightness, it increases your body's white blood cells called killer cells. This improves the immune system's first line of defense against infection.[11-12]

- [ ] Lowers blood glucose (sugar) levels, which enhance the function of your pancreas.[13]

- [ ] Releases dopamine and testosterone, which increase sexual function and brain function.[14,15]

- [ ] Releases growth hormone which burns body fat and heals connective and skeletal tissue.[16]

- [ ] Increases brain serotonin and dopamine, which are responsible for helping maintain mood balance.[17]

- [ ] Improves the functionality of your lungs, which helps prevent COPD.[18]

- [ ] Lowers blood pressure about as efficiently as Functional Cardio.[19] It improves kidney function by lowering blood pressure. High blood pressure is widely known for causing kidney failure, strokes, and heart attacks.

- [ ] Improves the function of your liver by preventing the buildup of fats in liver tissue.[20,21]

- [ ] Decreases visceral fat (fat that lies deep inside your body that can compress vital organs, blood vessels, and lymphatic vessels) and subcutaneous fat (fat that lies just beneath the skin that can negatively affect ones overall appearance and health).[22]

- [ ] Purges Dysfunctional Toxins (through sweat, burning of calories, and speeding up the elimination of food through your digestive tract) and lowers body fat, which improves immune functions and lowers the risk of getting cancer and other life-threatening illnesses.[23,24]

- [ ] Develops more skeletal muscle, which works in addition to smooth muscle to help squeeze lymph fluid through lymph nodes so Dysfunctional Toxins can be filtered.[25]

- [ ] Builds strong bones.[26]

- ☐ Improves balance and flexibility, and helps retain mobility in damaged joints.[27]
- ☐ Can be performed in a manner that does not produce a significant amount of harmful free radicals.[28]
- ☐ Reduces the risk of disease by improving the antioxidant system.[29]
- ☐ Strengthens the transverse abdominis that helps the colon excrete Dysfunctional Toxins.[30]
- ☐ Helps prevent an enlarged heart.[31]

Most of our clients come to us wanting to lose body fat, tone their muscles, and improve functionality in everyday activities without becoming injured in the process. Most are not signing up to become professional bodybuilders, power-lifters, or athletes. However, if they fall into that category, then we will train them in a different manner while still keeping safety our number one priority. Randomly bouncing around from one exercise to another doesn't constitute proper Functional Training. This form of Dysfunctional Training prevents specific adaptations from occurring. When specific adaptations are lacking, the training method becomes dysfunctional because the type-2 muscle fibers that are mostly responsible for providing muscle tone, strength, and improving functionality go unchallenged.

If you are a beginner or have pre-existing injuries, randomly switching from one Functional Training style or exercise to another before your body has a chance to adapt is a mistake. This increases your chance of becoming injured because you might run into an exercise that doesn't agree with pre-existing conditions. As a beginner, it also prevents a steady load on the muscles. A steady load on the muscles is needed to instruct the nervous system to become more efficient at recruiting the muscle fibers needed to lift more weight or perform more reps using a particular exercise. In order to make maximum progress, you must develop the necessary strength base by sticking to the same basic exercises for a few months. People with pre-existing injuries may have to stick with the same basic exercises indefinitely!

We often see people wandering around, looking at machines and free weights, trying things here and there, not doing them the right way, and then leaving after about an hour. Most people in the gym perform exercises improperly and in the wrong order. Many of the photos on the machines give unclear instructions or none at all. It's difficult to learn how to use machines and free weights in order to obtain maximum results and avoid injury. If you need assistance, we recommend that you hire a Functional Personal Trainer. Don't walk around without a plan and think you got a functional workout in.

Functional Alert: Without a functional workout plan your gym membership is useless!

Some people find it hard to muster up enough energy to come to the gym on a consistent basis after working all day. We have found that taking only one-quarter of a caffeine tablet or 1 cup of organic caffeinated coffee before Functional Training sessions awakens the brain and central nervous system, helps concentration, and decreases muscle pain while training. However, some people can't take caffeine because they experience side effects (e.g., anxiety and insomnia).[32] Stick to low dosages about thirty to sixty minutes before training sessions. Don't allow tiredness to keep you from enjoying your workouts when all it takes is a little caffeine and some upbeat music on your iPod to get you revved up to seize the moment. Functional Training is a break from a stressful day, a reward your body deserves!

Functional Alert: Functional Training is very effective at reducing fatigue and hunger, whereas going home and sitting on the couch makes you even more tired and hungry. You will have to experience Functional Training for yourself to understand how it increases energy levels and reduces appetite. If you neglect to incorporate consistent Functional Training into your lifestyle, you'll end up eating excess calories in order to try and find some extra energy just to make it through the day!

Free Weights vs. Machines

Whoever came up with the concepts that the tendons and ligaments are not strengthened with machines or that machines are not considered Functional Training because you don't have to balance the weight, was misinformed. The muscle and its tendons and ligaments act together as a functional unit! Free weights don't stimulate more muscle fibers than variable resistance machines as some claim, but they do recruit more connective tissue (tendons, ligaments, and fasciae) because the user has to stabilize the weight. A person's genetics (the amount of type-2 muscle fibers they are born with) is what determines how much muscle tone they can build, not whether they're using free weights or machines.

The improvements made in strength and athletic ability by machines is very similar to free weights. The difference between the two is small to none depending on the exercise.[1-5] Working each side of the body independently using dumbbells, weight machines, cables, and some body-weight movements can slightly help improve athleticism in some cases because both sides of the body are worked equally.

Functional Alert: Performing upper-body weight-training exercises while standing on one leg (e.g., the single-leg overhead press) is not sufficient for building the core or improving dynamic balance because it decreases forceful muscle contractions during upper-body exercises and it invites injury!

In some cases, free weights can be more versatile than weight machines since they allow for more variations in range of motion and don't hold you in a fixed position. But cable machines can allow for more variations than free weights. Cable machines and some weight machines allow you to keep constant tension on the muscle while putting less stress on the connective tissue and cartilage. With some weight machines (e.g., the preacher curl bicep machine) you don't get a chance to rest at the bottom or top position like barbell preacher curls. Therefore, the machine can work the muscles harder than free weights. On the other hand, some free-weight exercises are better than some weight machines for working the muscles more efficiently because they allow you to move more naturally.

Free weights work the connective tissue harder than machines, but it can also cause them to degenerate faster. So, it's a Catch 22! This is why some people try to use a combination of both and people with joint problems often have to steer clear of free weights and use machines, cables, and body-weight exercises.

Functional Alert: Always have a spotter on specific free-weight movements such as barbell bench press. If you fail to get the last rep on your own or a tendon tears, the weight will drop down suddenly and crush you. Several people die each year because they did not have a spotter!

The truth is that every single muscle in the body comes into play in a stabilizing role at some point, and it's basically the large muscle groups for each body part that are most responsible for stabilization of the joint. Tendons and ligaments are not stabilizing muscles, but they do help stabilize joints indirectly. Training in the proper manner using machines, cables, free weights, or body-weight exercises improve functionality!

Lower-Back Injuries

The greatest number of weight-training-related back injuries result from exercises in hyperflexion under a load, hyperextension under a load, and twisting movements under a load. In addition, excessive tightening of the iliopsoas muscle and tendon under a load during certain abdominal exercises (e.g., sit-ups) puts wear and tear on the discs and connective tissues.[1]

The lumbar hyperflexion exercise called dead-lifts, especially the stiff-legged version, is among the most dangerous because people often lose their normal inward curvature of the lumbar and cervical regions of the spine during the performance. A frequent error is to round the back and then rapidly jerk the weight up using the hips and lower back muscles to generate power. Lumbar hyperflexion, while lifting a weight rapidly, results in the load being shifted from the leg and back muscles to the posterior ligaments and the lumbar discs. As you lift or lower a weight to the ground, bend at your knees, not your waist, and use your legs to lift. Don't twist or round out your back while you're lifting or lowering the weight because this significantly increases the risk of hurting your back.

While performing regular deadlifts, you should keep the entire spine in proper alignment and focus on using the legs to lift the weight while keeping the core tight. Keep your back straight, not arched or rounded forward. Tightening up when lifting acts like a muscular corset to help keep your spine in proper alignment. Keep your feet spread shoulder width apart to give yourself a stronger foundation. In order to help prevent lower-back injury while performing exercises such as squats, never allow the lower back to arch inward while trying to keep the chest up too high because you are wary of bending forward.

Functional Alert: The power clean and jerk is a HAFT exercise recommended only for certain athletes. Straight bar deadlifts should be avoided by everyone because they put the body in an awkward position and cause lower back injuries. A Hex Bar should be used for those wanting to do deadlifts because it allows you to remain in a better anatomical position and takes strain off the lower back. We'd like to take this time to ask the "International Powerlifting Federation" to start using Hex Bars in their competitions in order to protect competitors' lower backs!

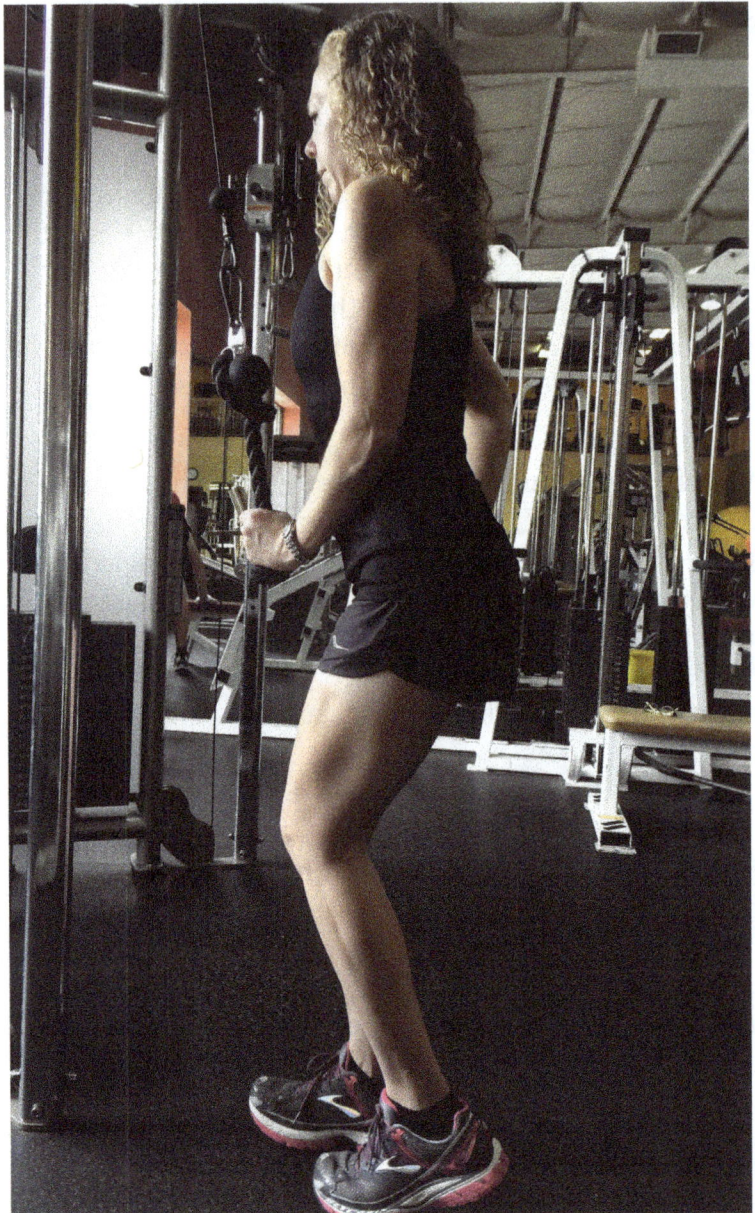

Katherine Lane

I was never an athlete in school or in my early adult life. I had good exercise and dietary habits, but I never considered being a sports competitor. In 2007 I suffered a severe back injury while lifting and twisting. I found out the hard way that the lower back isn't built for rotational movements under a load. I herniated my L5 disc and had fragments in the femoral nerve root. I lost most of the sensation in my right leg and I was in horrific pain. I elected to have a laminectomy to remove the fragments. I was immediately relieved of the leg pain, but I had a long recovery ahead of me to loosen up the tightness in my lower back and rebuild my core. Being unable to exercise for eight weeks, I gained weight and lost muscle composition. Once cleared by my doctor, I resumed my workout routine. In 2011 I began competing in local half Ironman races in Augusta, Georgia. I did not have exceptional overall finish times, but I completed the races. I was still lacking overall strength and my lower back was a limiting factor.

In 2013 I was introduced to Ronnie Rowland, a personal trainer at my local Gold's Gym. Upon meeting, Ronnie put me on the Functional Diet and Basic Functional Training. Next he began to teach me about functional anatomy! He taught me how to train mostly on machines to build my lower, middle, and upper core muscle. As he predicted, the left-over scar tissue from my back surgery did not irritate the nerve roots when I used certain machines in a controlled fashion. In addition, the machines have prevented the damaged L5 disc from protruding farther. This form of Functional Training has been necessary to prevent a spinal fusion surgery. I also learned how important strong hips/glutes are for stabilizing the lower back and improving my ability to balance. Body-weight Super Lunges have improved the shape of my glutes and my hip function. The smart work has paid off because I have less back pain and better posture!

Following the Functional Diet and incorporating Basic Functional Training, Rehabilitative Functional Training, and cardio, I started to transform my physical appearance. I gained muscle tone and lost over 15 lbs of body fat. I improved so much that in 2013, after Functional Training for 6 months, I finished the Augusta half Ironman 54 minutes faster than the previous year. Adding the proper Functional Training to my regimen has made me a much stronger athlete in all disciplines: swimming, cycling, and running! Continuing with my training plan, I finished the 2014 Augusta half Ironman in my best time of 5 hours and 34 minutes.

Having a structured plan consisting of Functional Training, swimming, cycling, and running, along with a Functional Diet (high protein, healthy fats, and lower carbohydrates), has transformed not only my physical appearance, but also my life! I have achieved so many accomplishments by changing to a functional lifestyle. I have now become a sub 2 hour half marathon finisher and won my age group in many local races. Basically, I have been able to turn a disability into an ability! I now have increased confidence in not only my appearance, but my performance as an athlete. I have used this confidence to propel myself further in life. My dreams have become reality and the proof is in multiple finisher medals and awards!

Functional Alert: The spine was not designed to twist while performing weight-loaded exercises (e.g., the standing cable twist, the standing rotational wood chop, and the lunge with twist). Rotating or twisting exercises are a great way to permanently injure your spine over time and should only be used by certain athletes who are willing to take a chance on getting injured. Strong core muscles brace your spine for stability, not twisting! The best core-building exercises to prevent unwanted motion of the spine are anti-rotation weight training exercises, anti-rotation body-weight exercises, and anti-rotation planks. These exercises are very important for building a strong core!

Hyperextension injuries to the spine often occur from arching backward in excess during exercises such as unsupported overhead presses, power cleans, bicep curls, rows, deadlifts, etc. Even the prone Superman exercise that is still being used by a few physical therapists has caused patients with a damaged disc (degenerative, bulging, torn, etc.) to get a herniated disc due to excess hyperextension!

Spinal discs are similar to different brands of tires. Some people inherit discs that are tougher and longer lasting. Other people inherit disc that wear out faster. One's structural alignment also affects the wear and tear on discs just like the alignment of a car's wheels affects the life of the tires. If the discs and tires are not properly aligned, they will likely show a slightly torn or bulging appearance. Tires with uneven wear won't handle as well or last as long as tires that are well maintained. Likewise, discs with uneven wear won't allow your body to maneuver as well or last as long as discs that are well maintained.

Functional Alert: Once discs are damaged, they will never be the same!

Hyperflexion injuries to the lower back commonly occur from abdominal exercises such as full sit-ups, especially with the feet hooked under a stationary object for support (e.g., GHD sit-ups performed by CrossFitters); reverse crunches with the hips coming very high off the ground (e.g., dragon flags); all forms of crunches, sit-ups, and hanging leg raises performed with a twist; and some abdominal machines. These injuries occur because the iliopsoas muscle and tendon contracts very hard, which dramatically increases compression on the lumbar spine.[2, 3] Those exercises also allows the hips to take over and can pull the pelvis out of alignment.

Functional Alert: Sit-ups are considered a Highly Advanced Functional Training exercise. They are recommended only for certain athletes (e.g., wrestlers and those involved in martial arts). Training your abs and neglecting to build up your glutes can increase compression force on the lower spine. In fact, direct ab work involving flexion of the spine often worsens a chronic lower-back condition deriving from disc problems!

Twisting exercises are often performed by gym members to try to work their oblique muscles and create a thinner waistline. However, building the muscles directly underneath the love handles pushes the fat outward, creating an even fatter appearance. In other words, the bigger your obliques are, the fatter you look! That said, building the obliques can help improve high-speed movements that require a lot of rotation (e.g., hitting a baseball). Therefore, those who are serious about excelling in certain sports may choose to make their obliques larger in order to slightly improve athletic performance.

Functional Alert: Twisting exercises won't trim the sides of the waist and should be avoided by people with bad backs.[4] People who are primarily interested in toning up and improving functionality should avoid these exercises! Focus on losing body fat and making the shoulders and lats wider. This will help the waist-to-hip ratio you inherited look smaller. Side planks on the elbow are much safer for building strength in the obliques than rotational movements. Furthermore, planks won't thicken the waist nearly as much as rotational movements!

We have trained a lot of people who had very bad lower backs (e.g., bulging disc, spinal stenosis, spondylolisthesis, scoliosis, bone spurs, scar tissue from prior surgeries, etc.). We have learned that the majority of these clients experience an increase in pain if they work certain parts of the lower core directly using exercises (e.g., crunches and hyperextensions) that involve the movement system of the core. We know that any form of deadlifts or standing over-head presses would be the absolute worst thing to do! In these particular cases, it's of the utmost importance to indirectly build the lower-core muscles as much as possible by working the stabilizing system of the core to help prevent unnecessary inflammation. This is accomplished with supported weight training exercises. Some clients do well with planks and static/or holds on a hyperextension bench. We also add some form of body-weight functional exercise to build the glutes. The goal is to build the lower-core without causing the tissues to swell and irritate local nerve roots of the lower back.

If the core isn't strengthened, there's a greater chance that the already injured disc and other surrounding discs will herniate. The odds are also greater that nearby vertebras will become subluxated (move out of their original alignment), causing pain and inflammation. This same rule applies to the cervical spine (neck). Many people with bad necks find that performing neck flexion, extension, and rotational exercises cause a substantial increase in inflammation and pain to the injured area. They have to use a more conservative approach for strengthening and toning the upper-core muscles that stabilize the neck. This involves building up the shoulders, upper back, and traps with weight-training exercises that don't irritate the neck. Isometric exercises for the front, back, and side of neck are great for strengthening the neck directly. Here are 3 great isometric exercises we recommend to our clients for strengthening the neck:

1. Static Extension—Place both hands against the upper back of your head and gently push your head backward for 10-15 seconds while resisting the pressure of your hands to move your head forward.

2. Static Flexion—Put both hands on your forehead and gently push your head forward and hold for 10–15 seconds while resisting the pressure of your hands to move your head backward.

3. Isometric Lateral Flexion—Place your left hand on the left side of your upper head. Resist the pressure to move your head sideways. Perform the same procedure on your right side.

During all isometrics neck exercises, make sure to tighten your neck muscles as you push your head into your hands. Your neck should remain straight throughout the performance of each exercise. It generally takes about 6 weeks to notice a reduction in neck pain. Performing isometric exercises twice a week, on non-consecutive days, is a good place to start.

Functional Alert: When your lower-core gets out of alignment, it increases the chance of your middle and upper-core slipping out of its proper alignment. All three parts of the core are interrelated and should be functionally trained with basic exercises!

The only joints that are not made for flexion and extension under any appreciable weight load are the facets joints of the back. They have little appreciable motion and were designed to be held statically while your trunk is being moved around by your limbs.

The discs are stiff shock absorbers that have no blood supply by the time you reach early adulthood. Therefore, if the discs were really moving all around, particularly under repetitive forces, they would break down rather quickly. With no blood supply to the discs, the body is unable to repair or heal itself, so disc degeneration occurs. When you bend over to pick up something off the floor, you bend mostly at your hips, not at your lower back or discs. The bottom line is, a weak core results in back pain, injury, and early degeneration. The wrong kind of core training (e.g., rotational movements) also results in back pain, injury, and early degeneration.

Ronnie: Please take care of your spine! By age 40 and beyond, more than 60% of people have disc degeneration at one or more levels. At least 25% of people younger than the age of 40 have disc degeneration at one or more levels.[5]

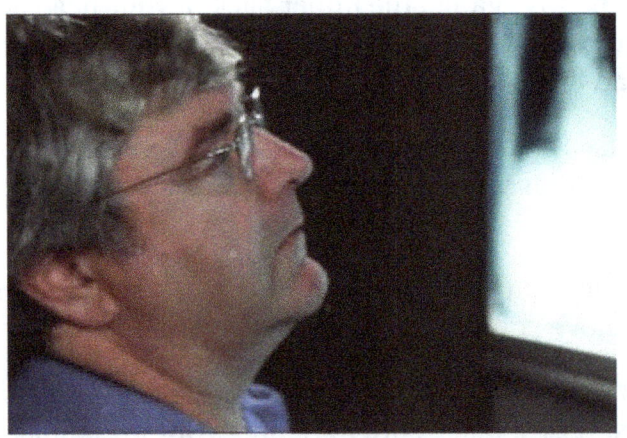

Dr. David H. McCord, M.D. Nashville Spine Specialist and Orthopedic Spine Surgeon. His pioneering work began in the early 1990's with the initial design of disc-cage replacements.

Ronnie Rowland has undergone 11 back surgeries. For most patients, that would result in lifelong pain and narcotic addiction. Instead, Mr. Rowland took matters into his own hands following his last surgery. He developed a program that is outstanding—almost unheard of. His success has been nearly miraculous.

Personally, I do not understand all of the details and intricacies of his training. Having practiced spine surgery for 23 years, Mr. Rowland's rehab program is the best I have witnessed. My only regret is that he is not located close to my practice. His outcomes speak for themselves. People with severe back problems who follow his rehab program will likely benefit and should not give up hope.

The added bonus is Mr. Rowland is not simply another academic trainer. He has lived the nightmares of constant, uncontrollable back pain, and many surgeries, and has first-hand knowledge of what it takes to help people get their life back.

Mr. Rowland is unique in this area of rehabilitative medicine. Most trainers are limited to their own didactic training and what they have read from textbooks. Mr. Rowland has actually lived and experienced the pain, disability, and emotional strain of severe back problems.

No person can develop such a successful program without first-hand understanding of what works and what does not.

Building up the Transverse Abdominis

The main function of the transverse abdominis is to compress the abdomen during functions such as keeping the core tight while lifting weights.[1] The transverse abdominis muscle works as a corset to help keep the spine in place. Functional movements involving the limbs of the body cannot be efficiently performed when the transverse abdominis is weak. Now you see why repeated bouts of weight training are so important for building up the deep core muscles that are harder to target!

Functional Alert: When you build the transverse abdominis you are strengthening the muscle that helps the colon excrete waste.

During every exercise, you should tighten or brace (not tense up) your abs as if you were getting ready to take a punch in the stomach. Brace your hips so that you feel tension all the way down to the bottom of your feet when they are firmly planted on a hard, stable surface. Your head should be looking straight forward: never up, down, or twisted. You must breathe properly during every exercise while keeping the entire core braced. In order to protect the spine and build the core, you must engage your core while performing every exercise. You must learn to use the muscles responsible for pulling the entire core into position, which helps stabilize your entire spinal column.

You can further strengthen the lower core by adding exercises such as planks, crunches, bench side crunches, and hyperextensions. We don't recommend that people with a lot of fat around their abdominals train abs directly with ab exercises that require movement. These exercises can cause an umbilical hernia (a protrusion of the abdominal lining requiring surgery) or a bulging disc from excessive pressure. Even fit people without back problems can develop hernias and back problems from doing low reps with heavy weight and/or explosive movements, or using improper form during ab exercises!

Avoid performing planks on an unstable surface such as a Swiss ball®/stability ball and suspension trainers/straps. Make sure your elbows and feet are always on a stable surface whenever you perform front and side planks! This prevents you from shrugging up or moving side to side, which puts the shoulders out of place. Allowing the shoulders to go out of place can cause pain and/or injury. If your shoulder hurts while performing planks properly, you'll need to avoid them altogether. If you want to make front planks more challenging, add a light-weighted plate on your lower back. Make sure to push the chest out while pulling the shoulders down and away from the ears. Furthermore, people with wrist, shoulder, and neck problems should avoid any form of planks that require using their hands for support. For example: side planks using their hand and the down dog to plank where the hands are above the head. The most common causes of pain/injury during these exercises are when the humerus presses into the shoulder joint and pinches the supraspinatus tendon and when excessive pressure on the wrists compress the median nerve, resulting in carpal tunnel symptoms.

Compound exercises (multi-joint exercises) involve large amounts of muscle and are highly effective for increasing muscle tone and functionality. Isolation exercises (single-joint exercises) allow for better targeting of individual muscles, enhancing muscle tone in specific regions, and improving functionality. Integrating both types of movements into your routine can have a synergistic effect that improves both muscle tone and functionality. The reward gained from weight training is that the stabilizing contractions of the core muscles are involved with all compound and isolation movements. In the strictest sense, any upper-or lower-body exercise used during intense Functional Training will make you tense your entire core because you are performing a static hold. This strengthens the stabilizers that hold your spine in place. Compound exercises with free weights, machines, and specific body-weight movements are particularly effective at causing your entire core to stay tight. Free-weight exercises are usually the most effective, but even isolation exercises on a machine, such as tricep pushdowns, still demand a considerable amount of core stabilization. A lot of competitive bodybuilders and powerlifters rarely do direct abdominal work, such as crunches and hanging leg raises, yet have phenomenal abs. Their abdominal development comes from stabilization during strenuous weight-lifting exercises. In other words, the core gets trained hard indirectly while lifting weights, just as the forearms do when gripping the bar on various exercises.

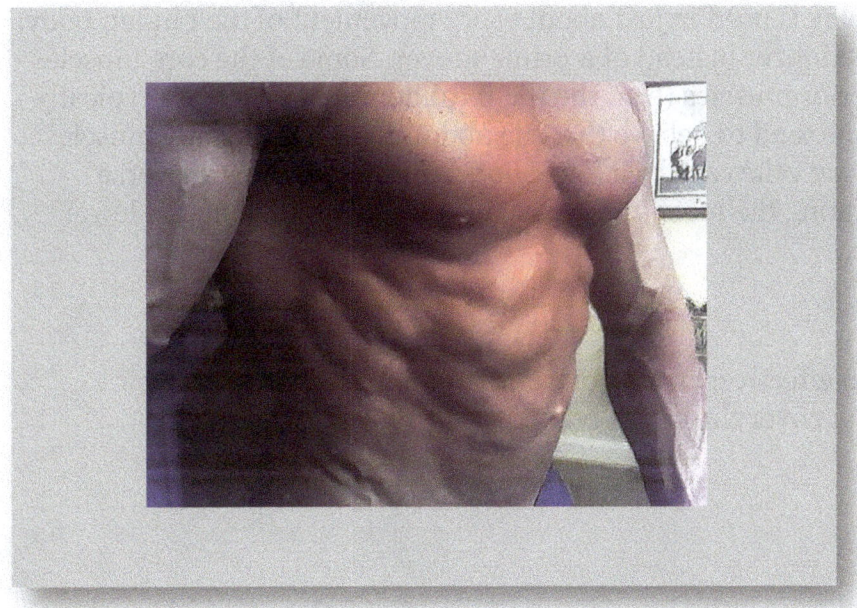

Photo of Ronnie's waistline without performing any direct abdominal training, such as crunches. They get enough stimulation from keeping the core tight while lifting weights!

Functional Alert: If you wear a weight-lifting belt, you should never give your abdominal muscles permission to shut off. There should be absolutely no talking during the performance of a Functional Set because it can disengage the core. Keep the abs tight at all times during a lift!

Your core is made up of every muscle in the body except your arms and legs. The core is made up of three different areas: (1) Your lower core holds your lumbar spine and pelvis in place, (2) your middle core holds your thoracic spine in place, and (3) your upper core holds your cervical spine in place.

Functional Alert: Your lower, middle, and upper core act together as a functional unit!

Your body relies on certain core muscles that attach to the spine to take the pressure off the discs and connective tissues. When the core muscles are weak or have an imbalance, then the stresses you endure every day will not be taken up by the core muscles in the way that's needed to protect the spine. If you have weak core muscles, the stress starts going to other structures such as the discs, facets, and ligaments. This leads to a lot of wear and tear. By keeping the core muscles strong and well-balanced, you take pressure off the discs, facets, and ligaments, making the spine a lot more durable.

Functional Alert: Back pain is the second most common health complaint! If you are obese, your chances of developing degeneration of the spine at an early age are significantly increased!

The entire core complex is used in just about every movement of the human body. Your core mostly acts as a stabilizer instead of a prime mover. Some of the core muscles are hidden beneath the exterior muscles (e.g., the rectus abdominis) which are typically trained for show. Most people tend to believe that the abdominals are the only muscles that make up the core. This isn't the case by a long shot! Building up the transverse abdominis and glutes are among the most important muscles for stabilizing the lower core, but not the entire core.

Functional Alert: You can effectively train your entire core by performing basic weight training exercises that cover the entire body!

Building up the Glutes

Weak glutes are very common because they are not efficiently activated in everyday activities such as walking. Glute dysfunction is brought about by pain, inactivity, and using improper exercises to try and make them functional. Weak glutes not only cause a saggy butt, they are also the number one cause of hip and pelvis instability, which triggers lower back pain and disc injuries! Throw in a bulging belly with those weak glutes and you have just compounded the problem. The hips are one of the most powerful joints in your body. Dysfunctions of the hip musculature due to weak glutes will rob you of your athletic performance and often cause a large number of painful injuries. Big muscles such as the glutes help hold you in proper alignment and improve balance. In order to have control of your body you need strong glutes. We have learned that compound leg movements (such as squats, leg presses, split squats, lunges, bench step-ups) that put your knee at about a 90-degree angle when you plant your foot on the ground, various forms of bridges (glute push-ups), and hyperextensions work synergistically with one another to build the glutes and maximize hip function. We can't emphasize enough how important it is to build your glutes! You can use a STEP Reebok® to make some of these exercises even more effective (e.g., an exercise Ronnie innovated called Super Lunges—lunges performed on a Smith Machine with the front foot on the STEP Reebok® and the back foot on the floor for balance only). Two of the most effective and user-friendly exercises to build your glutes are Swiss ball®/stability lunges and wide-stance Swiss ball®/stability ball squats. Strong legs and glutes are crucial for staying mobile as you get older, and they help improve your balance so that you have better functional stability. Falls are the second leading cause of accidental injury and deaths worldwide! [1]

Functional Alert: Make sure your feet are on a stable surface whenever you perform leg/glute exercises to help stabilize the lower core!

Functional Sets, Active Release Techniques, and Gentle Static Stretching

Functional Sets (work sets) combined with Self-Administered Active Release Techniques (deep-tissue massage) and gentle static stretching (approximately 5 seconds per stretch) can save you time, money, and unnecessary pain. Pain can arise from the joint itself or from the structures around the joint. Tight muscles and connective tissue compress nerves and can cause pain throughout the entire body. Your nerves are covered and protected with a coating of slick fascia that allows the nerves to slightly move during activity. If the fascia becomes sticky or hardened from a prior repetitive strain injury, it restricts the nerves from moving freely. This causes pain because the nerve gets pulled on as it travels through its normal route. Functional Sets, Active Release Techniques, and gentle static stretching in a variety of directions around a sticky, hardened fascia encourages it to break free, helping restore normal function of the nerve.

Many people develop pain in their joints as a result of tightness in muscles close to that joint. Tightness of a muscle occurs if a muscle imbalance is present or the muscle remains in an elongated/weak state from being inactive. If the muscle remains tight for too long, knots can form. Tight muscles and knots can be eliminated with Functional Sets, Active Release Techniques, and gentle static stretching! If a knot is allowed to harden over time, it can turn into scar tissue and shorten your range of motion. This weakens the connective tissues (tendons, ligaments, and fasciae). Aggressive static stretching should be avoided because it will further weaken the connective tissues. The more scar tissue that forms, the more difficult it is to remodel with Functional Sets, Active Release Techniques, and gentle static stretching. Remodeling scar tissue with Functional Sets, deep tissue massage, and gentle static stretching helps to align the collagen fibers that make up muscle and connective tissue, so they can return to a normal state. This realignment of the collagen fibers makes the scar tissue better able to tolerate the forces that are placed on it during activities. Scar tissue that can't be remodeled leads to a lifetime of chronic pain. Your goal should be to eliminate pain and restore motion, not stretch out your ligaments, tendons, and fasciae with aggressive static stretching. Functional Sets combined with Active Release Techniques and gentle static stretching are key for getting rid of knots in muscles. Although aggressive static stretching may feel good and it can temporarily take the edge off of muscle pain and stiffness, it causes loose connective tissue!

Functional Alert: Do not remodel an area that is severely swollen!

Active Release Techniques was developed and patented by a certified chiropractic sports physician, Dr. P. Michael Leahy.[1] It's somewhat painful, but it's much better and safer at breaking up knots and releasing tightness than static stretching. Active Release

Techniques is available through massage therapists, physical therapists, chiropractors, medical doctors, and certified athletic or personal trainers. The only drawback is the cost of sessions and the time that is required for attending the sessions. Therefore, when applicable, we recommend you self-administer Active Release Techniques on your own because it saves both money and time.

Self-administered Active Release Techniques can be done with various objects (e.g., foam rollers, wooden rolling pins, tennis balls, lacrosse balls, baseballs, and golf balls). You can perform it while lying on the floor or leaning against a wall. Let's use the lower back as an example: You start by lying on your back with the object under your lower back where it is tender. Raise your knees and rock your hips forward and backward to break up the knots. Another option is to lean your lower back against the wall with the object on the tender spot. Use your legs and body weight to apply force on the tender spot and roll up and down to break up the knots or muscle tightness. The legs are used to keep the object in place while you roll back and forth to massage the tender area to break up the tightness and knot. You can also have someone (e.g., a family member) who is educated about Active Release Techniques put their elbow on the knot and apply as much pressure as you can withstand in order to break up the knot.

Functional Alert: Active Release Techniques will not help get rid of cellulite! The best way to get rid of cellulite is by using a holistic approach: Functional Diet, Functional Training, Functional Hormone Replacement, and Functional Cardio!

We believe that a reputable chiropractor focuses strictly on limited treatment of neuromusculoskeletal problems that are connected with a mechanical problem. They can be extremely valuable when combined with the proper Functional Training. A chiropractor isn't going to be of much help if you don't strengthen the core muscles that hold the spine in proper alignment. Some people have to visit chiropractors on a regular basis to help correct misalignments of the spine or subluxations. A vertebral subluxation occurs when one or more vertebrae (bones of your spine) move out of position and irritate surrounding muscles and/or spinal nerves.

We have learned that some people can fix their own vertebral subluxations without having to visit a chiropractor. We refer to this as self-administered spinal adjustments. Never forget that no one knows your body like you do. Performing your own spinal adjustments saves you time and money! Here's how you can do it: Simply tape two balls together. Depending on your condition and sensitivity, you can use tennis balls, lacrosse balls, or baseballs. Lie on your back or lean against a wall (depending on your condition and sensitivity) and place the two balls that are taped together in a vertical position (up and down, not side to side). Then gradually apply pressure while lying on the floor with the knees up or while in a standing position with your back against the wall. You can roll back and forth ever so slightly to try to push the vertebra or vertebrae back in line. Another option is using a cut-off piece of foam roller or a wooden rolling pin approximately 5 inches in length to roll back and forth on the vertebrae that are out of alignment. Using these objects will put direct pressure on the vertebrae to help push them back into place. When you are able to push a vertebra back into place, you have successfully fixed a subluxation! You can find many videos on YouTube about how to use foam rollers and balls to loosen tight muscles and to fix subluxations. Be patient because it can require around 3 to 5 minutes of continuous pressure to get results. It is important not to roll over your bony areas (e.g., elbows, knees, and ribs). Roll in line with the muscles at a slow pace. When you roll over a painful area, you should stay primarily on top of this area, to get a release. If it's too painful to stay on top of this area, then decrease the pressure applied or work the area in close proximity.

Functional Alert: If injured sacroiliac joints (located at the base of your spine) are treated repeatedly by manipulation from either you or a chiropractor but the hips won't stay in place, the ligaments have most likely been permanently stretched. Functional Training exercises (e.g., lunges, squats, bridges, planks, and hyperextensions) that build muscle where the hips and lower back meet and in your abdominals, will help tighten loose ligaments and increase sacroiliac stability, given no aggressive static stretching is done afterward!

Overtraining

Overtraining is hazardous to your health. It depletes neurotransmitters that the muscles need to contract, which makes you weaker. Functional Training is like nutrition. In the correct amount for your genetic make-up, it's very beneficial, but in excess, it can be harmful! The key is to find the right level of Functional Training that challenges your body to maintain and increase fitness without over-stressing it. Overtraining significantly increases your chances of developing overuse injuries and weakening the immune system, which fights off life-threatening diseases![1,2] Overtraining is similar to not getting enough sleep in terms of the damage it can do to your body. You have to listen to what your own body can handle. Recovery is rarely about the actual muscles themselves, but rather how much the joints, connective tissue, and central nervous system can handle. While some degree of exhaustion after a workout is normal, extreme fatigue, headaches, irritability, chronic joint pain, and insomnia are signs of overtraining. Reduce the volume and/or intensity if you begin to feel overtrained.

Stress Kills

Chronic stress is public enemy #1![1,2] Functional Training helps us cope with the stress in our lives! Without Functional Training, the stress will eventually lead to an array of health problems.[3] Chronic stress also makes the skin, especially on the face, age faster because it upsets collagen production.[4] Unmanaged stress causes an increase in your appetite. It's not stress that makes us vulnerable to illness, aging, and body-fat gain, but how we react to it! The chemical release you get with Functional Training not only alleviates stress, but allows you to avoid becoming overly frustrated and depressed. When stress stimulates you to achieve your goals, it can be positive. However, when you bottle it up and become chronically frustrated and depressed, it's a killer! When under chronic stress, the body produces excess amounts of pro-inflammatory cytokines and free radicals. The blood vessels then narrow due to the excess production of white blood cells gathering on arteries, reducing blood flow and oxygen to the heart and other cells of the body.[5,6] It also increases nerve pain for those who suffer from chronic conditions such as fibromyalgia and neuropathy. Oxygen is the key to good health, and actively training your muscles increases oxygen levels in your body!

Functional Alert: People who don't exercise regularly have a large release of cortisol from mental stress while those who exercise regularly release only small amounts![7]

Cortisol is produced as a way to help the body respond to both physical and emotional stress. In stressful situations, cortisol provides blood sugar to the body in two different ways:

1. It strips amino acids from muscle tissue.[8]
2. It decreases insulin sensitivity by lowering the amount of blood sugar stored inside cells.[9,10]

Both ways provide a quick delivery of blood sugar to prepare your body for the fight-or-flight response caused by stress. When your body is in a persistent stressful state from a lack of Functional Training, cortisol is constantly gathering blood sugar.[11] This constant release of blood sugar leads to higher blood sugar, higher triglycerides, higher blood pressure, larger amounts of oxidized LDL cholesterol (the worst kind), and excessive production of white blood cells!

Functional Alert: Functional Training is the natural solution for lowering cortisol levels and promoting feelings of calm and relaxation in times of emotional distress. People who use alcohol to relieve stress are going in the wrong direction. Alcohol causes the body to release excess cortisol, excess pro-inflammatory cytokines, and excess free radicals that damage the tissues and organs![12,13]

Although intense Functional Training causes a temporary increase in cortisol, it ultimately helps reduce daily cortisol levels and the damage this hormone does to your body. Functional Training lowers blood pressure, blood sugar, and triglycerides, and improves immune functions and HDL cholesterol (the best kind) levels. Chronically elevated cortisol levels from stress lead to abdominal weight gain, type-2 diabetes, heart disease, and loss of memory functions (e.g., names, numbers, and words) and cognitive functions (ability to process thoughts).[14] Your brain depends on both circulation and its ability to direct information to nerve cells in order to process information. Chronic inflammation and oxidation in the brain throws off your equilibrium, making it hard to remain balanced while standing and walking. Cognitive impairments are cited as frequent causes of disabling and life-threatening falls.[15]

Healing the Brain with Functional Training

The gym is a place of healing! We are seeing an increased number of Posttraumatic Stress Disorder (PTSD) survivors joining gyms: people who have a lot of anxiety from memories of past traumatic experiences—war, natural disasters, life-threating medical experiences, motorized vehicle accidents, and violent physical and/or sexual attacks.[1] Continuous Functional Training helps manage PTSD. It reduces depression, anxiety, agitation, aggression, and increases cooperativeness. Functional Training allows PTSD sufferers to feel relaxed and to regain some control over their lives. They are focused on improving their body, not on their problems. Once people with PTSD get around the exercise equipment, they begin to loosen up. As time progresses, we see their self-confidence increasing. Eventually, we can see PTSD sufferers becoming more like the person they use to be before all the bad things happened. Working long-term with a Functional Personal Trainer who is down to earth and low key is a tremendous asset for trauma victims!

Going to the gym for Functional Training is the single most important long-term therapeutic choice you can make to heal the brain![2] Allow us to explain: According to newly published research by Dr. Jeffrey Meyer and collaborators from Canadian-based Centre for Addiction and Mental Health, higher levels of brain Monoamine Oxidase A (MAO-A)—an enzyme that breaks down serotonin and dopamine—are 35% higher in those with untreated depression.[3,4] Functional Training can significantly lower MAO-A levels and improve symptoms of depression.[5,6] This allows PTSD sufferers to take fewer prescription drugs or none at all.[7] It's not uncommon to see PTSD sufferers, especially vets who are over-medicated and can't function properly.

Functional Alert: Functional Training is more time efficient than cardio for relieving stress because large amounts of cardio are needed to adequately reduce stress levels, whereas it only takes small-to-moderate amounts of Functional Training. In addition,

Functional Training is healthier than cardio because large amounts of cardio cause excess free radical damage, whereas small-to-moderate amounts of Functional Training do not!

Learning to forge a mind-muscle link promotes renewed feelings of power. Functional Training replaces feelings of helplessness by empowering the person to take on new challenges in transforming their body. Functional Training and a Functional Diet teach people with this disorder to learn to trust themselves again and obey their brains' commands. Consistent Functional Training dramatically helps speed up the brain's recovery process. By combining the concepts found in **Functional Training with a Fork**, they can help rebalance the chemistry of their brains that has been altered by severe stress.[8-10] People with PTSD never forget the trauma they have gone through, but they can manage it with activities that have a personal meaning or goal.

Functional Alert: Functional Training not only helps alleviate PTSD, it can help prevent some cases!

Functional Training also helps heal people who are struggling with food addictions, drug addictions, obsessive compulsive disorders, attention deficit hyperactive disorders, oppositional defiant disorder, autism, family problems, financial problems, medical conditions, suicidal thoughts, etc. The concepts found in **Functional Training with a Fork** play a huge role in making people feel like their old selves again!

The suicide rate in the United States has been rising for all PTSD sufferers. It is an even bigger threat for military veterans because they want to disappear from the anger, flashbacks, survivor's guilt, and feeling that they no longer fit into mainstream society. Every 80 minutes, a veteran who has served in the U.S. military commits suicide. That's 18 veterans every day![11] It's very important that all PTSD sufferers seek professional counseling. According to various studies, it's common for veterans to reject counseling.[12] Having been trained to be self-sufficient, they believe they can fix PTSD on their own. In addition, they are often unhappy with the services provided by mental health professionals and don't trust them. It's very important to get enrolled in a reputable counseling program and stay with it! Furthermore, we believe all PTSD sufferers need to confide in those who have experienced similar trauma to whom they can relate. However, a depressed person speaking with another depressed person is not always good if there is not some third party or counselor to help them.

Functional Alert: Untreated PTSD has devastating outcomes for sufferers' functioning!

Equine therapy (working with a horse to build a bond) is a new treatment being used to try to help military veterans.[13] Unfortunately, the free 3-day program offered to veterans is not medically or clinically certified. We believe that equine therapy is great for the mentally and physically challenged. But we feel it's not effective for curing military veterans with PTSD. We and many others believe that allowing a veteran to build a bond with a horse over a 3-day period, then taking it away is like giving a traumatized child a dog for 3 days and then taking it back. We believe that could cause further trauma for some people with PTSD! After all, PTSD in military veterans often begins with a bond that has been broken (seeing their friends taken from them in battle).
We believe the only way equine therapy could be productive is if the veterans were allowed to remain with the horse on a continuous or permanent basis (as they do with service dogs), so the bond between them and the horse remains unbroken. There's no such thing as magically getting rid of PTSD.[14] Anyone who thinks otherwise has never experienced it.[15] Time doesn't always heal all wounds, but it helps you learn better coping skills.

Functional Alert: War takes its toll on every brave man and woman who fight for our freedom. Even the strongest people can get PTSD. It's not a sign of weakness. In fact, PTSD is a sign of great courage because it shows you were brave enough to endure the terror of war. We would like to take this time to thank the entire military for their service!

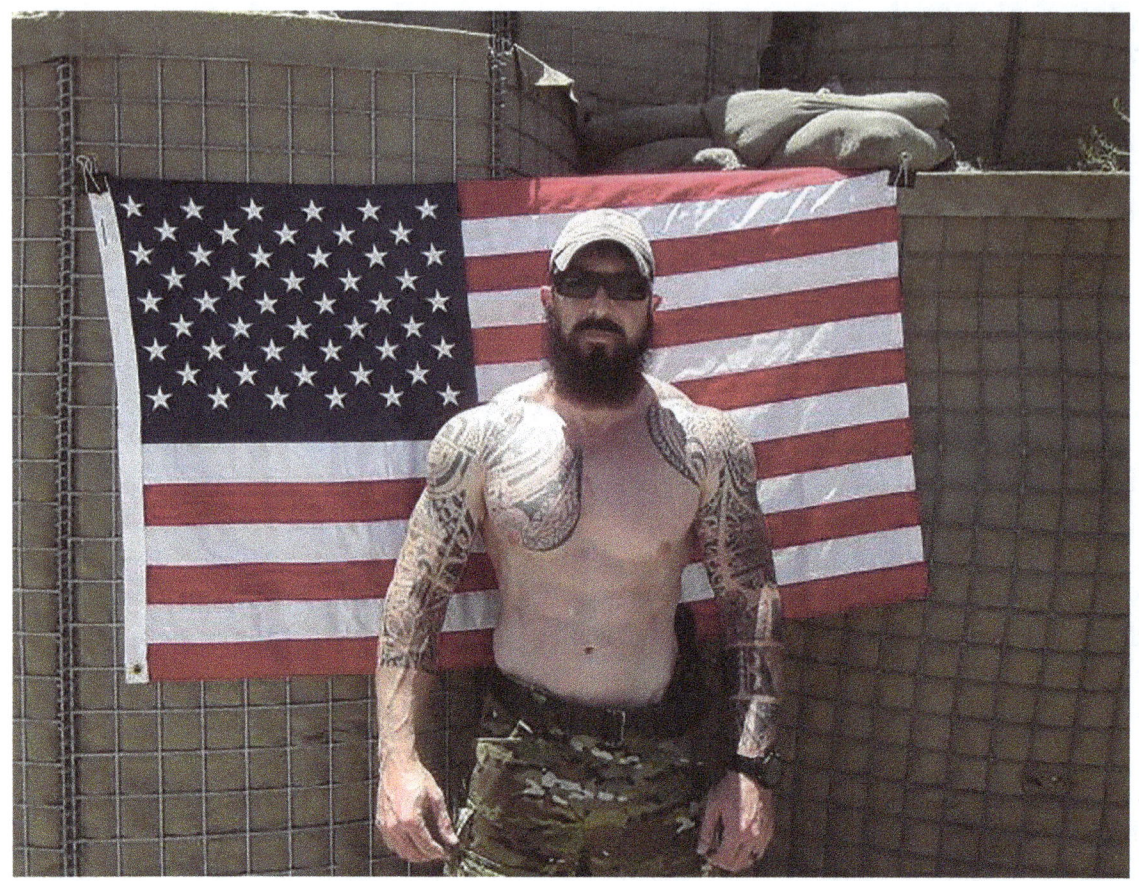

Lowell Koppert, U.S. Army Special Forces. Board member of Four Letter Word, www.flw.us (a non-profit organization for military veterans).

For someone suffering from PTSD or recovering from PTSD, Functional Training serves multiple facets. The most important one is that Functional Training is a productive outlet for focusing their energy and releasing their stress. For members of the military or former members of the military, it can also provide group interaction and camaraderie that they may be looking for (or may long for if they have left the military). And lastly, Functional Training provides and promotes a healthy lifestyle that will lead to quicker recovery and assist in preventing the individual's symptoms from returning.

Driving a Motor Vehicle

Driving a motor vehicle is the leading cause of deaths among Americans ages 1 to 34, and is the leading cause of long-term disability for everyone![16] Obesity and a lack of Functional Training are linked to a decrease in flexibility, slower reaction time, and poor cognitive abilities. All of these increase a person's chance of being in a motorized vehicle accident.

Functional Training with a Fork will have a major impact on your ability to safely operate a car. **Functional Training with a Fork:**

- Improves upper-body strength, making it easier to turn the steering wheel quickly and effectively.

- Enhances the ability to look over your shoulder to change lanes or look left and right at intersections to check for other traffic.

- Improves the ability to lean forward and side to side so you can see past the front and rear door frame (blind spots). This prevents pulling out in front of other vehicles and hitting them while changing lanes.

- Improves lower-body strength making it less difficult to move your foot from the gas to the brake pedal.

- Improves reflexes and the ability to make quick decisions.

- Enhances overall awareness and responsibility. This helps prevent distractions behind the wheel such as texting, speeding, and running red lights and stop signs.

- Reduces stress which in turn decreases one's desire to drive under the influence.

Functional Alert: Traffic fatalities and gun fatalities are among the major non-medical causes of death in the United States. According to MRI studies, Functional Training makes you smarter.[17] Functional Training is the key for decreasing non-medical deaths in America because it makes people smarter and improves their ability to manage feelings!

CHAPTER 3

The 7 Types of Functional Training

There are seven types of Functional Training. Your goals, age, and limitations should determine which type of Functional Training, or combinations thereof, you decide to incorporate.

Summary of the 7 Types of Functional Training

1. Slingshot Functional Training (SFT)

Slingshot Functional Training (SFT) is defined as the following: bodybuilding using Functional Sets or single-drop sets. It builds an "extremely high" degree of muscle tone and provides maximum body-fat loss over time and provides even more body-fat loss when Functional Cardio is incorporated separately. A minimum rest period of 60 seconds is taken between Functional Sets and single-drop sets.

a) The first type of SFT is performing around 14-20 Functional Sets weekly per major body part. Functional Sets are straight sets taken 1 rep shy of muscle failure in the 8-15 rep range.

b) The second type of SFT is using single-drop sets, performing around 7-10 single-drop sets weekly per major body part. This is a technique in which you perform an exercise using straight sets until 1 rep shy of muscle failure in the 8-15 rep range (Functional Set), then immediately reduce the weight load by approximately 10-30% for an additional Functional Set to be performed 10-15 seconds later.

2. Basic Functional Training (BFT)	
Basic Functional Training (BFT) is defined as the following: Functional Sets or single-drop sets. BFT is a step down from bodybuilding. It builds a "high" degree of muscle tone and provides a large degree of body-fat loss over time and provides even more body-fat loss when Functional Cardio is incorporated separately. A minimum rest period of 30 seconds is taken between Functional Sets and single-drop sets.	a) The first type of BFT is performing around 3-12 Functional Sets weekly per major body part. They are straight sets taken 1-2 reps shy of muscle failure in the 8-15 rep range. b) The second type of BFT is using single-drop sets, performing around 3-6 single-drop sets weekly per major body part. This is a technique in which you perform an exercise using straight sets until 1-2 reps shy of muscle failure in the 8-15 rep range (Functional Set), then immediately reduce the weight load by approximately 10-30% for an additional Functional Set to be performed 10-15 seconds later.

3. Advanced Functional Training (AFT)	
Advanced Functional Training (AFT) is defined as the following: supersets, a combination of Functional Sets and moderate intensity cardio, or a combination of single-drop sets and moderate intensity cardio. AFT is a 2-way circuit. AFT builds a "moderately-high" degree of muscle tone and provides a large degree of body-fat loss over time. AFT provides even more body-fat loss when various forms of cardio are incorporated separately. A minimum rest period of 30 seconds is taken between each cycle to allow your heart rate to lower.	a) The first type of AFT is performing around 3-12 supersets weekly per major body part. A superset is a technique where you perform two Functional Sets in a row using two different exercises. You perform around 3-12 supersets weekly per major body part. b) The second type of AFT is performing a Functional Set (straight sets taken 1-2 reps shy of muscle failure in the 8-15 rep range) and then immediately performing a cardio exercise to get your heart rate elevated to a moderate degree. You perform around 3-12 Functional Sets weekly per major body part. c) The third type of AFT is performing a single-drop set and then immediately performing a cardio exercise to keep your heart rate elevated to a moderate degree. Single-drop sets is a technique in which you perform an exercise until 1-2 reps shy of muscle failure in the 8-15 rep range (Functional Set), then immediately reduce the weight load by approximately 10- 30% for an additional Functional Set to be performed 10-15 seconds later. You perform around 3-6 single-drop sets weekly per major body part.

4. Highly Advanced Functional Training (HAFT)	
The first type of Highly Advanced Functional Training (HAFT) is defined as the following: drills, calisthenics, high-impact/high-force plyometrics, heavy kettlebell swings, Olympic lifts, hybrid martial arts, etc. Drills, calisthenics, and high-impact/high-force plyometrics build "very little" muscle tone. They provide "moderate" body-fat loss over time. Many forms of HAFT are much harder on the joints than other forms of Functional Training. The second type of HAFT is perfoming Functional Sets, single-drop sets, or supersets using free weights, machines, cables, and body weight. A minimum rest period of 1-3 minutes is taken between sets for small muscle groups and a minimum of 2-5 minutes between sets for large muscle groups. These sets build a "high" degree of power and muscle tone, and provide a large degree of body-fat loss over time. They provide even more body-fat loss when various forms of cardio are incorporated separately.	a) The first type of HAFT is training movement patterns to improve agility. b) The second type of HAFT improves explosive power and strength endurance by performing Functional Sets, single-drop sets, or supersets using free weights, machines, cables, and body weight.
5. Group Functional Training (GFT)	
Group Functional Training (GFT) is defined as weight-training performed in group classes, such as LES MILLS BODYPUMP™ Class, in some gyms. These classes will decrease body fat through burning calories, and build a "low" degree of muscle tone. These classes provide a "moderate" degree of body-fat loss over time.	GFT uses basic free-weight exercises such as squats, presses, and curls to tone the body.

6. Post-Catastrophic Functional Training (PCFT)	
Post-Catastrophic Functional Training (PCFT) is defined as Functional Training for those who have become less functional due to a catastrophic event. It builds a "moderate-to-high" degree of muscle tone over time. Body-fat loss varies depending on which type of Functional Training is used.	Most PCFT candidates are limited to BFT and RFT, but some can do supersets (AFT) and SFT.
7. Rehabilitation Functional Training (RFT)	
Rehabilitative Functional Training (RFT) is for rehabilitating injuries or preventing them. RFT slightly improves strength and endurance and it increases blood flow to the injured area. The vast majority of RFT exercises "will not" build any appreciable muscle tone and it's not designed for body-fat loss.	RFT includes gentle static stretching after a surgery, after an incapacitating injury, and during periods of inactivity; balancing; partial reps; isometrics; various Active Release Techniques, such as using foam rollers or tennis balls; performing slower reps; light weights; higher reps; and lower intensity with bands, free weights, machines, cables, and body-weight exercises for rehabilitating injuries or preventing them.

7 Types of Functional Training In-Depth

1. **Slingshot Functional Training (SFT)** is defined as the following: bodybuilding using Functional Sets or single-drop sets. It builds an "extremely high" degree of muscle tone and provides maximum body-fat loss over time and provides even more body-fat loss when Functional Cardio is incorporated separately. A minimum rest period of 60 seconds is taken between Functional Sets and single-drop sets.

   This form of Functional Training involves getting a maximum muscle pump while using heavy weights (the term "heavy" is relative) and great form. This type of training requires proper periodization to provide a slingshot effect. SFT is made up of two training phases: an 8-week reload and a 1-2 week deload. The reload is a high-volume training phase and the deload is a low-volume training phase. You continuously alternate between an 8-week reload and a 1-2 week deload. After 8 weeks of reloading, your body will need 1-2 week deloading to prevent overtraining of the joints, connective tissues, and the central nervous system. A deload consist of performing about half as many sets while using the same intensity, weight loads, and rep-ranges. It allows for catch-up growth to occur that was stimulated toward the end of the reload. After the 1-week, low-volume training phase is incorporated, your body fully recovers and allows maximum progress to continue. SFT is the most intense form of Functional Training because Functional Sets are taken 1 rep shy of muscle failure as opposed to 1-2 reps shy of muscle failure. The biggest advantage of using SFT is that it allows you to put forth your best effort in each set, for a longer period of time, which builds maximum muscle tone.

a. The first type of SFT is using Functional Sets (straight sets taken 1- rep shy of muscle failure in the 8-15 rep range) with free weights, machines, cables, or body weight. You should rest a minimum of 60 seconds between Functional Sets so heavy weights can be used in good form.

   Perform around **14 to 20 Functional Sets** weekly per major body part depending on how much muscle tone you desire, how much functionality you need, and what your joints and central nervous system can handle. You can train each muscle group once, twice, or three times per week on nonconsecutive days. Four to six days per week of weight training is optimal. Those who feel the need to do more than six days per week are not using their time wisely and are not training hard enough. Bodybuilders on a very tight schedule may be able to train only three days a week. You can perform less sets and higher-frequency workouts per each muscle group, or more sets and lower-frequency workouts per each muscle group. You have the option of performing fewer repetitions and using heavier weights for body parts that need more muscle tone, strength, and functionality. You also have the option of using higher reps and lighter weights for body parts you feel have already developed enough muscle tone. Keep the training intensity high regardless of the rep-range you decide to use in order to burn calories and prevent muscle loss. If you reach 15 reps and can continue, then do so. However, you will see the returns you get for your efforts slowly diminishing with each rep beyond 15. This means you need to adjust the weight load to stay in the 8-15 rep-range if you want maximum muscle tone and functionality for daily activities.

b. The second type of SFT is using single-drop sets. This is a technique in which you perform an exercise using straight sets until 1 rep shy of muscle failure in the 8-15 rep range (Functional Set), then immediately reduce the weight load by approximately 10-30% for an additional Functional Set to be performed 10-15 seconds later. You should rest a minimum of 60 seconds between single-drop sets to allow your muscles and heart rate sufficient time to recover based on the body part being trained. If your form starts to get careless, then it's time to drop to a lighter weight. These should burn like crazy!

Single-drop sets can be used with most exercises. We do not recommend using single-drop sets with compound leg exercises such as squats, lunges, and leg presses because it elevates the heart rate too much and causes excessive fatigue, which leads to overtraining the central nervous system and injury.

Perform around **7 to 10 single-drop sets** weekly per major body part depending on how much muscle tone you desire, how much functionality you need, and what your joints and central nervous system can handle. You can train each muscle group once, twice, or three times per week on nonconsecutive days. Four to six days per week of weight training is optimal. Those who feel the need to do more than six days per week are not using their time wisely and are not training hard enough. Bodybuilders on a very tight schedule may be able to train only three days a week. You can perform less sets and higher-frequency workouts per each muscle group, or more sets and lower-frequency workouts per each muscle group. You have the option of performing fewer repetitions and using heavier weights for body parts that need more muscle tone, strength, and functionality. You also have the option of using higher reps and lighter weights for body parts you feel have already developed enough muscle tone. Keep the training intensity high regardless of the rep-range you decide to use in order to burn calories and prevent muscle loss. If you reach 15 reps and can continue, then do so. However, you will see the returns you get for your efforts slowly diminishing with each rep beyond 15. This means you need to adjust the weight load to stay in the 8-15 rep-range if you want maximum muscle tone and functionality for daily activities.

Functional Alert: When performing Functional Sets and single-drop sets, always finish working an entire muscle group (e.g., the chest) before moving to the next body part (e.g., back). Likewise, when performing supersets (e.g., chest and back) always finish working both muscle groups before moving to the next two body parts.

Kathy: *My husband, Ronnie, is the Head Trainer. There are people across the world who consider him to be one of the best when it comes to body-fat loss, muscle toning, rehabilitation, and training around injuries. Ronnie also developed* **Slingshot Functional Training** *that is being widely used and has helped many bodybuilders, ranging from recreational to the professional level. He's also an expert in precontest dieting.*

Tricky Jackson, IFBB Pro Bodybuilder

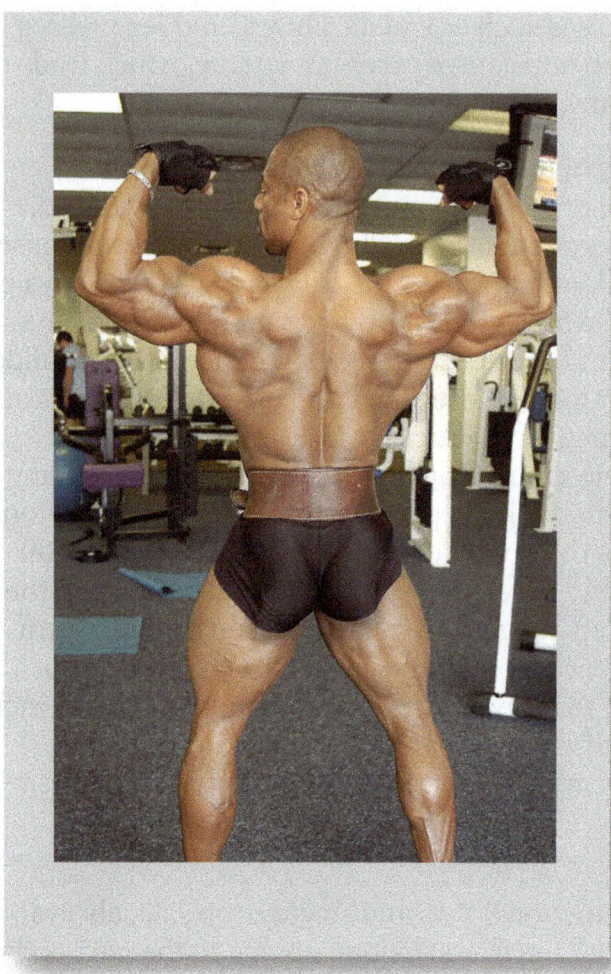

Photo taken by
http://www.mostmuscular.com/

*There's a lot of great bodybuilding routines to choose from and I have tried most of them. I prefer **Slingshot Functional Training** that was developed by Ronnie Rowland. He's been involved in the fitness industry for years and knows his craft. **Slingshot Functional Training** helped me obtain my pro card. The training system's 8-week reloads and 1-week deloads has taught me how to tweak things to make muscles grow beyond their normal capacity. For more details about how to become a better athlete in the fitness industry, I can be reached at www.trickyjackson.com.*

2. **Basic Functional Training (BFT)** is defined as the following: Functional Sets or single-drop sets. BFT is a step down from bodybuilding. It builds a "high" degree of muscle tone and provides a large degree of body-fat loss over time and provides even more body-fat loss when Functional Cardio is incorporated separately. You should rest a minimum of 30 seconds between Functional Sets and single-drop sets so heavy weights can be used in good form. The biggest advantage of using BFT is that it allows you to put forth your best effort in each set, which builds more muscle tone.

a. The first type of BFT is using Functional Sets (straight sets taken 1-2 reps shy of muscle failure in the 8-15 rep range) with free weights, machines, cables, or body weight. You should rest a minimum of 30 seconds between Functional Sets to allow your muscles and heart rate sufficient time to recover based on the body part being trained.

Perform around **3 to 12 Functional Sets** weekly per major body part depending on how much muscle tone you desire, how much functionality you need, and what your joints and central nervous system can handle. The more Functional Sets you perform, the more muscle tone and functionality you will obtain, given it doesn't hurt your joints or overtrain your central nervous system. You can train each muscle group once, twice, or three times per week on nonconsecutive days. Three to five days per week of weight training is optimal. Those who feel the need to do more than five days per week are not using their time wisely and are not training hard enough. People on a very tight schedule may be able to train only two days a week. You can perform lower-volume and higher-frequency workouts per each muscle group, or higher-volume and lower-frequency workouts per each muscle group. You have the option of performing fewer repetitions and using heavier weights for body parts that need more muscle tone, strength, and functionality. You also have the option of using higher reps and lighter weights for body parts you feel have already developed enough muscle tone. Keep the training intensity high regardless of the rep-range you decide to use in order to burn calories and prevent muscle loss. However, you will see the returns you get for your efforts slowly diminishing with each rep beyond 15. This means you need to adjust the weight load to stay in the 8-15 rep-range if you want maximum muscle tone and functionality for daily activities.

b. The second type of BFT is using single-drop sets. This is a technique in which you perform an exercise until 1-2 reps shy of muscle failure in the 8-15 rep range (Functional Set), then immediately reduce the weight load by approximately 10-30% for an additional Functional Set to be performed 10-15 seconds later. You should rest a minimum of 30 seconds between single-drop sets to allow your muscles and heart rate sufficient time to recover based on the body part being trained. If your form starts to get careless, then it's time to drop to a lighter weight. These should burn like crazy! Single-drop sets can be used with most exercises. We do not recommend using them with compound leg exercises such as leg presses, squats, and lunges because it elevates the heart rate too much and causes excessive fatigue, which leads to overtraining the central nervous system and injury.

Perform around **3 to 6 single-drop sets** weekly per major body part depending on how much muscle tone you desire, how much functionality you need, and what your joints and central nervous system can handle. The more single-drop sets you perform, the more muscle tone and functionality you will obtain, given it doesn't hurt your joints or overtrain your central nervous system. You can train each muscle group once, twice, or three times per week on nonconsecutive days. Three to five days per week of weight training is optimal. Those who feel the need to do more than five days per week are not using their time wisely and are not training hard enough. People on a very tight schedule may be able to train only two days a week. You can perform less sets and higher-frequency workouts per each muscle group, or more sets and lower-frequency workouts per each muscle group. You have the option of performing fewer repetitions and using heavier weights for body parts that need more muscle tone, strength, and functionality. You also have the option of using higher reps and lighter weights for body parts you feel have already developed enough muscle tone. Keep the training intensity high regardless of the rep-range you decide to use in order to burn calories and prevent muscle loss. However, you will see the returns you get for your efforts slowly diminishing with each rep beyond 15. This means you need to adjust the weight load to stay in the 8-15 rep-range if you want maximum muscle tone and functionality for daily activities.

Functional Alert: When performing straight sets and single-drop sets always finish working an entire muscle group (e.g., the shoulders) before moving to the next body part (e.g., arms)!

3. **Advanced Functional Training (AFT)** is defined as the following: supersets, a combination Straight Sets and moderate intensity cardio, or a combination of single-drop sets and moderate intensity cardio. AFT is a 2-way circuit that builds a "moderately-high degree of muscle tone and provides a large degree of body-fat loss over time. A minimum of 30 seconds is taken between each cycle to allow your heart rate to lower while performing these 2-way circuits.

Functional Alert: AFT is not a 3-way circuit. A 3-way circuit is HAFT used by certain athletes while participating in drills!

The biggest advantage of using AFT is that it allows you to maximize your workout time. Instead of performing only one exercise at a time that isolates one muscle, such as tricep pushdowns, you can do some other form of exercise, such as bodyweight squats between sets. When you struggle to find time to work out, do shorter workouts more frequently or perform longer workouts less frequently.

THE 7 TYPES OF FUNCTIONAL TRAINING

a) The first type of AFT is performing supersets. A superset is a technique where you perform two Functional Sets in a row using two different exercises. Nearly no rest is taken between exercises, only that which is taken to get in position for the second exercise. Only rest long enough to get your heart rate down before moving to the next superset. A minimum rest period of 30 seconds is taken between each cycle to allow your heart rate to lower. Each exercise is taken 1-2 reps shy of muscle failure in the 8-15 rep range.

    Supersets save time by reducing the rest interval between two exercises, and they elevate your heart rate more than straight sets. Supersets involve pairing exercises of opposing muscle groups such as chest and back, or different muscle movements such as; shoulders and biceps, chest and biceps, back and triceps, etc. When pairing antagonistic exercises, you're going to be able to maintain more strength during Functional Sets. However, supersets are not as effective for building strength and power as Functional Sets (straight sets taken 1-2 reps shy of muscle failure in the 8-15 rep range) due to a reduction in the amount of weight you can lift. This reduction is caused by fatigue due to less recuperation between Functional Sets. We don't recommend performing supersets with compound leg exercises such as squats, lunges, and leg presses because it elevates the heart rate too much and causes excessive fatigue, which leads to overtraining the central nervous system and injury.

    Perform around **3 to 12 supersets** weekly per major body part depending on how much muscle tone you desire, how much functionality you need, and what your joints and central nervous system can handle. You can train each muscle group once, twice, or three times per week on nonconsecutive days. Three to five days per week of weight training is optimal. Those who feel the need to do more than five days per week are not using their time wisely and are not training hard enough. People on a very tight schedule may be able to train only two days a week. You can perform less sets and higher-frequency workouts per each muscle group, or more sets and lower-frequency workouts per each muscle group. You have the option of performing fewer repetitions and using heavier weights for body parts that need more muscle tone, strength, and functionality. You also have the option of using higher reps and lighter weights for body parts you feel have already developed enough muscle tone. Keep the training intensity high regardless of the rep-range you decide to use in order to burn calories and prevent muscle loss. If you reach 15 reps and can continue, then do so. However, you will see the returns you get for your efforts slowly diminishing with each rep beyond 15. This means you need to adjust the weight load to stay in the 8-15 rep-range if you want maximum muscle tone and functionality for daily activities.

b) The second type of AFT is performing a Functional Set and then immediately performing a cardio exercise to get your heart rate elevated to a moderate degree. You perform around 3-12 Functional Sets weekly per major body part. Allow us to illustrate: perform an exercise such as a chest press in the 8-15 rep range stopping 1-2 reps shy of muscle failure (Functional Set). Immediately following your Functional Set you perform another exercise (e.g. bench step-ups) to get your heart rate elevated to a moderate degree. Allow your heart rate to lower and repeat the cycle (chest press and step-ups) again until you're ready to move to the next exercise or muscle group. Continue this throughout the entire workout. A minimum rest period of 30 seconds is taken between each cycle to allow your heart rate to lower.

You get your heart rate elevated to a moderate degree between Functional Sets by using exercises such as low-impact/low-force plyometrics on a stable surface, kettlebell swings that don't go above the forehead (above the head is considered a dangerous CrossFit® exercise that often damages the AC joint of the shoulder), low-impact calisthenics, various forms of step-ups on the STEP Reebok® or a bench, various lunge exercises, squats holding a medicine ball, sumo squats holding a dumbbell between the legs (some prefer performing these types of squats with the lower back on a Swiss ball®/ stability ball placed against the wall to take pressure off the knees and lower back), etc. If you reach 15 reps and can continue, then do so.

Functional Alert: We don't recommend incorporating an additional exercise (to keep the heart rate up) between Functional Sets while performing compound leg exercises such as squats, lunges, and leg presses because it elevates the heart rate too much and causes excessive fatigue, which leads to overtraining the central nervous system and injury. "We also recommend avoiding 3-way circuits because they are too fatiguing and counterproductive for building maximum muscle tone!"

Perform around **3 to 12 Functional Sets** (in addition to moderate intensity cardio exercises performed immediately after Functional Sets) weekly per major body part depending on how much muscle tone you desire, how much functionality you need, and what your joints and central nervous system can handle. You can train each muscle group once, twice, or three times per week on nonconsecutive days. Three to five days per week of weight training is optimal. Those who feel the need to do more than five days per week are not using their time wisely and are not training hard enough. People on a very tight schedule may be able to train only two days a week. You can perform less sets and higher-frequency workouts per each muscle group, or more sets and lower-frequency workouts per each muscle group. You have the option of performing fewer repetitions and using heavier weights for body parts that need more muscle tone, strength, and functionality. You also have the option of using higher reps and lighter weights for body parts you feel have already developed enough muscle tone. Keep the training intensity high regardless of the rep-range you decide to use in order to burn calories and prevent muscle loss. If you reach 15 reps and can continue, then do so. However, you will see the returns you get for your efforts slowly diminishing with each rep beyond 15. This means you need to adjust the weight load to stay in the 8-15 rep-range if you want maximum muscle tone and functionality for daily activities.

c) The third type of AFT is using an exercise to keep your heart rate moderately elevated between single-drop sets. This is a technique in which you perform an exercise until 1-2 reps shy of muscle failure (Functional Set) in the 8-15 rep range, then immediately reduce the weight load by approximately 10-30% for an additional Functional Set to be performed 10-15 seconds later. Immediately following your single-drop set you perform another exercise (e.g. bench step-ups) to get your heart rate elevated to a moderate degree. Allow your heart rate to lower and repeat the cycle (chest press, chest press, and step-ups) again until you're ready to move to the next exercise or muscle group. Continue this throughout the entire workout. A minimum rest period of 30 seconds is taken between each cycle to allow your heart rate to lower.

You keep your heart rate moderately elevated between single-drop sets by using exercises such as low impact/low force plyometrics on a stable surface, kettlebell swings that don't go above the forehead (above the head is considered a dangerous CrossFit® exercise that often damages the AC joint of the shoulder), low-impact calisthenics, various forms of step-ups on the STEP Reebok® or a bench, various lunge exercises, squats holding a medicine ball, sumo squats holding a dumbbell between the legs (some prefer performing these types of squats with the lower back on a Swiss ball®/stability ball placed against the wall to take pressure off the knees and lower back), etc. We don't recommend using them with compound leg exercises such as leg presses, squats, and lunges because it elevates the heart rate too much and causes excessive fatigue, which leads to overtraining the central nervous system and injury. If your form starts to get careless during single-drop sets, it's time to drop to a lighter weight. These should burn like crazy! If you reach 15 reps and can continue, then do so. However, you will see the returns you get for your efforts slowly diminishing with each rep beyond 15. This means you need to adjust the weight load to stay in the 8-15 rep-range if you want maximum muscle tone.

Perform around **3 to 6 single-drop sets** (in addition to moderate intensity cardio exercises performed immediately after single-drop sets) weekly per major body part depending on how much muscle tone you desire, how much functionality you need, and what your joints and central nervous system can handle. The more single-drop sets you perform, the more muscle tone and functionality you will obtain, given it doesn't hurt your joints or overtrain your central nervous system. You can train each muscle group once, twice, or three times per week on nonconsecutive days. Three to five days per week of weight training is optimal. Those who feel the need to do more than five days per week are not using their time wisely and are not training hard enough. People on a very tight schedule may be able to train only two days a week. You can perform less sets and higher-frequency workouts per each muscle group, or more sets and lower-frequency workouts per each muscle group. You have the option of performing fewer repetitions and using heavier weights for body parts that need more muscle tone, strength, and functionality. You also have the option of using higher reps and lighter weights for body parts you feel have already developed enough muscle tone. Keep the training intensity high regardless of the rep-range you decide to use in order to burn calories and prevent muscle loss. If you reach 15 reps and can continue, then do so. However, you will see the returns you get for your efforts slowly diminishing with each rep beyond 15. This means you need to adjust the weight load to stay in the 8-15 rep-range if you want maximum muscle tone and functionality for daily activities.

Functional Alert: When performing AFT, do moderate-intensity cardio, not high-intensity cardio after Functional Sets and single-drop sets!

SFT, BFT, and AFT allow you to use the proper rep-range and intensity, and to adjust the amount of work sets performed for each individual body part to give you defined shoulders and arms, strong lean legs, firm glutes, a tight core, etc. Choreography in each of these areas is specifically targeted so that, in the long run, you will build more muscle tone and achieve more fat loss. SFT, BFT, and AFT produce muscle overload, not to be confused with enhancing muscle endurance and building explosive power that mostly occurs with HAFT drills.

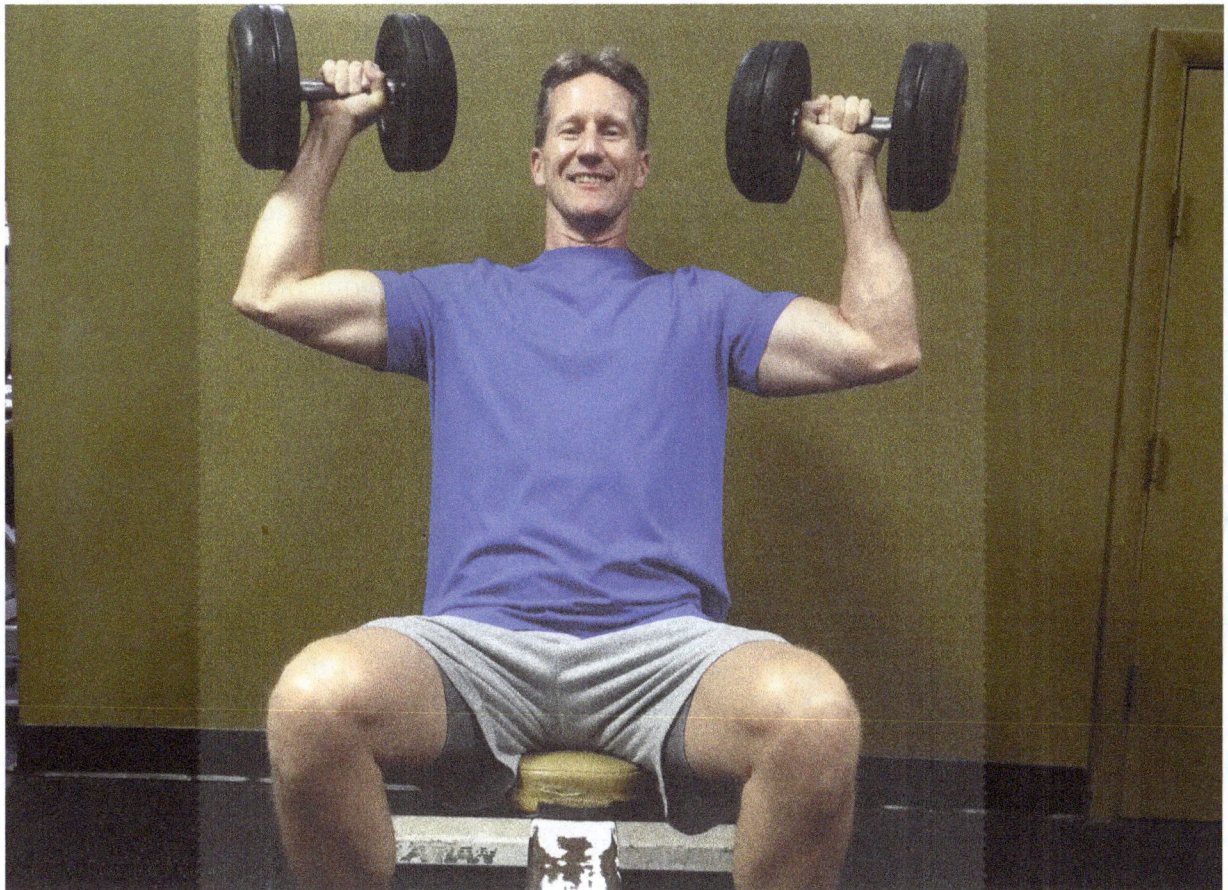

Bryan Mills, Patrol Lieutenant in S.C.

I am currently a Patrol Lieutenant in S.C. and here are some of my accomplishments: 1) Department's fitness award 12 times including the last 8 in a row. 2) Officer of the Year, 2004. 3) Distinguished Service Award 2014.

I've been a police officer and firefighter for 24 years, and health and fitness have played a big role in my career. I have tried different diets and exercise routines over the years, but eventually I learned that a Functional Diet accompanied with Advanced Functional Training (supersets using free weights and machines) was the key to my overall fitness and well-being. I've seen people lose weight on different types of diets, only to gain all the weight back when they stop. They don't understand that it is a lifestyle change they need in order to stay fit. I explain to them that maintaining a healthy weight is a simple process. All you have to do is balance the number of calories you take in with the number you burn. Then you add in some exercise to keep your heart and lungs healthy.

On the job, my fitness level has helped me in many ways. Some are obvious, and others you don't really think about unless you've actually performed the job.

Everyone has seen the police foot pursuits and scuffles while making arrests. Obviously being in good physical condition is going to help you there, especially if you have a foot pursuit ending in a scuffle. You need to have something left after the run to be able to get the handcuffs on the bad guy. A little less obvious is being able to stay alert and handle stressful situations at any time, even after being awake all night. A Functional Diet helps you stay awake and alert because your body is getting all the nutrients it needs, and Advanced Functional Training helps you handle the stressful situations by allowing you to control your breathing and slow things down. This gives you the ability to make clear, concise and correct decisions. One often overlooked part of police work is the fact that much of an officer's time is spent sitting in a patrol car or at a desk, and many officers develop back problems from this sedentary life. Regular exercise can help keep these problems from arising.

I am definitely a huge proponent of Advanced Functional Training and a Functional Diet. I encourage all of our officers, especially the younger ones, to be more aware of their eating habits and to exercise properly. It's not all about how much weight you can push. It's about living a long and healthy life!

4. The first type of **Highly Advanced Functional Training (HAFT)** is defined as the following: drills, calisthenics, high-impact/high-force plyometrics, heavy kettlebell swings, Olympic lifts, hybrid martial arts, etc. Drills, calisthenics, and high-impact/high-force plyometrics build "very little" muscle tone. They provide "moderate" body-fat loss over time. Many forms of HAFT are much harder on the joints than other forms of Functional Training. The second type of HAFT is performing Functional Sets, single-drop sets, or supersets using free weights, machines, cables, and body weight. A minimum rest period of 1-3 minutes is taken between sets for small muscle groups and a minimum of 2-5 minutes between sets for large muscle groups. These sets build a "high" degree of power and muscle tone, and provide a large degree of body-fat loss over time. They provide even more body-fat loss when various forms of cardio are incorporated separately.

a) The first type of HAFT is training movement patterns to improve agility.

b) The second type of HAFT improves explosive power and strength endurance by performing Functional Sets, single-drop sets, or supersets using free weights, machines, cables, and body weight.

Training movement patterns build less muscle tone than SFT, BFT, AFT, and GFT. Training movement patterns (e.g., high impact plyometrics and drills) provide moderate body-fat loss over time and are much harder on the joints than other forms of Functional Training. Leave these higher-risk forms of training for advanced athletes who are willing to take a chance on getting injured.

It should be noted that when it comes to muscle toning, high impact plyometrics and drills aren't a substitute for Functional Sets, single-drop sets, or supersets! HAFT that involves using only drills is usually too random in its exercise pattern to make any noticeable progress in muscle tone. This is because most drills are unable to break down the type-2 muscle fibers so they can grow back more toned. However, there are exceptions to the rule: If you were to perform a lot of box jumps in a series, you could stimulate the type-2 muscle fibers to a small degree and build a little more muscle tone in the legs/glutes. Drills such as these cause a lot of wear and tear on the discs, joints, and connective tissues! It's important to recognize that well-designed movement drills are not for muscle toning or body-fat loss, but rather developing the neuromuscular pathways that enhance athletic performance. They also improve one's conscious effort to react to various situations on the playing field.

What really disturbs us is when we see exercise programs that were originally designed for improved athletic performance (e.g., boot camp classes) paraded around as the cure for obesity and muscle toning! A lot of people have been misinformed and think that these forms of HAFT are their "get-toned-quick" ticket to a better body. The unfortunate outcome is that people of all ages are being subjected to higher-risk exercises that don't fall into the proper context of what they truly need to build muscle tone and improve functionality. The result is a lack of muscle tone, injury, and a dislike of exercise in general. We recognize that it's not done with malicious intent. However, it has reared its ugly head because people (some personal trainers included) are not being educated about what category of Functional Training is needed for each individual's needs.

The take-home message is that HAFT drills, calisthenics, and high-impact/high-force plyometrics burn calories, improves cardio health, endurance, and increases explosiveness. They are, however, an ineffective training system for the masses looking to get fit because they get fewer returns for their efforts and they're much harder on their joints, tendons, ligaments, fasciae, and discs. Only the people with an abundance of type-2 muscle fibers will see noticeable results in muscle definition from forms of HAFT, such as drills, simply because they are losing body fat and exploiting the type-2 muscle fibers they were born with. It's not because they are building any appreciable amounts of type-2 muscle fibers with drills. However, some forms of HAFT, such as Olympic lifts, do build a modest amount of muscle tone. Olympic lifts are not a user friendly way to shape your body and stay healthy.

Improving explosive power, strength endurance, and agility is the ultimate goal for enhanced athletic performance. Single-drop sets and supersets work well for athletes who are looking to build the most strength endurance (e.g., swimmers). Functional Sets (straight sets taken 1-2 reps shy of muscle failure in the 8-15 rep range) work well for athletes looking to build the most power (e.g., football players). When pure power is your goal (e.g., in a sport such as football), then we suggest doing your Functional Sets in the 8-10 rep-range while taking longer rest periods between sets. A minimum rest period of 1-3 minutes is taken between sets for small muscle groups and a minimum of 2-5 minutes between sets for large muscle groups. This allows your ATP levels to fully recover so you can lift heavier weights and build more power! Incorporate both compound and isolation exercises with heavy weights (free weights, machines, and cables) to thicken the muscles, ligaments, and tendons as much as possible without causing injury.[1-6] Performing repetitions within the 8-10 rep-range and long rest periods between sets will improve power by increasing your ability to send neurological impulses from your brain to your muscles.[7,8] Many sport injuries come from having weak muscles located at various points in the musculature. In order for athletes to remain flexible, they should add the proper amount of muscle evenly everywhere on their bodies and perform gentle static stretching and/or foam rolling after resistance training workouts in order to ensure a full range of motion.

Functional Alert: Powerlifting (1-5 reps) is not recommended for athletes (including football players) because it's too hard on the connective tissue and cartilage. Some football players think there is something special about training in the 1-5 rep range that powerlifters use. Powerlifters choose that rep range because they have to lift the weight only once in a competition. There is a little more neural drive with super-heavy weights, but powerlifters often permanently damage the connective tissues, joints, and discs, which makes them weaker over time. In the long run, you'll get better overall results by slightly increasing reps!

When using the second type of HAFT, perform around **3 to 20 Functional Sets, 3 to 20 supersets, or 3 to 10 single-drop sets** weekly per major body part depending on how much power, strength endurance, muscle tone, and functionality you desire, and what your joints and central nervous system can handle. You can train each muscle group once, twice, or three times per week on nonconsecutive days. Three to five days per week of weight training is optimal. Those who feel the need to do more than five days per week are not using their time wisely and are not training hard enough. Athletes on a very tight schedule may be able to train only two days a week. You can perform less sets and higher-frequency workouts per each muscle group, or more sets and lower-frequency workouts per each muscle group. You have the option of performing fewer repetitions and using heavier weights for body parts that need more power and strength. You also have the option of using higher reps and lighter weights for body parts you feel have already developed enough power and strength. Keep the training intensity high regardless of the rep-range you decide to use in order to burn calories and prevent muscle loss. If you reach 15 reps and can continue, then do so. However, you will see the returns you get for your efforts slowly diminishing with each rep beyond 15. This means you need to adjust the weight load to stay in the 8-15 rep-range if you want maximum muscle tone and functionality for daily activities.

You can't simulate a sport in the weight room! The Principle of Specificity says that to become better at a particular sport or skill, you must perform that sport or skill.[9] The only way to develop the muscle groups and balance required to ride a horse, for example, is to ride a horse! However, Functional Training in the gym will increase strength and flexibility, and provide the rider with a better foundation for muscle control and balance. Building strength and muscle tone in the legs/glutes, lower back, and transverse abdominis helps control pelvis stability and it increases flexibility! Squats, lunges, and step-ups that puts your knee at a 90-degree angle when you plant your foot on the ground are great exercises for building the legs/glutes. You should add weight as needed when you do these exercise to make them more difficult, but if you have knee problems you can do these exercises without any additional weight. The best exercises for the lower back are seated cable rows and hyperextensions. Building the transverse abdominis is best accomplished through repeated bouts of weight training using compound and isolation exercises, front planks on the elbows, and side planks on the elbow. All the exercises listed above help control pelvis stability, flexibility, and improves the rider's balance and center of control. It also enhances the ability to shift the hips to either side that's needed to signal the horse to move in a certain direction!

Likewise, in order to be a good golfer, you must play golf! What you can do in the gym to improve your golf game is focus on various compound and isolation exercises using good form. Building your upper back and shoulders improves speed and control of the club as you swing; building up the legs improves your balance so you can stay in the proper groove while swinging the club; and building the triceps and forearms provide additional power behind the club upon impact with the ball. Finally, building your core muscles (upper, middle, and lower) provides stability and power derived from the backswing to improve hitting distance. The upper core muscles/lats (sides and middle of your upper back) and lower core muscles (lumbo-pelvic-hip complex) play a major role in providing you with faster rotation and more explosiveness through impact. The strength of the legs allows the torso to promote club speed. Firing the hips, lats, and lower back in a synchronized manner leads to longer tee shots. Leg strength is your foundation in every sport for improving balance, flexibility, speed, and power!

Strength gained from compound and isolation exercises will help enhance overall performance as long as you don't overtrain a specific area. For example, you wouldn't want to put someone who jumps horses daily on the adductor machine for more than a few sets per week because their groin area is already being worked hard. Adding a lot of direct work to that particular area could cause overtraining and overuse injuries. A pulled groin muscle can range from mild to completely debilitating! The same rule applies to all sports.

There is a common misconception that performing speed reps under a load will train the muscles to react quickly in unexpected, real-world situations, which is how you protect yourself from injury. Plenty of athletes still do bizarre things, such as speed reps, in hopes of increasing athletic performance. This is wrong! It's important to know that speed reps under a heavy load actually do just the opposite over time by weakening the connective tissue. For instance, doing bench presses using very fast repetitions won't increase a boxer's punching speed as much as using normal cadence reps that keep the connective tissues protected. Another example is shadow boxing with dumbbells. Throwing punches while holding dumbbells does not improve power, speed, and endurance. This type of exercise is good for only one thing—injuring the neck, shoulders, and elbows! Furthermore, throwing punches while holding dumbbells will actually decrease your ability to punch by interfering with timing and mechanics. When a boxer hits a heavy bag or works on a speed bag, he is performing muscular endurance and techniques for improving speed and precision. This is referred to as training in a sport-specific manner. When he steps in the weight room it's time to switch modes! Teaching proper technique is the best way to improve punching power and speed, not lifting weights in a highly explosive manner. The second best thing you can do to increase power and speed is to focus on the type-2 muscle fibers when you are in the gym.[10] It's the muscle fibers being trained, not the speed of your repetitions, that make you bigger, stronger, and faster! You need to use moderate repetitions (8-15 reps) in good form in order to stimulate the type-2 muscle fibers without causing injury. This is the secret to avoiding injury and improving athletic performance for sports such as boxing.

Misinformed strength coaches have unintentionally hurt athletes by having them perform speed reps and high-impact movements under a load in order to try and max out their genetics. That form of training is like CrossFit®, not Highly Advanced Functional Training for improving athletic performance! There is no such thing as a training method that will allow you to overcome your genetic limitations. Speed reps are Dysfunctional Training and will only hinder your genetic abilities in the long run.

Functional Alert: Athletes should never jump with additional weight (e.g., dumbbells, barbells, and ankle weights) because it harms the joints, discs, and connective tissues!

Heavier training increases neural adaptations that help make people stronger. They also help make the tendons and ligaments a little thicker, but training too heavy damages them. Strong people owe most of their strength, speed, and size to genetics! They are born with thicker tendons and ligaments and have superior tendon attachments. The farther from a joint a tendon is attached, the more weight you will be able to lift and the faster you will be in sports. A long tendon insertion provides a tremendous advantage, providing you with better leverage. These traits are something you are born with and you can't change them significantly through any form of training!

Functional Alert: Genetics play the largest role in determining how much power and speed you will have on the playing field. Genetics can be a bitter pill to swallow!

Having a large frame and the way your muscles are inserted also play a role in how strong and fast you will be. A person with thicker tendons (connect muscle to bone), thicker ligaments (connect bones to other bones) and thicker fasciae (connect different muscles together and meet with tendons) will have more strength. The right kind of Functional Training strengthens connective tissue to a point, allowing you to become stronger, faster, and more flexible.

The thicker a ligament or tendon, the harder it is to damage. Tight ligaments and tendons are extremely important to their functioning! Once a ligament or tendon becomes stretched out, it's no longer capable of holding the joint together correctly. Friction starts to wear away the smooth cartilage causing arthritis and muscle weakness/imbalances.

We would also like to caution athletes about overuse injuries when combining HAFT with their sport. The last thing a coach wants is to lose an athlete in the weight room or during the performance of high-impact drills. Athletes can get injured more easily on the field and in the weight room when they overtrain.

As the body adapts to the excessive volume of weight training and drills, combined with intense sporting events, gains will stagnate, and joints often become negatively affected. If this occurs, your performance on the playing field will not be as good as it was before you began lifting weights and performing drills.

When athletes combine too many free-weight, machine, or cable exercises during the in-season, it's like adding plyometrics during a basketball season where a bunch of running and jumping is already being performed. This overlapping effect causes a lot of overuse injuries (for example, jumper's knee, torn knee ligaments, shin splints, sprained Achilles tendon, and plantar fasciitis). The right in-season program can help athletes continue training so they can remain conditioned and competitive. During in-season, you may need to train with weights only 1 to 2 times per week performing a very low-volume, full-body workout. This will help prevent delayed onset muscle soreness so it doesn't interfere with your performance. Delayed onset muscle soreness is caused by microfractures in the muscle cells, not lactic acid.[11] Lactic acid is the burning sensation often felt when actively training the muscles.

During the off-season, you can train each muscle group once, twice, or three times per week on nonconsecutive days. Three to five days per week of weight training is optimal. Those who feel the need to do more than five days per week are not using their time wisely and are not training hard enough. People on a very tight schedule may be unable to train more than twice a week. You can perform less sets and higher-frequency workouts per each muscle group, or more sets and lower-frequency workouts per each muscle group. You have the option of performing fewer repetitions and using heavier weights for body parts that need more muscle tone. You also have the option of using higher reps and lighter weights for body parts you feel have already developed enough muscle tone. Keep the training intensity high regardless of the rep-range you decide to use in order to burn calories. If you reach 15 reps and can continue, then do so. However, you will see the returns you get for your efforts slowly diminishing with each rep beyond 15. This means you need to adjust the weight load to stay in the 8-15 rep-range if you want maximum muscle tone and functionality for daily activities.

Functional Training is important for maintaining sports performance during the in-season, but it should be lower in volume than during the off-season. Whether you choose free weights, machines, cables, or body-weight exercises is up to you. Cardio should be dropped when playing sports if cardio efficiency is taken care of with the sport itself. All athletes, especially our youth, need to be made aware that overtraining can permanently destroy their athletic ability for the future and old injuries often come back to haunt them later in life.

5) **Group Functional Training (GFT)** is defined as weight-training performed in group classes, such as LES MILLS BODYPUMP™ Class, in some gyms. (This book has no affiliation with LES MILLS BODYPUMP™.).

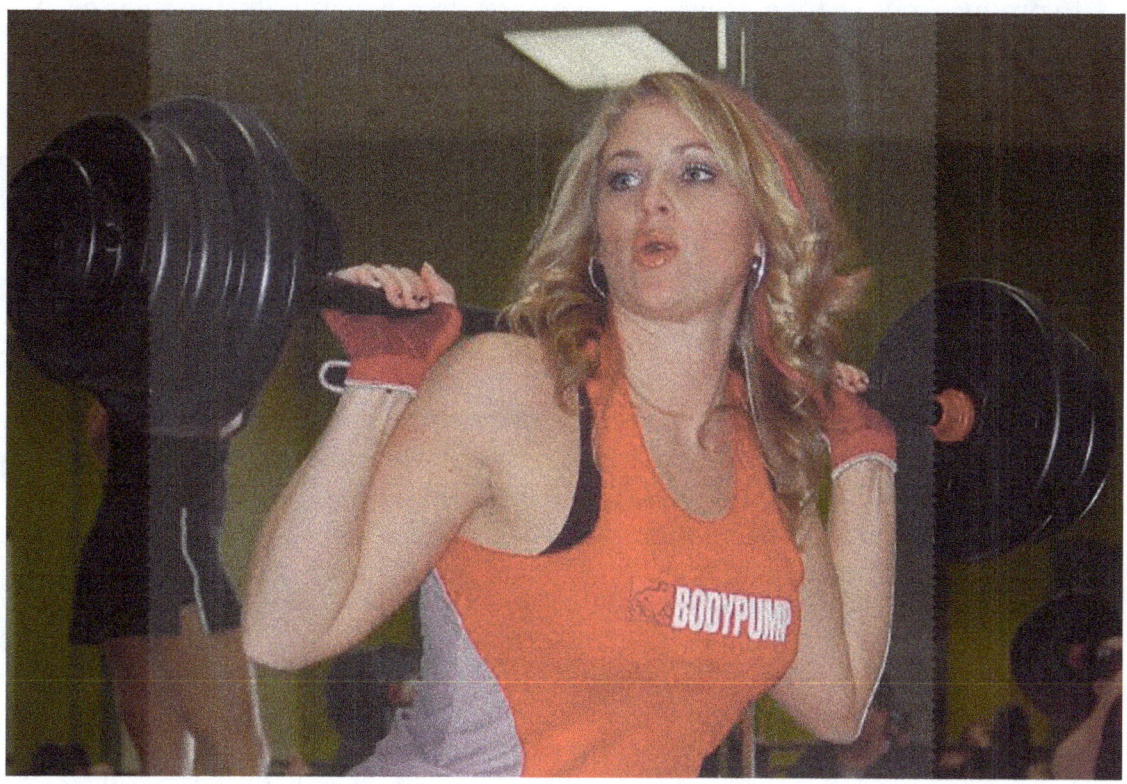

Amy Cross

In 2008, after having my daughter Savana, I joined Gold's Gym in North Augusta, SC, and attended my first Body Pump class. I was immediately hooked. This sent my life in an entirely new direction. Fueled by my love of group fitness, I became a certified instructor just a few months later. Over the course of 6 years, I trained and certified in four additional programs, became a certified personal trainer, and moved on to become the Group Fitness Coordinator for three Gold's Gym locations as well as the Program Director for Gold's Gym Personal Training. Being a part of the "change" leading the world to a fitter lifestyle has proven to be one of my biggest accomplishments!

A BODYPUMP™ class is generally one hour.[12] These classes will decrease body fat through burning calories, and build a low degree of muscle tone. It's easy to get comfortable using the same weights, which prevents future results. It's a lot more difficult to get toned doing higher reps. It's not uncommon for some people to get a temporary muscle pump during the class because of the increased blood flow to the muscles while performing high reps. This is only a temporary pump and may not produce any noticeable muscle tone for those who struggle with gaining muscle. This is because of the lack of stimulation to the type-2 muscle fibers that are needed to produce muscle tone. However, if you are already naturally muscular or have an abundance of dormant non-trained, type-2 muscle fibers waiting to be awakened, then these classes can build a noticeable degree of muscle tone. Even naturally muscular people can benefit by supplementing BFT and/or AFT with BODYPUMP™. This will allow them to stimulate muscles that aren't being worked in BODYPUMP™ due to limited exercise availability. Teaching Functional Training in a group setting can be very difficult. A good BODYPUMP™ instructor will have you concentrate on using good form.

With GFT you can train each muscle group once, twice, or three times per week on nonconsecutive days. Some people like group classes and some don't. GFT is a great option for people who refuse to train in the main part of the gym and otherwise wouldn't do any kind of weightlifting workouts at all. Three to five days per week of GFT is optimal. Those who feel the need to do more than five days per week are not using their time wisely and are not training hard enough.

People on a very tight schedule may be able to train only two days a week. With this form of training, we generally recommend higher-volume and higher-frequency workouts per each muscle group. Some classes are equipped to give you the option of performing fewer repetitions and using heavier weights for body parts that need more muscle tone, or using higher reps and lighter weights for body parts you feel have already developed enough muscle tone. Keep the training intensity high regardless of the rep-range you decide to use in order to burn calories.

Functional Alert: We consider all Zumba® classes, including Zumba® Toning, to be Functional Cardio, not Functional Training. Zumba® focuses on burning calories and on working the type-1 muscle fibers, not the type-2 fibers needed for muscle toning. We have found that you can't build muscle tone using a one pound dumbbell and performing a lot of repetitions with light weights at a low level of intensity. However, you can burn calories, which will help remove some fat off the muscles you were already born with. Losing body fat isn't building muscle tone, although some have equated it to muscle toning because of the fat loss. These same rules apply to classes such as spin class, kick boxing, etc. Always keep in mind that you can break down the smaller type-1 muscle fibers with cardio exercise and make them very sore, but when they rebuild you won't see any measurable muscle tone. You must put your efforts into breaking down the larger type-2 muscle fibers for increased muscle tone! You can't build any appreciable amount of muscle tone with various forms of cardio!

6) **Post-Catastrophic Functional Training (PCFT)** is defined as Functional Training for those who have become less functional due to a catastrophic event. There are more than 6.8 million people living outside of institutions using assistive devices, such as wheelchairs, scooters, crutches, canes, and walkers.[15] It's highly important for people who have experienced a catastrophic event to train with weights in order to create more effective ways for building muscle that they still can use. PCFT helps them become much more functional during daily activities, and their digestive system functions a lot better. Building muscle tone with PCFT speeds up their metabolism, which helps purge their bodies of Dysfunctional Toxins that would otherwise just sit there. We have found weight machines, cables, dumbbells, and body weight to be highly effective for PCFT. The rep-ranges and exercises used will be based on each individual's limitations and goals.

Most PCFT candidates are limited to BFT and RFT, but some can do supersets (AFT) and SFT. You can train each muscle group once, twice, or three times per week on nonconsecutive days. Three to six days per week of weight training is optimal. Those who feel the need to do more than six days per week are not training hard enough. People on a very tight schedule may be able to train only two days a week. You can perform less sets and higher-frequency workouts per each muscle group, or more sets and lower-frequency workouts per each muscle group. You have the option of performing fewer repetitions and using heavier weights for body parts that need more muscle tone, strength, and functionality. You also have the option of using higher reps and lighter weights for body parts that have a pre-existing condition or areas you feel have already developed enough muscle tone. Keep the training intensity as high as you can without causing further injury in order to burn calories and improve cardio. If you reach 15 reps and can continue, then do so. However, you will see the returns you get for your efforts slowly diminishing with each rep beyond 15. This means you need to adjust the weight load to stay in the 8-15 rep-range if you want maximum muscle tone and functionality for daily activities.

7) **Rehabilitative Functional Training (RFT)** is defined as gentle and brief static stretching after a surgery, after an incapacitating injury, and during periods of inactivity; balancing; partial reps; isometrics; planks; various Active Release Techniques, such as using foam rollers or tennis balls; performing slower reps; light weights; higher reps; and lower intensity with free weights, machines, bands, and body-weight exercises for rehabilitating injuries or preventing them. RFT slightly improves strength and endurance and it increases blood flow to the injured area and it's not designed for fat loss. It also enhances motor coordination after sustaining an injury by improving proprioceptive information (sensory receptors commonly found in muscles, tendons, and joints that give your brain feedback about the movements and position of the body).[13] Improving proprioceptor feedback makes a difference when

you have an injury and need to rehabilitate it. If, for example, you neglect to rehab an injury such as a sprained ankle, it's easier to injure it a second time because you get a weaker feedback from proprioceptors in the joints and muscles, therefore weakening your ability to know where your foot is in relation to the ground.

Functional Alert: The vast majority of RFT exercises will not build any appreciable muscle tone!

RFT, like physical therapy, can make your pain worse if it's not performed properly. While rehabbing an injury, exercises should be added gradually to see how your body responds. For example, let's say you are having shoulder pain in your supraspinatus tendon that travels beneath the acromion process that extends laterally over the shoulder joint—in other words a rotator cuff injury. You decide to perform some direct rotator cuff exercises on the cable machine at the gym. You start out with the following exercises to further strengthen the rotator cuff muscles beyond what basic shoulder exercises can do: internal rotation, external rotation, bilateral extension, diagonal plane exercises, prone horizontal abduction, and lateral rotation abduction. The problem with such an approach is that excessive irritation can occur and you won't necessarily know which exercise is causing your pain to increase! Therefore, it's important to start out using only a couple of exercises and see how you do before adding an additional exercise the following week. If you perform the wrong direct rotator cuff exercises or use too much intensity, volume, or frequency, excess swelling of the supraspinatus tendon and subacromial bursa sac can occur. Not only will this cause your shoulder pain to become worse, it can eventually create scar tissue, bone spurs, and bursitis! When scar tissue develops, it causes soft tissue to thicken and become biomechanically weaker.[14] It can also cause pain by irritating surrounding nerves.

The key to successful rehabilitation is to incorporate the proper exercises in a controlled fashion and allowing any small amount of swelling/irritation that may occur to leave before training again. We have found that performing direct rotator cuff exercises twice a week (e.g., Monday and Friday) to be plenty under most circumstances. In some cases, once a week is sufficient, especially for maintenance. It's important to know what is best for your body. Others function better not performing any direct rotator cuff exercises at all and find that direct rotator cuff exercises can cause further damage, leading to surgery. Some find that they experience less shoulder pain by using only basic exercises for the shoulders (e.g., overhead cable shoulder presses, leaning one arm cable lateral raises, and reverse cable flyes). Then, there are those who can only work their rotator cuff muscles indirectly with chest and back exercises.

Functional Alert: Training intensity is low to moderate. RFT builds the least amount of muscle tone, but it helps stabilize and lubricate the joints. It provides minimal body-fat loss over time!

What really disturbs us is when we see exercise programs that were originally designed for rehab purposes paraded around as the cure for obesity and muscle toning! A lot of people have been misinformed and think that RFT is their "get-toned-quick" ticket to a better body. The unfortunate outcome is that people of all ages are being subjected to incompetently administered exercises that don't fall into the proper context of what they truly need to build muscle tone and burn body fat. The result is a lack of muscle tone and a dislike of exercise in general. We recognize that it's not done with malicious intent. However, it has reared its ugly head because people (some personal trainers included) are not being educated about what category of Functional Training is needed for each individual's needs.

RFT, performed correctly, should be performed one to three days per week on non-consecutive days per body part. We recommend lower-volume and lower-frequency workouts for muscle groups that easily become inflamed. This will help reduce the buildup of inflammation in the joints and connective tissues. For body parts that you are not rehabbing, you have the option of performing SFT, BFT, or AFT using fewer repetitions and heavier weights in conjunction with RFT. You also have the option of using higher reps and lighter weights or fewer sets with lower reps for non-injured body parts you feel that have already developed enough muscle tone. For example, if you have knee problems, stick to higher reps, lower weights, and less intensity when training legs. However, you can train with lower reps, heavier weights, and higher intensity for upper-body parts if they are healthy. Keep the training intensity high for uninjured areas in order to burn calories. Cardio should be performed separately with RFT.

CHAPTER 4

Dysfunctional Training (DFT)

Dysfunctional Training (DFT) is defined as improper training methods. We are here to warn you of the great falling away in the fitness industry by those who have taken the term Functional Training out of context and turned it into Dysfunctional Training!

Here are five examples of DFT at its worst:

1. CrossFit®

   The CrossFit® industry has done an unbelievably good job of marketing an incredibly dangerous form of exercise to the masses. Their followers are under the delusion that they are reaping tremendous benefits from their efforts. CrossFit® is a fitness company founded by Greg Glassman.[1] It has 4,500 gyms across the world.[2] We believe CrossFit® is a "high-risk sport" like football. We don't believe it's a sustainable exercise program for people looking to improve their overall health and functionality. In fact, we believe most CrossFit® exercises are worse than not exercising at all because of the potential orthopedic problems that will most likely occur.

   What is CrossFit®? It is performing a lot of technically hard movements as fast as you can and/or lifting as much weight as fast as you can.[3] CrossFit® is basically a competition where you try to do more reps and weight than the other participants. This makes it extremely dangerous! Form gets thrown right out the window and becomes worse as participants start to fatigue. We believe a more accurate name for CrossFit® is WhiplashFit! CrossFitters make their muscles contract with greater intensity by maximally stretching them. When the connective tissue is stretched to a great degree, its muscles contract to an equally intense degree. When coupled with the huge shift in momentum, this causes the connective tissue (tendons, ligaments, and fasciae) to tear on a microscopic basis. Do an Internet search on YouTube for CrossFit® kipping pull-ups and you'll get the picture. CrossFitters just trying to get fit will become dysfunctional rather than functional. Collected data shows that 73.5% of CrossFitters have sustained an injury during training and some have required surgery.[4] The end product for participants in CrossFit® can be a vicious cycle of dysfunction, degeneration, and chronic pain. Their checklist of results include getting injured and developing arthritis, degeneration of the spinal disc, scar tissue, and hypermobility of the joints.

Functional Alert: Exercise should be about what gives you results and makes you more functional!

CrossFit® gyms are popping up everywhere and most of the CrossFit® exercises make no sense to us from a biomechanical standpoint. We can find something dysfunctional with just about every CrossFit® movement. They focus on dangerous exercises, using highly explosive form, that provide little in return: kipping pull-ups (which is basically just their way of showing others the correct way to perform an incorrect pull-up), handstand push-ups, hand-release push-ups, high box jumps, explosive sit-ups on ab-mats, overhead kettlebell swings, sumo deadlift high-pulls, clean and jerks, deadlifts, flipping big tires, etc. Performing Olympic lifts for reps with intensity, is showing a lack of knowledge regardless of your level of development!

Functional Alert: We enjoy watching the CrossFit® games on TV. Likewise, we enjoy watching motocross. However, it's wrong to say that either sport is a sustainable lifestyle of fitness. We believe CrossFit® is a sport like motocross, not a functional way to become fit, and whether you decide to participate is your choice. Unfortunately, the majority of people who participate in CrossFit® are not doing it for sport. They are doing it to try and get functionally fit! Some people have mistaken CrossFit® for AFT/CrossTraining!

We hope the CrossFit® exercises are nothing more than a fad that will soon end. Functional Training is making people stronger and keeping them away from doctors. CrossFit® exercises, on the other hand, are sending people to chiropractors and to surgeons who specialize in spine, shoulder, knee, hip, ankle, wrist, elbow, and hernia repair. We consider CrossFit® to be Dysfunctional Training because it continues to permanently injure a lot of people. Many insurance companies are now beginning to ask gym owners if they allow CrossFit® in their gyms before they insure them. In the near future, gyms that promote CrossFit® may not be able to get insurance and if they do, their premiums will be high. Gym owners who care about the well-being of their members shouldn't allow CrossFit® in their gym!

Functional Alert: If you are a police officer, fire fighter, military personnel, etc., who needs more strength and endurance to pass a Physical Fitness Test for employment, then you need to be using Slingshot Functional Training (SFT), Basic Functional Training (BFT), Advanced Functional Training (AFT), or Highly Advanced Functional Training (HAFT) depending on what's required to pass your test. On the other hand, Crossfit® (the use of super high-impact/fast-paced circuits) is very likely to disable you and cause you to become unemployed!

Dysfunctional Training

We are amazed at the number of people who are joining CrossFit® gyms thinking that they are the answer to losing body fat and toning up fast. They are taking huge risks in trying to acquire their goals. We think there is a major problem when the simplest, safest, and most potent functional exercises are right in front of people, and they are off searching for something new, hoping it will give them better results! Overcoming boredom and pushing yourself can be easily fixed without joining a CrossFit® gym or doing CrossFit®. Functional Training is your ticket! CrossFitters have been deceived into believing harder work is better than smarter work. In all fairness, CrossFitters aren't the only people who have bought into the myth that you need to "train till you puke"!

Functional Alert: Most of the movements being promoted in CrossFit® gyms as Functional Training are actually doing just the opposite by decreasing people's ability to function in everyday activities!

At the very least, CrossFit® instructors should have their trainees learn more about risky Olympic moves before allowing them to compete and then have them reduce the intensity and frequency until time to compete. This is what powerlifters do. Olympic moves were designed to improve explosive strength and stability, not to be performed in high repetitions like CrossFitters are doing. High-rep Olympic lifting in CrossFit® is extremely dangerous because these exercises were never designed to be a speed movement against the clock. Sacrificing form in exchange for a less muscle toning movement for the sole purpose of beating the clock is Dysfunctional Training at its best and has no business being peddled as Functional Training!

Functional Alert: Young people hear stories of the aches and pains they will have to face when they get older, but many don't take them seriously. We are here to warn you that CrossFit® can result in some of the worst pain imaginable: lumbar spinal fusion and degenerative disc disease! [5, 6]

We realize that controversies are a natural part of exercise science. However, controversies are not always a result of legitimate evidence, but instead reflect the perceived need to distort evidence. Most of us have been victims of false advertising. You can't believe everything you see on infomercials, billboards, and the Internet, and in magazine ads. For example, the moves with most CrossFit®-style workouts are not easily mastered, and it's a brutally painful and dangerous way to train. Most people don't enjoy it, and it's not user-friendly on the body, especially for those with pre-existing injuries or medical conditions, or who are over the age of 30. Few are capable of sticking to it long-term. CrossFit® is the perfect program for overtraining the joints and central nervous system. People train to the point of exhaustion and sometimes become nauseated.

Functional Alert: We have met some very kind and sincere people who began their fitness endeavor using CrossFit® because it looked like fun and they thought it was a short cut to losing body fat. They liked the group mentality and the potential motivation gained by posting their workouts for others to see. Their fun stopped when the injuries began to outweigh the benefits!

Frequent bouts of super-intense exercise, such as CrossFit®, are associated with changes in the function of immune cells. It's far worse for those who already have a weakened immune system, but even those with a strong one can eventually fall prey to immune system dysfunction. For up to three days after an intense workout such as CrossFit®, a flood gate can stay open allowing Dysfunctional Toxins, such as viruses and bacteria, to assault your immune system.[7] The most noticeable signs of chronic inflammation and immune system dysfunction are a decrease in white blood cell count and antibodies, which are needed to fight off infections and warn other immune defenses. When white cells and antibodies decrease, upper-respiratory colds, viruses, and bacterial infections increase![8-9]

Functional Alert: A CrossFit® training session is comparable to a bodybuilder's once-a-week leg-training day in terms of the fatigue it generates. Everybody who has trained their legs like a pro-bodybuilder knows what it's like to experience fatigue for a day or two after the workout is complete. This is why the vast majority of professional bodybuilders only train their legs once a week. But CrossFitters usually train 4-5 days per week. It's easy to understand why many are damaging their central nervous systems and immune systems! [10]

Another concern with CrossFit® is how it can negatively affect your immune system by causing an overproduction of pro-inflammatory cytokines and free radicals from excessive type-1 and type-2 muscle tissue damage.[11-16] The end result is chronic inflammation and oxidation. This causes a lack of oxygen inside the body's cells which can result in disease. It has been found that interleukin-1 (a group of cytokines that regulate the immune system) and tumor necrosis factor-alpha (a cytokine causing cell death) are produced in excess when excessive tissue destruction and inflammation occur.[17-19] Cytokines are proteins responsible for causing your immune system to produce antibodies to fight against Dysfunctional Toxins. The body needs a healthy production of cytokines to amplify the functions of the immune system. Functional Training helps accomplish this very thing! On the other hand, CrossFit®-type exercise is notorious for over-stressing the immune response and depleting antibody reserves, especially as you age. This causes damage to the internal organs.

Functional Alert: Functional Training does just the opposite of CrossFit® by improving the functions of the immune system, organs, and making one more resistant to injury!

A Functional Diet, combined with Functional Training and Cardio, is the key to rapid results that are sustainable, not CrossFit®! CrossFit® is the kind of exercise you perform if you don't want to be functionally fit! CrossFit® doesn't even fall into the same category as SFT, BFT, or AFT which incorporate lifting weights with intensity for safely improving muscle tone, strength, flexibility, and endurance, and safely eliminating body fat.

We are convinced that CrossFit® throws out misinformation regarding exercise science to the general public to promote its selling points. CrossFitters often claim you can get better results by committing to their gyms. The truth is that mainstream CrossFit® workouts have incorporated a lot of training methods that we, as Functional Personal Trainers, would never use because of the high injury rate we have seen over the past few years. That said, a few of the exercises being used by CrossFitters (e.g., the sled push and burpees) are fine for certain athletes because they are considered Highly Advanced Functional Training. However, the majority of CrossFit® exercises are counterproductive for athletes looking to improve long-term athletic performance. The reason Highly Advanced Functional Training has been around for so long is because it actually works and the risk of becoming injured is much lower than CrossFit®!

People involved with CrossFit® in order to lose weight and stay in shape often become militant (competitive and aggressive) thinking their way is the best way. Many are getting permanently injured because they have been misled. Some even brag about their injuries and how they push themselves until they vomit. Most CrossFitters brag about their workouts because they feel as if they have something to prove.

Functional Alert: Even when CrossFitters do everything right in terms of preparation and using proper technique during exercise, they still get injured on a frequent basis. For many CrossFitters, their injuries will last a lifetime!

Not only are some of the exercises themselves risky, but performing while extremely fatigued during an intense circuit, increases the risk of injury even further. Injuries sustained during CrossFit® workouts also result from overuse. People with pre-existing injuries are put at even greater risk. Years of training improperly will unevenly lengthen and shorten ligaments around the joints and spine, causing movement and subluxation, which is when one or more of the bones of your spine move out of position and put pressure on the spinal nerves. For example, performing exercises such as the power clean and jerk and deadlifts in an explosive fashion stretches out ligaments in the sacroiliac joint in the lower part of the back. This allows the nearby vertebrae and discs to easily slip out of alignment, thus, causing subluxation of the vertebrae and possible disc herniation, spinal stenosis, spondylolisthesis, facet joint disease, piriformis syndrome, etc. Eventually the ligaments can stretch to the point of putting pressure on local nerve roots and the spinal cord causing excruciating pain that often runs down the lower extremities.

Another example is stretching out the ligaments that keep the facet joints in proper alignment. The facet joints provide stability to the vertebral column. They are almost completely immobile and are coated with a small amount of cartilage. When the facet joints become inflamed or out of place due to a subluxation or spondylolisthesis (forward slippage of one vertebra upon another), it causes surrounding muscles to go into severe spasms. In addition, the cartilage inside the joint eventually wears out; it becomes arthritic and develops bone spurs. In most cases, a sudden injury from lifting in an explosive fashion causes permanent damage to the cartilage within the facet joint and the supporting ligaments. This causes recurrent episodes of dislocation of the joint and a stiff and painful lower back and/or neck.

Safety is #1 in our book! We are already starting to see countless people who have had both minor and major injuries, including torn tendons, cartilage, ligaments and herniated disc causing debilitating back and neck pain, and surgeries from CrossFit®. While recovering from a surgery, you won't be able to train and will lose any progress you had previously made in the gym. If you make a decision to do CrossFit® as a "high-risk sport," then that is your choice, but we ask that you are honest with others and don't promote it as a safe and sustainable form of fitness. It's sad when you see a person who has never been injured experience a first-time injury that causes them to live in chronic pain for the rest of their lives because they never fully recovered. The bottom line is—the risk of getting permanently injured with CrossFit® far outweighs the benefits!

Some instructors are constantly having their clients perform different and dangerous exercises (without any rhyme or reason) in order to keep them confused in hopes they will never be able to do it on their own. These instructors wrongly believe that this provides them with a steady source of income. This is one of the greatest sins in the fitness industry today! Unfortunately, a lot of people are going to waste a lot of money and have chronic pain down the road from performing useless and dangerous exercises like the types used in CrossFit®. They use poor form, choose unsafe exercises, change exercises constantly (putting themselves at risk for finding one that doesn't agree with their biomechanics), and perform high-impact exercises, and often arrange them in improper order, putting the discs and connective tissues at risk. They train way too explosively, as opposed to using a slow, steady pace, which is just asking for an injury because they are unloading the muscle, thus allowing the stress to be placed on the connective tissues and cartilage.

Functional Alert: You can't make the human body stronger by training it in a manner that eventually makes it weaker. The proof is there and we must let it be known. We can't let these dangerous training fads go unchallenged and watch others suffer needlessly. It's time we Functional Personal Trainers stand up for what is right, clear the air, and take control of the fitness industry!

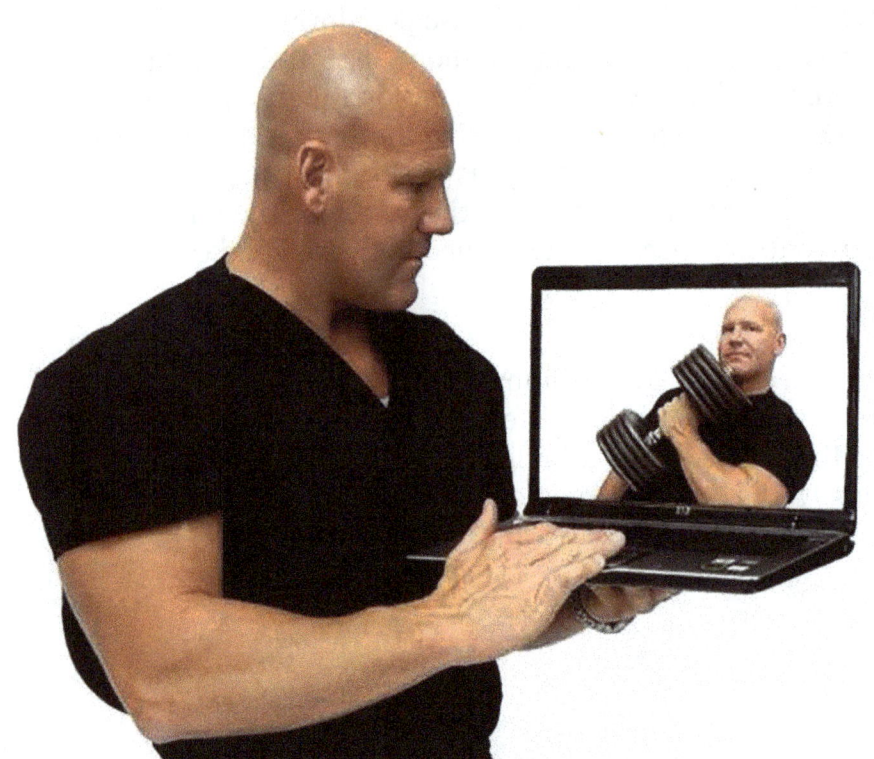

Dr. David T. Ryan, DC is the current Co-Chairman, medical committee, Arnold Sports Festival. (Former assistant strength and conditioning coach, the Ohio State University.) International author for multiple fitness media including Muscle and Fitness, Fitnessbodybuilding.com, Labrada.com. Trainer of several Olympic and professional athletes. Cecil Award-National Arthritis Foundation. Dr. Ryan can be reached at Northern Woods, 6040 Cleveland Avenue, Columbus, OH 43231, telephone #614-890-7952.

CrossFit® has taken the country by storm. Massive amounts of marketing are luring in newcomers. The major problem associated with CrossFit® is the lack of overall screening for individuals who want to participate in their program. A majority of the people entering CrossFit® are healthy young individuals. Unfortunately, some of these people have never had any athletic training and are expected to challenge themselves and perform at levels far beyond their abilities. They end up with significant overuse injuries and other trauma.

Without a doubt, the most technically challenging lift is the power clean and jerk. The snatch is almost immeasurable on how difficult it is to perform correctly. The Chinese, who are considered some of the best weightlifters in the world as a team, practice using a broomstick for years before weight is added. CrossFit® encourages individuals who don't have proper court training to use as much weight as they can while performing this move. I personally have seen hundreds of injuries from using this format. I have been training for over 40 years. I wouldn't even conceive of trying to do power cleans without using a step protocol to enter into such an activity. The effects on your body can be devastating. On the minor side, overuse injuries occur;

on the major side, problems, such as Clay-shoveler's fractures, are very common as a direct result of swinging kettlebells or performing power cleans incorrectly. I believe that it's always best for people to enter into basic bodybuilding formats. Massive amounts of injuries are recorded every week due to improper exercise technique and excessive volume. Basic bodybuilding formats enhance controlled movements in basic weightlifting and should be carried on for some time prior to beginning explosive activities such as those found in the CrossFit® protocol. I consider CrossFit® to be the home of rogue fitness, and do not recommend it as a fitness lifestyle.

2. Exercises Performed on Unstable Devices Such as a BOSU®ball

A lack of understanding has led to erroneous training methods in the fitness industry, such as standing on a wobbly BOSU®ball while lifting weights in order to try to work the small stabilizers of the knee and the core or to improve balance. The BOSU®ball consists of a black side that is completely flat and can lie flat on the ground. The opposite side is a blue cushiony ball. Although the BOSU®ball is good for a few things such as performing crunches, we believe incorrect use can result in serious injury: Standing, balancing, and lifting weights on the blue cushiony part of a BOSU®ball is dangerous. Standing, balancing, and lifting weights on the flat black end is extremely dangerous! Look at the flat, black end of the BOSU®ball. It has a disclaimer that says "Standing on this side is not recommended." Why? First, you could fall and get hurt. Second, it's very unstable and can stretch out the tendons, ligaments, and fasciae, which invites injury to the spine, hips, knees, and ankles. Third, exercises performed on unstable devices account for 70% less muscle force output and 44% less muscle activity than stable surfaces.[1]

Let's begin with the knee. The BOSU®ball myth states that your joints have these small stabilizer muscles to keep the knee joints in place. The myth teaches that these small stabilizing muscles are stimulated more when you balance the weight you are lifting while standing on a BOSU®ball. For those who don't fully understand physiology it might sound correct, but for those of us who do, we know it's simply not true. Let's take a look at the anatomy of your knee and get to the bottom of this myth. There are several muscles that affect knee movement. Located above the knee are the four large muscles of the quadriceps. Then we have the large glutes/abductors and the thigh adductors. We also have the three large muscles of the hamstrings. We want you to understand that all of the muscles just listed are large muscles, not small muscles. Therefore, there are no small stabilizing muscles that help support the knee! These large muscles are there for joint stabilization and to help your body move through various ranges of motion during daily activities and sports. Tendons and ligaments are not stabilizing muscles, but they do help stabilize joints indirectly. When you exercise your legs on a hard, stable surface using compound movements with free weights, machines, or specific body-weight movements, you are training all the muscles, ligaments, and tendons that support the knee joint! This same argument holds true for the other joints in your body.

Standing on an upside down BOSU®ball does not improve one's ability to balance during daily activities or sports. Functional tests of balance focus on maintenance of both static and dynamic balance. It's important to note that maintaining Static Balance is defined as "your ability to hold a position without moving." It's not the same as Dynamic Balance, which is defined as "your ability to maintain your balance while in motion, such as walking, running, skiing, gymnastics, and all other sports."[2] A person who stands on a wobbly BOSU®ball will improve only his ability to stand on the ball and nothing more. When you train actively on a stable surface or in a sport-specific manner, it improves balance and motor skills for activities in everyday life and athletic skills. Training on a stable surface also helps with proprioception (the body's ability to sense movement within joints and joint position). Proprioception lets us know where our limbs are without having to look. The BOSU®ball might make the exercise feel harder, but it won't make your muscles work as hard. The uncontrollable wobbling leads to overstretching of the tendons, ligaments, and fasciae causing hypermobility in the joints. This actually causes a decrease in proprioceptive information![3]

Functional Alert: Building strong legs on a stable surface and preventing neurological conditions through Functional Training and a Functional Diet is the key to having better balance! In other words, if you have weak legs and/or a neurological condition, you will experience balance difficulty!

Studies have shown there is no difference in core activation between standing on an upside down BOSU®ball and the solid ground while lifting equal weight loads![4-6] The ball made the exercise more difficult and dangerous to perform, but it didn't make the core muscles work harder. In fact, lifting weights on an unstable surface eventually weakens the core over time by stretching out the ligaments that bind the sacroiliac joints together tightly! Loose ligaments increase motion of the vertebrae in the lower back, allowing them to slip out of alignment easier. It also decreases stability of the pelvis. A large study among elite soccer players found that training on an unstable surface increased major injuries, such as ACL tears.[7] Even standing on an upright BOSU®ball (blue cushiony part facing up), makes you more prone to knee injuries, ankle sprains, hip sprains, and sacroiliac joint dysfunction due to the lower extremities twisting in an awkward way and stretching or tearing ligaments. Jumping onto either side of a BOSU®ball is just asking for an injury because you can easily twist the ankles, knees, hips, and lower back or fall off and get injured. The bottom line is, lifting weights or exercising while standing on an unstable object is not functional because it increases your chance of herniating a disc or tearing connective tissue from head to toe! Furthermore, you won't be able to lift as much weight on an unstable surface. This decreases your ability to build muscle tone and strength, which in turn, decreases your functionality during daily activities and sports.[8] Studies have also shown that training on unstable devices decrease agility, speed, and jumping ability![9]

Functional Alert: In 2009, a woman fell off an unstable BOSU®ball and got injured while working under the supervision of a Planet Fitness personal trainer. The woman had to have one hip surgery and three wrist surgeries. She won a $750,000 settlement against the gym because the judge said that the waiver she had signed was impossible to enforce![10-12]

3. **Improper Exercise Selection**

Using improper exercise selection can cause an injury! We don't have the space in this book to explain all the improper exercise selections and techniques so we will examine a few. An example of performing exercises out of proper order is CrossFit®. We have watched CrossFitters engage in the power clean and jerk exercise, which fatigues their lower back, before proceeding to deadlifts. Performing exercises in the improper order invites injury to the lower back because it decreases stabilization. CrossFit® gives the chiropractors and spine surgeons a lot more business!

We wouldn't have clients with bad discs in their lower back perform kettlebell swings, plank twists, deadlifts of any form, free-weight squats with a loaded bar across their shoulders. Neither would we have them do crunches, hyperextensions or free-weight exercises while in a standing position, especially lifting overhead. We wouldn't have them bend over and lift from the floor or perform twisting movements and unsupported rows, curls, etc.

Functional Alert: We recommend that people with back/neck and shoulder problems avoid suspension trainers/straps (e.g., the TRX Suspension Trainer) because they are unstable and often worsen one's condition!

Performing twisting exercises on the floor (e.g., seated twist with a medicine ball and lying torso twist) can damage the spine and should be avoided by everyone. This is because the lumbar region has very little ability to rotate and the facet joints take the extra pressure. This often leads to facet joint syndrome (the joints in the back of the spine degenerate and cause pain and stiffness). Standing rotational exercises provide a little more functionality for some athletes and are safer than rotational movements performed while lying or sitting on the floor.

Training for sports can demand using some of the higher-risk exercises. Medicine ball throws and slams are Highly Advanced Functional Training exercises used to improve explosiveness for sports such as volleyball and tennis. These rotational movements are not user-friendly for athletes who are prone to shoulder or spine problems. Consistent use of the spine, rotator cuff tendons, and cartilage can cause damage and chronic pain in the long-term. People who are primarily interested in toning up and improving functionality should avoid these exercises!

Functional Alert: Throwing or slamming a medicine ball has little to no carry-over effect for anything applicable to activities of daily living!

The cable wood chop and the medicine ball wood chop are weighted device rotational movements used to directly build the obliques and enhance athletic performance; for example, swinging a baseball bat. These exercises should be used sparingly by certain athletes and performed under control using strict form and light weight for higher reps (15 reps and above). It's important to note that some rotational exercises will actually decrease your ability to swing a bat by interfering with mechanics and timing. For example, swinging a baseball bat with a weight attached on the end would cause your muscles to fire differently and affect the timing and mechanics of your swing.

You must target the muscle you are trying to build! For example, if you want to build the legs, your mind must be focused only on that body part. You can't target the legs if you are simultaneously working other body parts (e.g., the shoulders). All leg work and shoulder work should be performed separately during Functional Sets in order to sufficiently improve muscle tone and overall functionality! Combining multiple weight-training exercises into one exercise (not to be confused with supersets) is a new form of Dysfunctional Training! Performing two weight-training exercises simultaneously (e.g., performing dumbbell squats (stronger exercise) and dumbbell shoulder presses (weaker exercise)—won't sufficiently stimulate muscles). This is because the weaker exercise prevents you from lifting enough weight and using enough intensity to sufficiently work the muscles in the stronger exercise. Therefore, you shouldn't simultaneously perform dumbbell squats and dumbbell shoulder presses during Functional Sets. Each exercise should always be performed separately during Functional Sets in order to sufficiently build muscle tone and improve functionality. However, performing two weight-training exercises at the same time can be used between Functional Sets in order to keep the heart rate elevated during the performance of AFT (Advanced Functional Training). We believe that the concept of performing two weight-training exercises at the same time during a work set was invented to sell fitness books and magazines and to trick people into thinking that they are doing some form of cutting-edge Functional Training. Functional Personal Trainers will not have their clients perform two exercises at the same time during a Functional Set!

Functional Alert: Always use common sense by choosing exercises that offer the least risk while providing the most benefit. A lot of people have been injured in gyms performing exercises just because they looked like fun or because that's what they've always done. They forgot that their primary objective was to not get injured while getting functionally fit!

4. **Improper Functional Training Methods**

Using Functional Training methods out of their proper context can cause an injury! For example, you wouldn't use certain forms of HAFT (Highly Advanced Functional Training) such as high-impact plyometric (e.g., box jumps) and rotational movements (e.g., horizontal wood chop) for muscle toning and fat loss. All areas of the body are a very individualistic thing. Some people get injured much easier than others due to their structure. You know your own body better than anyone, but a Functional Personal Trainer can help you make the right choices for improving functionality. The ideal training program is to incorporate exercises using free weights, machines, cables, and bodyweight if health permits. You may find that free weights are harder on your joints and tendons for some exercises while machines and body-weight exercises are harder for other body parts. Tendon and joint pain can result from not being in an anatomically correct position for your particular body on any exercise. The movements that work best for one don't always work for someone else.

You need to pay careful attention to how your connective tissues and joints feel on various exercises for different body parts. It can vary greatly among individuals. Making only small adjustments in one's feet or hand positions, and/or range of motion can be all that is required to be able to perform an exercise without experiencing joint and connective tissue pain. A Functional Personal Trainer can be of great value in these particular situations because they have the ability to put your limbs in the proper anatomical position.

Keep in mind, there will always be a few genetically gifted individuals who can take an enormous amount of impact on their joints, tendons, ligaments, fasciae, and discs and be okay for most of their lives. However, odds are great you are not one of them! More people fall into the average to below-average toughness category than the above average. People with smaller frames, tendons, and joints, as well as people over the age of 35, usually fall into the below-average toughness category. In most cases, healthy joints, tendons, ligaments, fasciae, cartilage, and discs should last a lifetime and never need repair or replacement unless someone is in an accident or uses Dysfunctional Training methods.

Tendonitis is the most common form of injury sustained during exercise. Fortunately, it can be prevented and treated to full recovery in almost all cases. Tendonitis usually starts out as a small pain in a joint, so people tend to try and work through the nagging pain. Left untreated, tendonitis can progress into tendonosis, which may decrease functionality for a lifetime. Once the tendons are compromised, damage carries over into the joint itself, which can permanently damage cartilage and lead to painful arthritis. We have learned that most people who are already experiencing tendon pain can often still perform exercises by using the cable machine, given the proper exercise selection, volume, and form.

Tendon wraps can dramatically decrease tendon pain during work sets, but they shouldn't be used during very light warm-up sets or what we refer to as Functional Stretching. Tendons need some light high-rep work without wraps to allow more blood to reach them before working out intensely. A wrap absorbs a lot of the additional stress instead of the tendons when lifting heavier weights, so it prevents them from breaking down and becoming weaker. Wraps need to be adjustable, such as Velcro, to remain tight during each Functional Set. We use adjustable tennis elbow wraps to help prevent tendonitis of the elbows and biceps. In order to be effective, the wrap must be tightened down hard during Functional Sets to provide the needed support, just like when a person tightens up their weight-lifting belt for a heavy set of squats. Then the wrap must be loosened between sets to allow blood to flow back into the muscles and tendons. Elastic wraps that can't be tightened during Functional Sets are not going to give you enough support. If you don't have to release them between sets, wraps are not really supporting or protecting tendons! However, there are supports that don't need to be loosened between Functional Sets. For example, Tiger Paws Wrist Supports. We highly recommend these for anyone who experiences wrist pain during exercise or wants to prevent future wrist problems. Tiger Paws keep your wrist straight and prevent wrist strain/pain. We believe they have made other wrist supports for resistance exercise obsolete. Another one of the best products ever invented for weightlifting is Versa Gripps®. We believe this product has made standard weight-lifting gloves obsolete because they can be used interchangeably as super-grippy weightlifting gloves or as lifting straps that don't slip or cut into the wrist. They prevent the grip from giving out so the targeted muscle can be fully stimulated. They also help protect your hands from becoming damaged.

5. Obsession

Obsession is a form of Dysfunctional Training that can destroy relationships, families, and marriages. Some people have the mind-set that the gym always comes first in their lives. They can end up in a vicious cycle where all they do is work out and eat an inadequate amount of calories. This isn't healthy, nor is it an effective way to find relief from their insecurities or feelings, because it causes them to become isolated from others.

We firmly believe that everyone who is serious about getting into shape and becoming more functional must make a lifestyle change, but we also firmly believe that moderation is the key! We have seen people become so obsessed that they get burned out and stop training altogether.

Functional Alert: You can't fill a void by creating another void!

CHAPTER 5

Functional Muscle Fiber Training

The information in this chapter is the most important ever written regarding which muscle fibers need to be targeted in order to obtain muscle tone. We are born with different types of muscle fibers, each responding in a different way to exercise. Human muscles contain a mixture of both fast twitch (type-2 muscle fibers) and slow twitch (type-1 muscle fibers).[1] Your genetics determine if you are born with more type-2 fibers or more type-1 fibers and how many of each one. Most people find out that some muscle groups have more type-2 fibers whereas others have more type-1. The only way to find out, other than having a muscle biopsy, is to work out with weights using reps of 8-15 and see how your body responds.[2]

It's often impossible to look at someone and tell how many type-2 fibers they possess. We have a lot of people who look about the same size when in a non-trained state. However, after Basic Functional Training for 3-6 months it's not uncommon to watch one person surpass another in gaining strength and muscle tone. This is because they have more dormant type-2 fibers, which don't appear until they are trained. Genetics plays a much larger role than most realize when it comes to how fast and how much muscle tone and strength you will be able to gain. Some people really struggle to gain muscle tone and strength because they lack type-2 muscle fibers. These same people often have an abundance of type-1 fibers and are better at endurance sports. The majority of people will fall somewhere in the middle.

Functional Alert: Some people have certain muscles with a lot of type 2-muscle fibers and other muscles with a lot of type-1 muscle fibers. Some people have certain muscles with a lot of both type-1 and type-2 fibers and other muscles with little of either!

Function of Type-2 Muscle Fibers

Fast twitch type-2 muscle fibers are most responsible for giving your body muscle tone, explosive power, and strength. They enable you to sprint fast, balance, punch with great power, and lift heavy weights. If you want to run faster, punch harder, get stronger, have better balance, or develop measurable muscle tone, you have to build your fast twitch fibers![3] It's absurd though to think that just because you go out and start running sprints, you will automatically develop the body of a sprinter. It will never happen if you weren't already naturally muscular and born with a lot of type-2 muscle fibers.[4, 5] This is because type-2 muscle fibers are much larger in size than type-1 fibers.[6]

Functional Alert: Some people are born with an abundance of both types of muscle fibers. These are the athletes who can excel during events such as triathlons and still keep good muscle tone. These lucky people have plenty of type-1 fibers to sustain them through a lengthy race and enough type-2 fibers to help them power their way through barriers!

We have found that using sets of 8-15 reps are best for stimulating the type-2 muscle fibers that produce muscle tone and improve functionality. Anything lower than 8 reps is getting into power lifting and puts too much strain on the discs, connective tissues, and joints. Repetitions higher than 15 will still stimulate the type-2 fibers and create muscle tone and strength, but you get fewer returns for your efforts as the repetitions go above 15. Eventually you reach a point where it turns into cardio and you are working mostly the type-1 fibers instead of the type-2 fibers.[7] Cardio increases the oxidative capacity of muscle, whereas Functional Training in the 8-15 rep range promotes muscle tone and strength by increasing the volume of contractile proteins in the fibers.[8-10] Furthermore, when you are working the type-2 fibers in the 8-15 rep range, you are also stimulating your type-1 fibers.[11] As soon as you can go past 15 reps using good form, it's time to raise the weight for the next Functional Set.

Functional Alert: Never lose sight of the fact that regardless of how you gain measureable muscle tone, it will be mostly type-2 related growth, not type-1!

Type-2 muscle fibers tone up more than type-1 muscle fibers and produce a more pronounced "afterburn effect" (post-exercise calorie burn) during the rebuilding process.[12] Therefore, high-intensity weight training is more effective than high-intensity cardio sessions if your goal is body-fat loss! Furthermore, researchers at Boston University School of Medicine have found that increasing muscle tone by increasing the size of your type-2 muscle fibers decreases overall body fat.[13] Type-2 fibers are also more responsible for keeping the body hydrated when you drink plenty of fluids. Hydration is one of the most under-rated habits you can have to remain healthy. You can train your type-1 fibers for long periods (e.g., a triathlon), making them so sore it takes several days for the muscles to recover. However, doing so won't cause any appreciable muscle tone due to their small size.[14] Type-2 muscle fibers decrease in number as you get older, causing your body to gradually shut down.[15] Therefore, it's important to continue to stimulate the type-2 muscle fibers as you age to prevent dysfunction on both the inside and the outside of the body. Building the type-2 muscle fibers through Functional Training increases your functionality, joint stability, metabolism, hydration, circulation, oxygen, feel-good chemicals, and nutrient uptake, and is responsible for the elimination of more Dysfunctional Toxins.

Functional Alert: Building the type-2 muscle fibers through Functional Sets is the most effective exercise for boosting the metabolism and losing stubborn body fat![16]

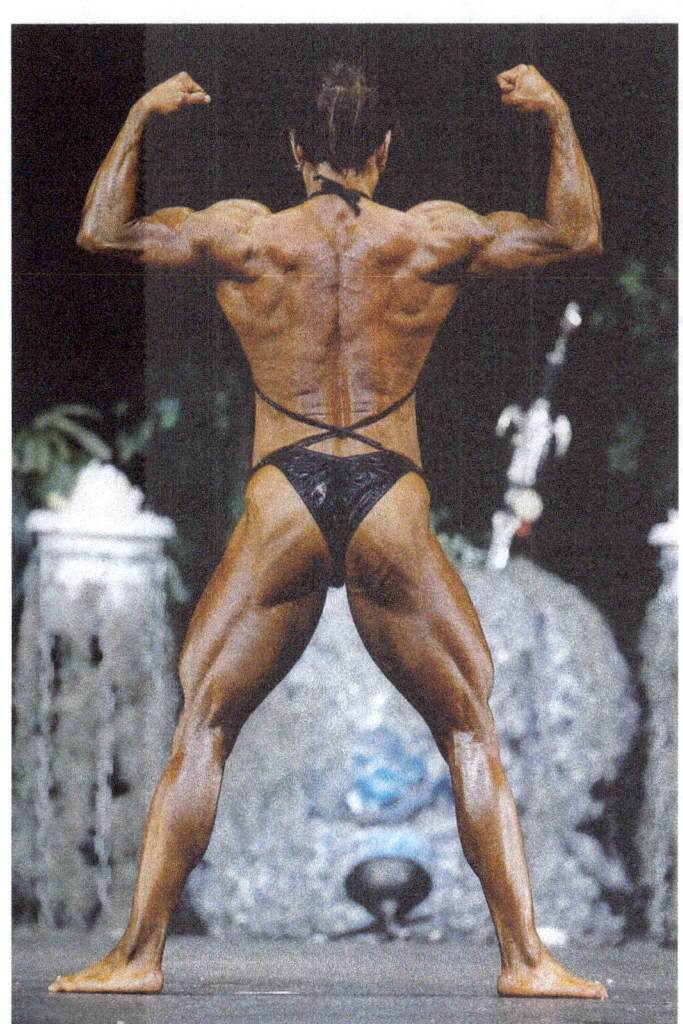

Photo taken by http://patrickcollardstudios.zenfolio.com/

Kathy Rowland: *I was born with an overabundance of type-2 muscle fibers throughout my entire musculature, especially my legs. This influenced me to become a bodybuilder. I love Slingshot Functional Training!*

Function of Type-1 Muscle Fibers

Slow twitch type-1 muscle fibers are mostly responsible for giving your body endurance, which allows you to keep going through long, physically demanding sporting events.[17] If you are born with an abundance of type-1 fibers and few type-2 fibers, don't expect to have a great deal of muscle tone, speed, and the power of a sprinter or bodybuilder. You are more cut out for running long distances. Type-1 fibers won't grow to any appreciable degree regardless of what you do, and the slight amount they can grow is also stimulated with intense Functional Sets that cause type-2 muscle growth. The abdominal and lumbar-back regions are best trained with high reps (above 15 reps) and static holds because it's safer for the spine and places less emphasis on the type-2 fibers. When you train the lower back and abs with heavy weights and low reps, you put yourself at risk for injuring the spine. Furthermore, if you are one of these people who were born with an abundance of type-2 muscle fibers in the abdominals, you will develop super-thick abs (which can cause protrusion of the belly). If you want flatter abs, you need to focus on the type-1 muscle fibers using light weights and high reps with various forms of crunches, planks, or by allowing your weight lifting routine to build them through repetitively tightening up the core during Functional Sets. Remember, diet plays the most important role in obtaining flat abs!

Functional Alert: When the smaller type-1 muscle fibers repair themselves after a hard work out, they don't grow enough to show any appreciable gains in muscle tone!

Functional Muscle Toning

What's preventing most people from getting toned? When we hear people complain that they just can't get toned, we know it's because they are neglecting to sufficiently stimulate their type-2 muscle fibers using Slingshot Functional Training (SFT), Basic Functional Training (BFT), or Advanced Functional Training (AFT)! In other words, they are working out in a way that trains the fibers in a dysfunctional manner instead of a functional manner. Building muscle tone and strength isn't just about picking weights up and putting them down. You can't just combine several intense exercises and string them together into one long, difficult circuit, resulting in a very high heart rate, and expect to gain maximum muscle tone or not risk injury in the process!

Trying to combine more than two exercises within a circuit is too much on your plate when trying to achieve maximum muscle tone, strength, and functionality. If you can do more than two exercises in a circuit, you are not training with enough intensity! You must fully work a particular muscle group with intensity before jumping to the next one. In other words, you can't build maximum muscle tone by doing a set for chest, then a set for quads, then a set for biceps, then a set for back, then going back to chest and repeating the sequence all over again. You must complete your entire chest workout to fully stimulate the type-2 fibers and gain muscle tone before moving to the next body part. Every single body part needs to be treated this way regardless of whether you are following SFT, BFT, AFT, or GFT.

You must break down the type-2 fibers to get toned muscles! With each subsequent work set or Functional Set performed for a specific body part following the first set (8-15 reps taken 1-2 reps shy of muscle failure), the type-1 muscle fibers tire out earlier in the set and the type-2 muscle fibers start working harder. By the time you have finished around 3 sets, the type-1 fibers (endurance fibers) begin shutting down much earlier in the set and the type-2 fibers (muscle toning fibers) are mostly being used to lift the weight.[19] Once 3 to 20 work sets per body part have been performed, depending on which body part you are training and how much muscle tone and functionality you desire, both the type-1 and type-2 muscle fibers will be adequately stimulated. You need to push the limits while knowing there is a point of diminishing returns.

Functional Alert: In order to learn how to properly implement BFT and AFT, you must first learn basic bodybuilding formats using low volume and not taking work sets to muscle failure!

There is one truth regarding muscle tone, strength, and functionality: You have to lift heavier weights and/or perform more volume with a lot of intensity! This is referred to as a progressive overload. A progressive overload was developed by Thomas Delorme, MD.[18] A progressive overload is best accomplished by gradually increasing Functional Sets as you become stronger while not exceeding a specific amount of Functional Sets weekly for each muscle. For example, 12 sets for triceps and 12 sets for biceps weekly would be about the maximum amount needed for arms when implementing BFT and AFT. The minimum amount would be 3 Functional Sets per major muscle group once a week. Functional Stretching (warm-ups sets) are not included as Functional Sets.

Functional Alert: When performing 12 sets weekly for a body part (e.g., the quads) it can be split as follows; 12 sets performed once a week, 6 sets performed twice a week, or 4 sets performed 3 times per week!

Functional Stretching and Functional Sets

There are numerous weight-lifting injuries each year because people neglect to warm up properly. You will always need to do warm-up sets (starting out with a lower weight and intensity while working on a machine or using free weights), what we refer to as Functional Stretching, for each body part. Functional Stretching, before performing Functional Sets, is very important for preventing injuries. As you begin an exercise, you must warm up gradually with Functional Stretching by using lighter weights and lower intensity. Gentle static stretching is not effective for preventing injury during the performance of your Functional Sets.

Areas that have been injured in the past need more Functional Stretching (warm-up sets) in order to prevent pain during work sets or reinjuring the area. Actively stretching the muscles through gentle Functional Stretching will pump blood to an area, lowering the chance of a soft tissue or joint injury. Aggressive static stretching (stretching the muscles to the point of discomfort while the body is not moving and holding that position for approximately 15-30 seconds) actually decreases the blood flow within your tissue creating lactic acid buildup and increasing the chance for injury! [19]

Most people do their Functional Stretching incorrectly. They move the weight too fast or use loose form, not allowing the muscles, fasciae, ligaments, tendons, and cartilage to get fully warmed up before intense Functional Sets. Warming up by performing cardio doesn't sufficiently prepare your muscles, ligaments, tendons, and fasciae, for resistance training. Static stretching and cardio cannot take the place of Functional Stretching. It is important to not be aggressive in your Functional Stretching. You need to actively stretch the muscles in a gentle, controlled, and slow manner during Functional Stretching (warm-up sets)!

Functional Stretching is required each time you change over to training another body part. For example, if you just got through training the biceps and are moving to triceps, you'd need to perform at least one set of Functional Stretching (warm-up set) before training your triceps with Functional Sets (work sets). You don't need to do Functional Stretching for the next exercise for the same body part because that muscle group will already be warmed up. For example, when you get finished doing tricep pushdowns, you can go immediately to overhead tricep extensions without performing a set of Functional Stretching.

Functional Alert: Everyone should avoid training to muscle failure because it leads to arching, twisting, excessive straining, and using other muscle groups to move the weight. You should also avoid training beyond muscle failure (e.g., forced reps and heavy negatives). Excessive training intensity is widely known for causing injury and overtraining! You can only break down so much muscle tissue in a work set. Creating more muscle cell damage by employing beyond failure training methods (e.g., forced reps and heavy negatives) create a scenario were over-training of the Central Nervous System, joints, and connective tissue will outpace muscular damage. Therefore, it's always better to add more work sets than train beyond muscle failure in order to increase strength and produce muscle growth!

Performing Functional Sets (straight sets using good form taken 1-2 reps shy of muscle failure in the 8-15 rep range) is the standard method for arranging your weight-training workouts in order to stimulate the type-2 muscle fibers when incorporating SFT, BFT, AFT, and the second type of HAFT! Functional Sets require you to perform a number of work sets for a given body part while using about the same number of repetitions and weight. For example, for your first chest exercise, 3 Functional Sets while using the decline chest press machine would include:

Functional Stretching (warm-up sets)	
1st warm-up set (Functional Stretching)	15 repetitions of decline chest press using 20 pounds
2nd warm-up set (Functional Stretching)	12 repetitions of decline chest press using 30 pounds
Functional Sets (work sets)	
1st Functional Set (work set)	15 repetitions of decline chest press using 60 pounds
2nd Functional Set (work set)	12 repetitions of decline chest press using 60 pounds
3rd Functional Set (work set)	10 repetitions of decline chest press using 50 pounds
3 Functional Sets (work sets)	

Functional Alert: Functional Sets are for building muscle tone, strength, and functionality. Cardio exercises and Highly Advanced Functional Training (HAFT) drills are not Functional Sets! For example, using battle ropes, swinging kettlebells, and stepping on and off a STEP Reebok® is not going to be good enough when trying to increase muscle tone in the legs or build a better butt. In order to be considered a Functional Set, you must keep constant tension on the muscle throughout the duration of the set, use a great deal of intensity, and use plenty of resistance. In order to stimulate muscle tone, you must break down the muscle you are trying to target with multiple Functional Sets before moving to the next muscle group. Exercises such as kettlebell swings and step-ups are designed to keep the heart rate up between Functional Sets during Advanced Functional Training (AFT). During Highly Advanced Functional Training (HAFT) low step-ups and kettlebells can be used to improve agility, but they are not considered Functional Sets!

Here's a list of some of the best basic exercises to use during Functional Sets to build muscle tone, strength, and power in order to enhance overall functionality as well as athletic performance.

Exercises for Muscle Toning and Functionality

Chest/Core
Bench press using barbells, dumbbells, cables, machines, and the Smith Machine
Slight-decline bench press using barbells, dumbbells, cables, machines, and the Smith Machine
Low-incline bench press using barbells, dumbbells, cables, machines, and the Smith Machine
Upper-Back Width/Core
Medium-to-wide grip over-handed lat pulldowns to the front of the neck with cables and machines
Medium-to-wide grip over-handed pull-ups to the front of the neck with bodyweight or assisted pull-up machines
Upper-Back Thickness/Core
Rows using various grips with cables and machines
Traps/Core
Shrug exercises with dumbbells, plate-loaded machines, and the Smith Machine
Shoulders/Core
Overhead shoulder press with dumbbells, cables, machines, and the Smith machine
Leaning side lateral raise (one arm at a time) with dumbbells and cables
Reverse flyes with cables
Biceps and Core
Curls with barbells, dumbbells, cables, and machines

Triceps and Core
Tricep pushdowns with cables using ropes, bars, and single handles
Tricep overhead extensions with cables using ropes, bars, and single handles
Dips with bodyweight, plate-loaded machines, and assisted dip machines
Quads/Glutes/Core
Wide-stance squats with Smith Machine (feet placed farther forward than you would in a regular freeweight squat)
Swiss ball®/stability ball squats holding dumbbell between legs (feet placed further forward than you would in a regular freeweight squat)
Lunges with dumbbells, plate-loaded machines, Swiss ball®/stability ball, and Smith Machine Super Lunges using the STEP Reebok®
Wide-stance leg press
Various forms of bridges
Hamstrings and Core
Leg curls
Calves and Core
Toe presses with the leg press machine
Lower back/Core
Hyperextensions
Abs/Core
Crunches with BOSU®ball and machines
Reverse crunches or hanging leg raises with bodyweight
Forearms and Core
Standing barbell wrist curls behind the back
Reverse barbell wrist curls (pre-loaded barbells work best)

Functional Alert: You should always use bodybuilding formats/training splits to structure your functional workout routine. If you perform too many Functional Sets per exercise, you run the risk of overuse injuries and hindering your body's ability to recover. On the other hand, if you don't perform enough Functional Sets per exercise, you run the risk of not providing enough stimulus required to signal your muscles to make the changes you desire. We usually recommend 3-10 Functional Sets per exercise and 1-5 exercises per body part!

Aggressive Static Stretching

Aggressive static stretching before weight training is counterproductive because muscular performance decreases when you loosen the ligaments and tendons, making them less capable of engaging.[20-21] This is because they are largely involved in transferring muscle power to your skeletal structure. Stretching a cold muscle with aggressive static stretching not only reduces power, it increases the risk of straining, pulling, or tearing a muscle. Aggressive stretching also leads to fascial scarring and adhesion.

Functional Alert: Active Release Techniques and gentle static stretching help increase blood flow to inflamed/sore areas, which promotes recovery, whereas aggressive static stretching restricts blood flow and actually promotes delayed onset muscle soreness by causing further damage to the muscles!

Active Release Techniques and gentle static stretching is performed to release bound-up fascia (connective tissue that surrounds muscle fibers and connects to bones, muscles, and organs). If there's no significant muscle imbalance, Active Release Techniques and gentle static stretching can help alleviate pain in tight muscles (trigger points) and connective tissues that get bound up in sticky, hardened fascia.

Bound-up fasciae restrict range of motion. Functional Sets, Active Release Techniques, and the proper static stretches in a gentle manner can help release fasciae that get bound up from inactivity so they glide more easily. This prevents neighboring muscles from sticking together. However, in cases where there's a muscle imbalance, gentle static stretching and Active Release Techniques won't cure muscle tightness and pain! Tight, painful muscles are primarily caused by muscle imbalances and/or degeneration rather than a lack of gentle static stretching and Active Release Techniques. When a muscle imbalance occurs, you will have two opposing muscles that fight back and forth in a tug of war to pull the tension to their side. The muscle that is strongest wins the tug of war match. Gentle static stretching and Active Release Techniques doesn't fix the root cause of the problem because the problem is a weak muscle being overpowered by a stronger opposing muscle! For example, trying to gently stretch out tight or sore hamstrings that are being overpowered by strong/tight hip flexors is not going to cure the tightness or pain, even though it may feel good in the process. In order to cure the pain, you will need to gently stretch and unbind the hip flexors, performing Functional Sets using compound exercises for the quads/glutes (e.g. squats) and then you need to work on building up the hamstrings with Functional Sets (e.g., leg curls) to help strengthen and shorten the weak/elongated muscle (hamstrings). Perform your leg curls after your hip flexors have been stretched out with compound exercises for the quads/glutes. Then the tug of war between the opposing muscles will become more evenly matched. This will help take the excess pressure off the weak and elongated hamstrings and its ligaments, tendons, and fasciae. Performing aggressive static stretches for a hamstring that has already been pulled tight or elongated by an opposing muscle is only going to make the problem worse! It will also put you at risk of tearing the hamstrings or its connective tissue.

Functional Alert: Gentle static stretching and Active Release Techniques won't cure chronic pain caused by degeneration.

Some muscle imbalances can't be completely cured by building up the weak muscle because the muscle imbalance is being caused by degeneration (e.g., scar tissue, bone spurs, calcium deposits, and loss of cartilage or disc height) which leads to loose ligaments and joint problems. For example, when the ligaments that attach to the sacroiliac joint become loose from degeneration and/or aggressive stretching, it causes the pelvis to rotate and leads to hip, back, and knee pain. Therefore, the last thing a person with degenerative disc disease would want to do is stretch out the ligaments even farther or avoid building muscles to help tighten the ligaments as much as possible. In these particular cases, you need to correct the muscle imbalance to the best of your ability without causing further damage. You'll also have to learn to cope with the pain and activity restrictions.

Gentle static stretching and foam rolling alone won't usually cure common ailments such as Piriformis Syndrome (a neuromuscular disorder that occurs when the sciatic nerve is compressed). This is because Piriformis Syndrome is caused by the shortening or lengthening of the muscle due to altered biomechanics of the low back and pelvic regions. This means Functional Training is what's truly needed to help realign the uneven piriformis muscle so pain will disappear! Things you can do to prevent Piriformis Syndrome are: Don't exercise in unnatural positions (e.g., some yoga stretches, and certain Pilates and resistance training exercises). Don't exercise on uneven surfaces (e.g., upright BOSU®balls and upside down BOSU®balls). Avoid lunging forward during stretching, exercising, and sports.

You have to be very careful with static stretching because when you stretch the muscles you also stretch the connective tissues (ligaments, tendons, and fasciae). It's common for people to stretch their ligaments, tendons, and fasciae too much and experience joint dysfunction and pain later in life. As personal trainers, we've seen a lot of injuries, chronic pain, and joint problems from aggressive static stretching that was taught by some well-meaning, but uninformed, yoga and Pilates instructors, athletic coaches, physical therapists, and doctors.

Functional Alert: Have you ever slept wrong on your pillow (stretched your neck muscles in an awkward position) and woke up with neck pain? Have you ever experienced back pain from bending over (over-stretched your back muscles) during yard work? This is from overstretching the connective tissue!

Adding the proper amount of muscle evenly everywhere on your body and preventing degeneration is the key to having more flexibility, not static stretching! Flexibility refers to your muscles whereas hypermobility refers to your ligaments, tendons, and fasciae. When your ligaments, tendons, and fasciae stretch, they behave elastically during just the first small bit of the stretch. However, if they're stretched beyond that point, they can stay at that new length. This is what we refer to as having loose ligaments, tendons, and fasciae. Loose ligaments, tendons, and fasciae can no longer stabilize your joints and are a major source of chronic pain and injury for a lot of people!

Functional Alert: Don't overstretch your connectors!

As you age, aggressive stretching is even more harmful because you lose some of the muscle that helps hold joints in place. As you get older and/or suffer a back injury, your discs will flatten (degenerate) and leave you with loose ligaments that attach to the sacroiliac joint or SI joint. This allows the pelvis to rotate and the vertebrae to subluxate more easily. It can also cause weakened discs to protrude or herniate. The last thing you want to do is aggressive stretching, which can make the condition worse or cause a devastating back injury!

Unstable joints cause increased strain on nearby muscles, fasciae, ligaments, tendons, cartilage, discs, and nerves. Overstretching your ligaments, tendons, and fasciae is easy to do with static stretching or lifting weights and performing bodyweight exercises in exaggerated ranges of motion. Due to their biomechanics, some people's muscles can safely stretch farther than other people. Even a little pain, when stretching the muscles is the body's way of saying STOP!

We highly recommend that you stay away from all forms of exercise that aggressively stretch the muscles or cause you to get in awkward positions. For example, some of the mainstream yoga stretches and Pilates exercises engage the body in positions that are unnatural for the human body. To be safe in yoga and Pilates you need to maintain natural postural alignment and joint function. Don't blindly perform some of the traditional stretches, poses, and exercises that can permanently injure you. If you decide to do yoga or Pilates, find a good instructor who has eliminated some and modified most of the stretches, poses, and exercises that are being taught by mainstream instructors. They realize the importance of protecting you and themselves. A good instructor understands that the wrong kind of exercising, stretching, and posing actually weaken the core by permanently stretching out its connective tissues. A good instructor will tell you what was once thought to make the core stronger, actually does just the opposite over time by weakening the core and making you more prone to joint pain and injury!

Functional Alert: Both participants and instructors of mainstream yoga and mat Pilates (who engage in aggressive stretching) often end up with a saggier posture and loose, flat butts. This is caused by connective tissues that have been overstretched and remain loose. Your goal should be to have good posture and a tight, round butt!

Just because your muscles can stretch through a particular range of motion doesn't mean it's safe to stretch or load your ligaments, tendons, and fasciae throughout that full range. Furthermore, just because it feels good at the time to aggressively stretch out a tight, elongated muscle, you shouldn't do it! Ligaments and fasciae are much easier to permanently stretch out than tendons. When tendons become loose, it's a sign they have been torn. When a ligament and fascia is overstretched, they lose their ability to recoil. The elasticity leaves and you become less functional as a result.[22-24] There's no such thing as lengthening a muscle with any form of exercise or stretching, but you can permanently stretch out the connective tissue![25]

Functional Alert: Aggressive stretching binds you up!

The lumbosacral joint (L5-S1), shoulder joint, knee joint, hip joint, and facet joints (entire spine) need tight ligaments, tendons, and fasciae to maintain stability for proper joint function. Ligaments, tendons, and fasciae need to be tightened by building the stabilizing muscles, not overstretched with static stretching, exercises in unnatural positions, or exercises under a load that are taken through excess ranges of motion. Dull aches and sharp pains in the same area are often signs that you are overstretching during exercise.

Loose ligaments in the lower back, neck, hips, and knees are the number one cause of pain and degeneration in those areas! Even though aggressive stretching might feel good at first, it further elongates weak and tight muscles that are being pulled at length. You should exercise the weak, elongated muscles, with Functional Training in order to strengthen and tighten them! Adding a lot of gentle static stretching, in addition to Functional Training (which already actively stretches the muscles and fasciae in a gentle manner), is often redundant and a complete waste of time! In addition, foam rolling classes are what's needed to help alleviate muscle soreness and inflammation in the soft tissues because it increases blood flow.[26]

Functional Alert: Loose ligaments, tendons, and fasciae are often misdiagnosed as Fibromyalgia!

It's common for people to overstretch their ligaments, tendons, and fasciae in traditional yoga and Pilates classes, unaware that it will cause lower back, neck, shoulder, wrist, ankle, knee, and hip problems in the future.[27-33] Dr. Michelle Carlson, an orthopedist who specializes in injuries or ailments involving muscles, joints, and bones, recently wrote an article about this problem, entitled "Yoga Injuries On The Rise In Women." [34]

Exercising and stretching in body positions that do not simulate real-life function eventually leads to misalignment, chronic pain, and surgical repairs. 'I'm seeing an increasing number of patients who have muscular strains or aggravated degenerate discs after attending Pilates classes because they thought it would help with their back problems,' says Dr. Stewart Tucker, an orthopaedic spine surgeon at the Royal National Orthopaedic Hospital, London.[35]

Ronnie: *I rarely recommend floor exercises to clients who have had back or neck surgery, especially spinal fusion. All floor exercises and most static stretches make my pain level increase. I think a lot of people who have never had severe back or neck problems don't understand that many exercises performed on the floor (e.g., many of the floor exercises performed in traditional mat Pilates and yoga) are actually counterproductive. Anytime you fully extend your legs while lying on your back or in a seated position (e.g., the Can-Can exercise and the Open Leg Rocker) it puts you at risk for injuring the spine. Performing exercises such as roll-ups, spine twists, and criss-crosses is just asking for more pain and another spine injury! These types of exercises often cause excess flexion for people with bad backs/necks and most don't translate to everyday activities that back/neck pain sufferers need to remain functional. Furthermore, most people with back/neck trouble work all day in a seated position over a computer—so I see no value in having them perform a lot of flexion exercises. In addition, you can overtrain the connective tissues of the core just like any other muscle. The bottom line is don't injure your spine or weaken it with these awkward, so-called core-building exercises!*

CHAPTER 6

Muscle Toning vs. Bulking

The information in this chapter is the most important ever written regarding muscle toning versus bulking. The most common complaint we hear from males is that they can't get big enough muscles or enough strength. The most common complaint we hear from females is about having too much body fat or saggy skin. The fact is, we are not all meant to look the same, just as we are not all cut out for the same occupation or sports. For example, some of us can look like bodybuilders; most cannot. A 6-foot, 6-inch basketball player has a chance to make it to the NBA; one who is 5-foot tall cannot hope to reach that level. It's very important that you learn to accept your body's characteristics and type so you can reach realistic goals. In the gym, some people will progress much further and faster than others. We have seen it happen thousands of times and it's not just a training routine design, diet, effort, or dedication. It's a matter of genetics and there is nothing you can do but accept it and work hard to reach your potential. Follow the principles we have laid out in this book and you will make the best of your God-given genetics.

Ronnie: *Throughout the years, I learned to be secure with my genetics. It was a real struggle at first. Most people don't understand how much genetics play a role in one's ability to gain muscle tone and strength. I have had some very genetically gifted male clients come into the gym and surpass my overall strength and muscle size in less than a year of steady training—and I have been doing this for more than thirty years!*

Kathy: *Ronnie has worked his calves hard most of his life and they will never get big, but his arms are huge! We have seen a lot of men who worked out very hard for years, yet they could never get bulked up with muscle even though they had a large amount of testosterone (which leads to an increase in fat-free muscle mass). You might be wondering how this could happen. The answer is, they simply weren't born with enough type-2 muscle fibers!*

You can't always tell by looking at someone in a non-trained state who has the most type-2 fibers. We have taken two different people who looked about the same and put them on the exact same workout and diet. Sometimes one person can eventually add a lot of muscle tone due to having a lot of type-2 muscle fibers, while the other can gain only a very small amount of muscle tone due to a lack of type-2 muscle fibers.

Ronnie: *Thanks a lot, Kathy, for rubbing it in my face about having puny calves! Kathy is right though about my calves and my arms. My dad has big arms and small calves. I inherited a lot of type-2 muscle fibers in my biceps and triceps. However, I was born with very little muscle tissue in my calves, so there isn't a lot there to work with. We still get a lot of clients (both male and female) who are under the false impression that they're calves are big because of some form of exercise they did when they were younger. What they fail to realize is that muscles shrink very fast once you stop training them with the same kind of intensity, and it's really their genetics, not the exercise they performed years ago, that made their calves big. I played just about every sport under the sun and continue to train my calves hard and heavy today, yet they never grow larger. They are, however, a little more toned. Unlike the thighs, calves are a very dense muscle group. If you are a female and have large muscular calves, those puppies are there to stay!*

I think that a lot of women are afraid to lift heavier weights because they think it will create the exact opposite look they are trying to achieve. The bottom line is that they are not going to look like bodybuilders by accident. The all-natural female bodybuilders are a select few who are known for being way above average in their ability to gain muscle. They train with a lot of volume using heavy weights and great intensity. They have to seek it out and train hard for it—and have the right genetics. I want to be clear that the vast majority of females don't have the genetics to be bodybuilders. It's incomprehensible to me that about half of the females I meet think that it's possible for them to look like a bodybuilder.

Some women who have an abundance of type-2 fibers in certain areas (usually their legs) can get bulkier than they desire. When a female appears bulky, it's usually because she is eating a diet that is too high in calories for her metabolism.

I have seen cases where no amount of exercise or diet would completely lean out women's bulky legs, but they can make them smaller. The reason is their genetic make-up—they hold a lot of body fat in that area. I would like to point out that big, muscular legs are not the same as legs that hold a lot of body fat. I have worked with many females who were under the false impression they had big, muscular legs, but in reality, their legs looked bulky from holding body fat in that area. In other words, their leg muscles weren't really big. I can usually tell because their legs are much weaker than they appear to be. (A female with big muscular legs can squat a considerable amount of weight using good form.) You may be a female with a small midsection, but you struggle losing body fat in your legs. It's the same scenario as guys who have small legs, yet struggle to lose that last bit of fat from their midsection. A good point to remember is that our bodies need a little fat for good health. I believe it's best for females and males to accept their bodies for what they are capable of achieving rather than trying to change them into something that isn't possible from a genetic standpoint.

It's much healthier to have big legs than a big midsection. Legs are the largest muscle group in the body, which means training them for muscle tone will dramatically increase the metabolism and sex drive, improve insulin sensitivity, help purge Dysfunctional Toxins from the body, and improve circulation and hydration. Compound leg exercises, such as squats, lunges, and leg presses, are among the best exercises for strengthening the entire posterior chain, which includes the more difficult areas to tone for most females (glutes, inner thighs, and hamstrings). Performing multiple sets of squats, lunges, and leg presses burn more calories than mainstream cardio routines because you are training your largest muscle group in a way that requires more oxygen, training intensity, and effort. An added benefit is that they give you a body that is much more attractive to the opposite sex.

Functional Alert: It should come as no surprise that the females with the nicest glutes are usually the ones who can squat, lunge, and leg press the most weight using proper form with great intensity and plenty of volume, while staying in the 8-15 rep range. These females also have an abundance of type-2 muscle fibers in their glutes and they're body-fat levels are relatively low!

Squats build the core better than just about any other exercise. Sometimes a female has to choose between having bigger legs/glutes or more cellulite in those areas. Heavier lifting and the proper diet are the best options for reducing cellulite if one's testosterone levels are in balance.

There are plenty of endomorphic (naturally heavy) females at the gym who can build the same amount of muscle tone if not more than ectomorphic (naturally thin) females. However, the endomorphs will have more trouble building as much visible muscle tone because they have higher body-fat percentages. Some endomorphs hate their thick legs, but when they learn to eat right and train right, their legs take on a much better shape. They learn that a Functional Diet, Slingshot Functional Training (SFT), Basic Functional Training (BFT), or Advanced Functional Training (AFT), and Functional Cardio will have an even bigger impact than genetics in determining whether their muscles will be covered with fat or have a more defined look.

Most males tell us they would rather have a female with larger legs and round glutes than a female who loses size in her legs at the expense of losing her butt. We've also seen females who could not simultaneously keep shredded abs and a nice round butt. We think some women's magazines have distorted females' perceptions about what most men think looks attractive. Most guys think alike! They're not looking for stick-thin females who starve themselves and only do cardio. They like sculpted buns of steel. Guys also like women with sexy abs, but a nice butt can make women look very appealing. So our advice to you is: Get to work on those legs/glutes, ladies! Both you and your man will reap the benefits.

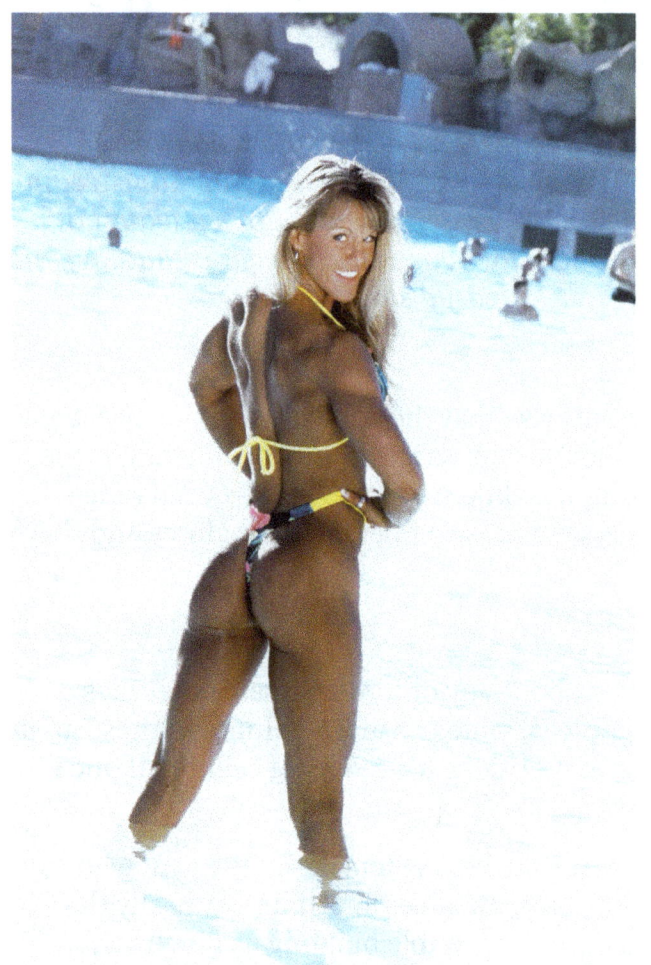

Shannon Meteraud, IFBB Pro Figure and Fitness Model- displaying her *sexy* glutes!

There is beauty to be brought out in all female bodies by implementing **Functional Training with a Fork**! To the females who have smaller legs or bigger legs, it doesn't matter if you carry a little more fat around your midsection than the next girl. You can strive for perfection in your workouts, but perfection isn't obtainable. Men are not looking for perfection; they are looking for true beauty. True beauty is the only thing that is attainable and that is accomplished by getting the best body you can for your body type while not making yourself miserable in the process and having a great attitude. Outward beauty is worthless without inner beauty. It takes both to have true beauty!

Training Myths

It's a myth that high repetitions using lighter weights make your muscles long and sexy, whereas heavier weights using lower repetitions make your muscles short and bulky. The shape of your muscles is determined at birth. When they grow bigger, their shape will become exaggerated whether you use lighter weights or heavier weights to make it happen. In other words, either a muscle grows or it doesn't, and the rep ranges used to get them to grow won't determine their final shape. Genetics always determine their final shape! Diet is what makes you lean, but lifting weights in the 8-15 rep range is the most effective way for the masses to build that lean, sexy sculptured look for their bodies.

MUSCLE TONING VS. BULKING

Losing body fat and gaining muscle tone is usually more difficult for females than males. If we could do one thing for females involved in fitness, it would be to give some clarity as to what many want and what they are not getting. One of the most common concerns of our female clients is fear of bulking up, and their concern is a legitimate one. They often wonder, If I train with heavy weights, will I look huge like a bodybuilder? The answer is no if they follow our Functional Training methods!

Many females join the gym thinking that low-intensity forms of exercise or various types of cardio (e.g., the stair stepper) are the key to a toned lower body. Nothing could be further from the truth! You need to perform squats, lunges, leg presses, and leg curls while using SFT, BFT, or AFT in order to gain muscle tone in the lower body and lose the most cellulite possible. It's hard work, but the training sessions are short-lived and you feel energized afterward. Group Functional Training (GFT) can also work if the weight loads are heavy enough, adequate volume is performed, and enough intensity is applied. The proper selection of Functional Training is a must for building muscle tone and helping get rid of saggy skin and cellulite. To fix loose skin and cellulite to the best of your ability, you must perform a lot of Functional Sets with the proper exercises, and lift heavy weights with great intensity using great form! Females in particular are guilty of lifting too light and stopping too soon in a work set. This is the primary reason they struggle to get the muscle-toning results they want. By training intensely while using compound exercises such as squats for the legs, problem areas like the glutes will gradually improve as skin tightens.

Functional Alert: Too much cardio eats away at type-2 muscle fibers (fast twitch), especially, in the legs and glutes.[1,2] This muscle loss causes skin to become loose and cellulite to rear its ugly head!

Females wanting to build muscle tone are doing a great disservice to themselves by focusing on easy, non-productive workouts that don't work! These so-called "feel-good" workouts are nothing more than a placebo effect. If you really want results, let your personal trainer know you want SFT, BFT, or AFT. Always remember to tell your personal trainer you want to lift heavy in the 8-15 rep range using good form, adequate volume, and great intensity (according to your limitations and strength capabilities) while placing primary emphasis on compound exercises and secondary emphasis on isolation exercises so that you can build maximum muscle tone, lose maximum body fat, gain maximum strength, and improve functionality!

Functional Alert: Not getting results is a classic reason people give up. Be prepared to get in the gym and train hard if you really want results!

Muscle tone is the new sexy for females. Weight training for females became popular during the 1980s. Today, females have a new perspective on what type of body looks attractive—one with more muscle tone and less body fat.

Females frequently bypass the heavy dumbbells and machines fearing that manly muscles might result from any training with heavier weights. Often we see women lifting light weights or performing bodyweight floor exercises that are at an extremely low to moderate challenge level. Let us be clear: that isn't the answer to getting a toned body! It's also a common misconception that lighter weights performed for a high number of reps (e.g., 20-25) won't tone the body. Lighter weights and high reps will increase muscle tone if you train with enough intensity, volume, and frequency. However, higher reps don't build as much muscle tone as lower reps (e.g., 8-15). When some women move out of the light-weight range, they often ask us this question, "Will lifting this heavy weight make me bulky?" Our answer is always the same: "Women won't bulk up when training with heavier weights if their training volume and diet are adjusted properly in accordance with their genetic makeup, because they don't have as much testosterone as their male counterparts." Females produce about 13 times less testosterone than males.[3]

It's very common to look around the gym and see females doing 10 reps with a weight when they could be doing 15-20. They have been misinformed that this is what it takes to tone the muscles. The problem with such training is that they are wasting their time performing exercises that are lacking in enough intensity to properly develop the muscles, tendons, and bones or improve strength and burn body fat. Some have asked us, "Couldn't we get the same improvements by doing extra sets with low intensity?" The answer is absolutely not! You might see a little improvement performing more sets with less intensity. However, you will make much better improvements and spend less time in the gym by using Functional Sets!

Having lower testosterone decreases muscle mass by decreasing the amount of muscle protein synthesis in the body. Testosterone leads to an increase in fat-free muscle mass. Testosterone, an anabolic hormone, has also been found to limit the effects of cortisol (a hormone that eats away muscle). Lower testosterone in females allows cortisol to break down muscle and bone, increase body fat, and cause mood swings and inflammation.[4] This can result in high blood pressure, high cholesterol, high blood sugar, and a slower metabolism. This is the primary reason that females with the same body types as their male counterparts (e.g., endomorphs who have a slow metabolism) can't consume as many calories without gaining body fat.

As Functional Personal Trainers, we have learned it's easy to get comfortable seeing a certain type of look, and if we are not careful, it starts to alter our perception. We have also learned the need to be highly focused on a female's genetics, body-fat levels, and desires. If a female client says, "I don't want to get bulky muscles," we listen! As Functional Personal Trainers our job is to ask her what that means to her. A good approach is to have her show us pictures of what body types she likes and dislikes. Each female has a look she wants and the term "too much or too little muscle tone" is subjective. She has her personal reasons, and it helps us to determine the best course of action. As Functional Personal Trainers, we make the necessary adjustments in training and diet to meet each female's wants and desires. The majority of females (age isn't a factor) will pick out the photo of a female who competes in figure competitions as opposed to bikini or bodybuilding. Males these days (age not a factor) usually choose photos of physique competitors instead of top-level bodybuilders. Obtaining these types of bodies usually requires a lot of intense weight training in the 8-15 rep range, healthy testosterone levels, normal genetics, and a high-protein diet.

Ladies, please pay close attention to what we are about to say: If you are one of the select few genetically gifted females who has the ability to gain some muscle bulk, then simply replace the amount of heavier work sets for any body part you feel is getting too big with lighter weights and more reps (e.g., 20-30 reps)! Don't ease up on the intensity or volume because you will lose too much muscle tone and not burn as much body fat during your Functional Training sessions. If you want to lose a lot of muscle tone in a particular area, simply stop training it for about eight weeks to allow it to shrink back to its non-trained state. Then begin training using higher reps and lighter weights. It's that simple!

If you are a female who desires to gain less muscle tone and wants to get a cardio session in as you lift weights, then your best option is AFT! You will still want to place more emphasis on weaker body parts or trouble spots, such as the triceps (back of the arms) and glutes. Many opt to continue with SFT or BFT on a permanent basis as opposed to using AFT, especially those who are over 35 years of age, have pre-existing injuries, or struggle to gain muscle tone. Many people with injuries and who have a hard time gaining muscle tone do better performing cardio separately from weight training (preferably after weight-training sessions, not before) instead of implementing it into their training sessions.

Bodybuilding

Bodybuilding is muscle toning taken to the extreme! Bodybuilding requires training with more volume, and/or intensity. Bodybuilding or Slingshot Functional Training causes a considerable amount of type-2 muscle fiber breakdown, which builds large muscles in people who have a lot of type-2 muscle fibers. Our mainstream male and female muscle-toning programs require using less volume and sometimes less intensity than our male and female bodybuilding programs. The end result is a strong and toned physique. Remember, a Functional Set involves using great form and stopping 1-2 reps shy of muscle failure. Muscle failure is the point where a repetition fails due to inadequate muscular strength. Functional Sets will add muscle tone and strength and help prevent overtraining and becoming injured. This increases your functionality both inside and outside the gym. The muscle tone most females desire is just a small growth in the size of the muscles. Most have to work really hard to obtain it!

One of the complaints we get from some female clients is that someone told them that their metabolism will increase for each pound of muscle they build. However, they don't want to build a lot of muscle! In some cases, genetically gifted females are willing to give up the extra metabolic boost to appear less toned. Since these females prefer not to gain as much muscle tone, we have them perform more reps with lighter weights so it doesn't break down the type-2 muscle fibers as much. It's a personal decision between the trainer and their female client. That's why it's called personal training!

Struggling to Develop Muscle Tone

Whether male or female, some people have trouble with developing muscle tone. It can be much harder than people think! Bulking up with muscle takes about 3-6 months for a female if she has the genetics. Remember, all it takes to shrink an area back down to its original non-trained state is to stop training it for a while. Let us assure you that most females should have no fear of getting too bulky "musclewise" from using heavy weights during Functional Training. As explained earlier, the bulky look in females usually comes from eating too many calories, not from lifting heavy weights! Some people get the term "muscle bulk" mixed up with "fat bulk" but they are not the same. A pound of fat weighs the same as a pound of muscle, but a pound of fat takes up a whole lot more space than a pound of muscle! Think of how much space is taken up by a huge five-pound pile of feathers. Those feathers represent body fat. Now think of how little space is taken up by a small five-pound brick. That brick represents muscle. Body fat usually produces the bulky appearance in females, not lifting heavy weights!

The majority of females who think they are gaining muscle bulk are not! Most never get lean enough to see the muscle that is actually underneath their body fat. This same rule applies to males who intentionally try to bulk up eating tons of calories. When body-fat levels are too high, muscle definition will be hidden and muscles will push up on fat, making people look bulkier in street clothes.

Everyone is born with a certain amount of fat cells and muscle cells. Fat cells can increase from birth through teenhood. The more fat cells you accumulate, the more fat cells you have to deal with. This makes it extremely important that kids don't allow themselves to gain excess body fat because it's going to make it harder for them to lose body fat when they reach adulthood!

As an adult, fat cells don't increase in number. When you gain weight, your fat cells expand in size.[5] Likewise, when you gain muscle, your muscle cells expand in size. Muscle cells don't replace fat cells. When you lose body fat and gain muscle, the fat cells shrink and the muscle cells overpower. When you lose muscle and gain body fat, the muscle cells shrink and the fat cells overpower. If you gain fat and muscle at the same time, you will expand both, giving you a bulky appearance!

> **Kathy:** *Looks and body types are very subjective. People can find all kinds of things attractive. If you want to look sexy, then lift weights and work on losing body fat. A plumping effect can occur in some females when they first start weight training due to muscle pushing on fat. Don't worry about it because it will leave once the workouts and diet burn away the fat, leaving you with sleek, toned muscles!*

We have learned that regardless of whether you are male or female, diet plays a larger role than genetics in terms of losing body fat. Many gym goers who are leaner consume food that is at the higher end of the Functional Food Spectrum and lower in calories! Likewise, those that look more bulky are usually the people who don't pay as much attention to their diet and eat larger quantities of food on the lower end of the Functional Food Spectrum. Most of the leaner people go home and eat something like baked chicken breast and a salad after working out whereas the heavier people go to restaurants and eat fattening food.

It takes a lot of work and great genetics to obtain bulky muscles. It doesn't take a long time to build a little muscle under the fat and achieve a plumping effect. What some women don't realize is this is only a temporary effect, and if they keep lifting and continue with their diet, they will shrink down in size while having a higher muscle-to-fat ratio after only 3-6 months. They will also have a faster resting metabolism post-workout and a faster active metabolism when working out with weights. We have seen many females train with weights and lose inches and fit into smaller sizes of clothes, yet they lose only small amounts of weight on the scale. How could this be? The answer is, they gained muscle tone while simultaneously losing body fat. On the other hand, we have seen females who have stopped training with weights, yet their weight remained the same. How could this be? This answer is, they gained body fat while simultaneously losing muscle tone.

Gaining muscle bulk for an intermediate or advanced lifter requires consuming more calories than your body needs to maintain its weight. We have found that if you are already lean (these rules apply to both male and female), your muscles won't grow to any appreciable degree without a surplus of calories around the first six initial months of proper weight training! Muscles grow at a snail's pace after the first three months of training. After approximately one year, muscle gains level off and it becomes extremely difficult to add any additional muscle tone. To lose body fat, you need to consume 500 fewer calories per day than your body needs to maintain its weight. To build new muscle, your body needs energy and nutrients to enhance protein synthesis. In other words, if you are already lean, you will need to consume an additional 500 calories per day to make a measurable amount of muscle tone once you get past the first 3-6 months of training. The vast majority of males and females who have already been lifting weights don't have to worry about bulking up if they are dieting down to lose body fat. When they are in a calorie deficit, their ability to build muscle tone and strength is compromised. However, beginners on a weight-training and nutrition program geared toward fat loss can simultaneously build muscle and lose fat for approximately six months because their bodies are not accustomed to any form of weight training.

Functional Alert: We use the word muscle toning in this book so everyone can relate. The definition of toning is to build lean muscle so you will become firmer and leaner. In both male and females, a toned look comes from a combination of less body fat, denser muscle growth from training the type-2 muscle fibers, and consuming plenty of protein and water. The problem with many programs is that they teach you to get toned using techniques that don't work. For example, you can work out with one pound dumbbells and do hundreds of reps every day, but you will never develop any appreciable muscle tone beyond what you started with prior to lifting weights. Obtaining a pump and getting a burn in the muscles doing high reps, light weights, and low intensity doesn't make the muscles get toned! We believe some of the classes offered at many local gyms (e.g., Zumba® Toning) causes some body-fat loss, but we don't believe they produce any measurable muscle tone. In fact, these classes can reduce muscle tone if the proper form of Functional Training is not performed in addition to Zumba®. The bottom line is, you must consistently perform Functional Training in order to build and maintain muscle tone!

Approximately 4-8 lbs of newly built muscle is required to achieve the shaping and toning that most females desire. Most low-intensity exercise programs touted in many women's magazines, which guarantee a flatter tummy, reduced hips and thighs, and toned arms are only going to allow you to gain about one pound of muscle, if that.

No one knows the exact numbers, but it's our estimation that every pound of muscle you have on your body in a non-trained state (before you begin lifting weights) burns only around 6 calories or so per day.[6] That isn't a lot! But here's the good news: For every new pound of muscle you gain after you begin weight training, we estimate you will burn on average around 35 calories according to studies performed by Tufts University.[7] It's important to understand that it's not the 1 lb of muscle itself that burns the additional 35 calories, but the workouts required to sustain the 1 lb of newly built muscle. This means it takes only 4 lbs of new muscle to burn an additional 140 calories per day. Again, the extra calories burned are from workouts required to build and maintain that new muscle. That is what we refer to as actively trained muscle. We have noticed it takes only 4-8 lbs of newly added muscle to have a significant impact on a female's metabolism. We can't make this point strongly enough. Adding 4-8 lbs of actively trained muscle can completely turn your lives around, ladies! Likewise, 10- 20 lbs of actively trained muscle can completely turn your lives around, gentlemen!

We are of the opinion that the caloric burn derived from building and maintaining 8 lbs of muscle is equivalent to about 40 minutes of moderate-intensity cardio on the treadmill, 7 days a week, 365 days a year! Now you know why most of these male bodybuilders who work out to maintain their newly built muscles can get by with eating more calories and not get fat. For those of you who have friends who exercise 7 days a week on a piece of cardio equipment such as a treadmill, you can say:

> *I burn just as many calories, if not more as you do by only training with weights three times per week because I have built up my lean muscle mass! Furthermore, the treadmill workouts leave me bored, tired, hungry, and craving sugar, while the weight-training workouts leave me feeling challenged, exhilarated, and less stressed and craving protein and fibrous, plant-based food, which enhance my metabolism even further due to their thermogenic effect during digestion. I am toning and re-shaping the muscles throughout my entire body, but you are doing nothing to tone up your muscles and your skin. In addition, your body is going to become very saggy.*

Proper Exercise Form for Males and Females

For males and females, performing a correct lift should take about 1-2 seconds on the lifting phase and 2-3 seconds on the lowering phase to obtain maximum results. Slower reps are best for Rehabilitative Functional Training (RFT), not muscle toning! Lifting heavier weights with intensity is not the only requirement to build optimal muscle tone. You must use great form. When training for muscle tone, a Dysfunctional Set is defined as stopping too early in the set (lacking intensity) or training beyond muscle failure while rocking your body to generate momentum.

Muscle toning and power lifting are not the same! Power lifters use very fast repetitions because their primary objective is moving as much weight as possible, not stimulating their muscles. When we refer to lifting heavy weights we are also talking about using impeccable form. This is a very hard concept for some people to accept, especially males. Heavier is better only if you can keep the muscles under tension by lifting the weight in proper form. At this point, it's safe to add more weight if it doesn't hurt your joints. Once you can perform more than 15 repetitions of an exercise, it's a good time to increase the weight unless you are in rehab mode or you want to have less muscle tone and just burn calories. Increase your weight by the smallest possible increment in order to spare your joints over the long haul. It's up to each individual to find out which rep-range best fits their needs.

Functional Alert: A common mistake made by rookies is bouncing the bar off the chest to complete a few reps during a bench press. You should not bounce the bar off your chest during the bench press!

The form you use in the gym is what separates you as a muscle toner from people who just lift weights! Poor form using too heavy of a weight takes some of the stress off the targeted muscle group and puts a lot more stress on the vulnerable joints, ligaments, tendons, and fasciae. When momentum comes into play (e.g., CrossFit®), it takes some of the load off the actual muscle group being targeted and puts a lot more on the connective tissue and joint at the beginning and end of each repetition. To gain muscle tone without tearing up your joints you must take the most precise, educated, scientific approach possible! We have learned that some people, due to their superior genetics, can get by with a lack of training knowledge and still reach a decent level of development. However, maximum muscle toning in a safe manner can only be achieved when you fully concentrate on the muscle being trained. You must control the weight! Always lower the weight slowly since you are working the same muscles as when you are lifting. Controlling the negative phase during the lift produces more muscle tone, enhances functional strength, and decreases muscle and connective tissue injuries, more so than performing positive lifting only. Controlling the negative also helps build up resistance to future injuries. Unfortunately, many people in the gym cheat themselves by dropping the weight instead of controlling it on the negative phase. If you are slamming weights in the gym, it's a sign you are not controlling the weight during the lowering phase. This means you are trying to lift more weight than your muscles can handle! This form of training damages your body and the expensive gym equipment the owners purchased with their hard-earned money. We ask that you be respectful of your body and other people's property. The lifting phase should be performed with a smooth explosion—not with bouncing, jerking, swinging, and throwing weights like they do in CrossFit®.

Functional Alert: Don't CrossFit® it!

Ask yourself this, What am I trying to accomplish in my workouts? Remind yourself which muscle you're working and focus on that muscle. It's easy to do chest presses and work your front deltoids more than your chest. Don't take the easy way out! When training for muscle tone your #1 goal is to make the exercise harder, not easier as many people in the gym are doing so they can lift more weight to impress their peers or stroke their ego, rush to get their workouts done, or avoid feeling the muscles burn. Trying to beat your personal record every time you enter the gym should never be your #1 goal as this will lead to poor form, over-straining, and injury. The most effective approach for muscle toning is actually a very mentally tough way to train. Instead of taking the path of least resistance, you want to develop a "strong mind-to-muscle link," which requires taking the path of most resistance, muscle pain, and effort. Your muscles will burn more and you will have to train your brain to push past the pain barrier. That is how you get toned muscles and maximize your endorphin high! Most people have to re-train their brain to learn to lift properly because they were never taught correctly in the beginning.

Functional Alert: You must learn to embrace muscle pain, not avoid it!

Approximately 75% of everyone in the gym take the path of least resistance! Unfortunately, the majority of people never develop the kind of muscle tone they are capable of because of this training error. We see so many frustrated people who can't develop the muscle tone they desire yet are often nursing a nagging injury from lifting too much weight with improper form. The largest single factor preventing people from reducing the amount of weight they lift is their ego. Males in particular (age not a factor) really tend to struggle with this concept. The professional bodybuilders you see in muscle magazines have given a lot of males an inferiority complex. The fact is that men in these magazines are freaks of nature. Even the above-average male could never get that big or strong regardless of what he did. If you are concerned about what other people in the gym think in regard to how much weight you are lifting, then you have an ego problem! Never forget that walking around the gym with extreme muscle tone is far more impressive to both males and females than bouncing a super-heavy weight off your chest a couple of times while a spotter helps you in the process. In addition, just because you have the genetic capability to lift a very heavy weight (e.g., bench pressing a lot of weight) for a couple of reps doesn't mean you should. It's common for people to rupture tendons in their genetically gifted body parts when training with super-heavy weights. This is a result of the muscles becoming stronger than the tendons can support! The shoulders, biceps, triceps, and pectorals are among the most common muscle groups to experience a tendon rupture. As we get older, the blood supply to the tendons and ligaments decreases, resulting in weaker tendons and ligaments.

Functional Alert: Ego lifters (bodybuilders and athletes included) will make better gains by reducing the amount of weight they are lifting by about one-third. There's a limit to how strong everyone can get. That limit is usually reached within the first year of training. Consistency is the key to making continued progress once you've maxed out your strength potential, not trying to lift heavier weight and/or using poor form to get more reps!

Another problem is that most people shorten the range of motion in order to lift more weight. They totally miss out on the extension (the gentle stretch) and the contraction (the intense squeeze). Your primary objective must be to find ways to increase tension on the muscles, not decrease it. During the performance of every repetition you must stretch the muscle without overdoing it and squeeze without locking out the joint. The secret is never to allow the muscles to relax during the set while still allowing for a peak contraction.

Allow us to illustrate: While working your chest using a decline barbell bench press, the top position provides little resistance on the chest because the triceps take over. If you want maximum overall chest growth, you need to keep tension on the chest for the entire duration of the set. Locking out your joints or taking small rests between reps will unload the chest muscles and reduce the amount of tension and intensity the muscles will be subjected to. You don't want to do this because it allows oxygen to come back into the muscles between reps. When you pause at the top or bottom of each repetition, you are inviting injury because you are taking tension off the muscles and putting it onto the joints and connective tissues. The next time you train your chest, use no pause or momentum whatsoever while squeezing the muscle at the top. It will give you a burn and pump you won't soon forget. You will feel more muscle pain while training in this manner and instead of making your joints and connective tissues weaker, you will make them stronger because you are able to work with less weight and better form to get the job done. Never take the path of least resistance when toning the muscles and strengthening the connective tissues. When you do, you cheat yourself!

Bad Pain

One of the biggest mistakes people make is trying to work through bad pain! We are referring to joint, ligament, tendon, and fascia pain, not muscle pain. You need to stop an exercise immediately upon feeling a sharp painful twinge, even if it's your favorite exercise. This goes for rehab exercises as well. For example, if you are performing leg presses and you feel a sharp twinge in your knee, stop using them. If you fail to do so, you can cause an injury that can take months to get over—and even longer as you get older. If you develop an injury, it's imperative that you rest, use ice, and allow inflammation to leave before you begin rehabbing in a controlled fashion. We know resting is one of the hardest things for most people to do after becoming injured because exercise is very addictive, but in these particular cases, the term "no pain, no gain" doesn't apply!

Functional Alert: Sometimes rest is the only cure!

It's very common for people to ignore bad pain when doing certain exercises. They think the toned muscles they will get are worth the discomfort. The flat bench press using free weights is a good example. This exercise is notorious for causing shoulder pain in some people. People need to understand that the exercises that cause them the most harm (hurting in a bad way) will not, in the end, lead to building sustainable muscle tone and functionality. All too often, we have seen them get to the point where they can't do those exercises at all due to excruciating pain stemming from chronic inflammation.

You must listen to your body because the best muscle-toning exercises allow you to do the most work with the least pain. Some body parts may require replacing free weights for machines, or machines with cables. The muscles get toned by "time under tension," not whether you are performing an exercise such as bench press with free weights versus a machine. Choose the exercises that spare your joints so you can build and maintain more muscle tone and functionality over the long haul. Being forced to take time away from training will only set you back! If you happen to develop chronic inflammation or get injured, simply work on your other body parts until you are healed. Also, don't be surprised if the pain reappears while performing an exercise that initially caused an injury, even after you have let it heal. That is your body's way of letting you know to steer clear of that particular exercise!

Functional Alert: If you are experiencing joint pain, it's a sign you are lifting too heavy. It's amazing how many people ignore this obvious fact instead of reducing the weight!

Rest Time between Functional Sets

The amount of rest needed between each Functional Set will vary to some degree. For gaining maximum muscle tone, moving too fast between Functional Sets when employing SFT, BFT, and AFT isn't appropriate for training the type-2 muscle fibers that are required to develop a toned body. Moving too fast between Functional Sets is a totally different scenario than supersets, which require bouncing back and forth between two muscle groups; for example, chest presses—then immediately to lat pull downs—rest until you feel recovered—then back to chest presses—then lat pull downs again—and so on. With supersets you don't have to wait 30 seconds before going from chest to back because you are simultaneously working different body parts.

ATP (adenosine triphosphate) is the chemical that cause muscles to contract so you can lift the weight.[9] Your ATP levels must be replenished before further muscle contractions can occur. ATP supports very brief, high-intensity activities, such as Functional Training. If you fail to give your body enough time for ATP levels to recover, you won't be able to lift enough weight to break down the type-2 muscle fibers and develop maximum muscle tone, strength, and functionality. This means you will experience ineffective workouts! If you forfeit rest between Functional Sets, you reach cardio failure, central nervous system failure, and ATP depletion before reaching good muscle failure (1-2 reps shy of muscle failure). You will be too exhausted to effectively work your muscles, and then too sore later to want to continue the training regimen. Experience has taught us that you need a minimum of a 30-second rest between the same body parts being trained in order for ATP levels to recover. However, 10-15 seconds is all that is needed between single-drop sets because you are making a reduction in weight.

CHAPTER 7

Functional Cardio

Functional Cardio is defined as the amount of moderate-intensity, steady-state cardio needed for your body type in order to do four things: (1) improve heart efficiency, (2) experience fat loss without muscle loss, (3) avoid overstressing the central nervous system and immune system, and (4) avoid causing joint and connective tissue pain.

We would like to set the record straight about cardio by letting you know the truth. We have worked with many people over the years and by far their most common desire is to replace body fat with muscle tone. However, fat and muscle tissue are composed of two entirely different types of cells. You can burn fat and build muscle, but you can't turn fat into muscle! When fat is lost and muscle tone is increased, muscle simply replaces the area where fat used to reside.

Many people have been told that cardiovascular exercise is the key to losing body fat and becoming more toned. However, that is wrong! Think about it: When a 150-pound person walks at a fast steady pace on a treadmill (10-degree incline) for 30 minutes at a moderate intensity, they burn approximately 200 calories. That is all! It requires around 90 minutes to burn off a large serving of fries from a mainstream fast-food restaurant. Clearly, diet is far more important and convenient for losing body fat than endurance-type exercise. Regardless of your body type, we feel that if you need a ton of cardio for body-fat loss when following a diet, then your diet isn't a Functional Diet or you are trying to lose too much weight in too short a period of time.

You need to burn an additional 3,500 calories to lose a pound of body fat. If you weigh 150 pounds and perform 40 minutes of moderate-intensity, steady state cardio 6 days per week, you will burn roughly 1,800 calories (300 calories x 6=1,800 calories) a week. That's still about a half a pound of fat per week. That adds up to approximately two pounds of additional fat loss per month. This means that cardio will help you lose body fat faster than diet alone!

Functional Alert: Functional Cardio can help get rid of that stubborn lower-belly flab when you combine it with a Functional Diet and Functional Training!

However, there's one thing that cardio doesn't eliminate: your appetite! The more cardio you do, the hungrier you will get because your blood sugar drops. It gets even worse if you do cardio in the morning in a fasted state before breakfast. You will burn some calories, but you may be tempted to eat twice as many calories afterward, which will make you gain body fat. You have to train your mind as well as your body. If you can't control the increased hunger pangs from doing cardio in addition to the cardio workout you get from Functional Training, then Functional Cardio should be kept to an absolute minimum or avoided altogether!

Functional Alert: We don't recommend fasted cardio on an empty stomach (first thing in the morning before breakfast). Fasted cardio lowers your training intensity, it burns more muscle, and it causes a rapid drop in blood sugar, thus causing you to be hungrier and eat more calories afterward. Fasted cardio also causes the body to release excess amounts of pro-inflammatory cytokines and free radicals. Always have a small meal composed of protein and carbs before morning cardio to prevent a rapid decline in blood sugar and to prevent feeling miserable both during and after your workouts. Furthermore, consuming some protein before working out increases glutathione (the master antioxidant) levels, which can help combat free radical damage that occurs during cardio workouts!

Most people overestimate how much they burn and say, I did cardio today so I can overindulge on junk food. How many times have you faced a food temptation and thought, I performed a lot of cardio today, so it's okay to eat bad today? Or thought, I will eat bad now and work out extra hard tomorrow to burn it off? If that sounds all too familiar, this is one of the reasons why you are struggling to lose body fat and are having bouts of low energy. The extra energy required for your body to digest all that additional food leaves you feeling tired, sluggish, and sick to your stomach. We refer to this as a "food hangover" because it has similarities to that of an alcohol hangover in terms of how it poisons the body!

Functional Alert: Cardio doesn't burn nearly as many calories as most people think!

It's a scientifically proven fact that muscle proteins are broken down and used for energy during cardio exercise to varying degrees. The amount of muscle that gets broken depends on eight things:

1. How well you are fueled before cardio sessions. Cardio on an empty stomach causes more muscle loss, which slows down your metabolism.

2. The duration of each cardio session. The longer you do cardio, the greater your chances of using muscle protein for fuel. It also increases free radical damage and cortisol levels.

3. The training intensity used during each cardio session. The more intensely you train, the faster glycogen stores will become depleted and start tapping into muscle protein for fuel.

4. How often you do cardio. The more often you do cardio, the higher your odds of overtraining and releasing excess cortisol, which results in muscle loss and immune system dysfunction.

5. How much spare body fat you are carrying. The less body fat you have, the earlier your body will tap into muscle protein for fuel.

6. The amount of cortisol your body releases. Some people release more cortisol than others when performing cardio, which causes them to lose more muscle and maintain more belly fat.

7. Your testosterone levels. Those with the least amount of testosterone will lose muscle faster during cardio because testosterone prevents muscle breakdown.

8. The amount of type-2 muscle fibers you have to spare. People who have more type-1 fibers lose muscle tone faster during cardio than people with more type-2 fibers.

Functional Alert: There's a point you reach when performing cardio where your body begins using less body fat for fuel. At this point, the body begins using muscle tissue as its primary fuel source!

Excessive or Dysfunctional Cardio can cause as much loss of muscle as it does body fat in some people, and sometimes more, even though the scales show you weigh less. It's an illusion! People think they are losing all body fat because the scales show they are losing weight, but that isn't always the case. They are often losing a considerable amount of hard-earned muscle tone! It's the reverse scenario of some off-season bodybuilders who bulk up and often gain more fat than muscle, even though the scales show they weigh more. Again, it's all an illusion! They think they are putting on mostly muscle weight because the scales show they are gaining weight, but it's not the case. Cardio is a very individualistic thing. Your genetics, Functional Training Program, and diet will determine how much muscle tone you can keep while doing a lot of cardio. For the average person, cardio is responsible for roughly 10% of body-fat loss before it starts reducing muscle tone. Keep in mind, a 10% body-fat loss is still a substantial amount!

Skinny fat people who are diagnosed with diabetes are twice as likely to die as overweight people with more muscle tone who are diagnosed with the same disease.[1] This means you should never do only cardio! You also need to incorporate some form of Functional Training to build muscle tone.

Dysfunctional Cardio

Dysfunctional Cardio (Excessive cardio) is more stressful than a lower-calorie diet. The nervous system fatigue associated with Dysfunctional Cardio encourages you to eat more calories in order to have enough energy to function during daily activities. Decreasing calories, instead of increasing cardio, makes it easier to lose body fat because you have less of an appetite. In today's busy world, it's more practical for people to limit caloric intake than to spend extra time doing cardio to burn calories. There is a point of diminishing returns with all things, including cardio. Adding too much cardio and/or overdoing the intensity causes chronic inflammation and oxidation. It eventually slows down your metabolism and causes dehydration by decreasing your type-2 muscle fibers. Dysfunctional Cardio drains the central nervous system and encourages overuse injuries. It usually causes you to become stressed and irritable afterward because it increases cortisol, which breaks down muscle tone and decreases testosterone levels.

Functional Alert: Experience has taught us that after more than 60 minutes of moderate-intensity, steady-state cardio, the body begins to break down muscle tissue!

You will achieve a more efficient calorie deficit by implementing a reasonable balance between calories consumed and calories burned with Functional Exercise (Functional Training and Functional Cardio). Dysfunctional Cardio ignites ravenous hunger pangs for sugar carbs, which is very unhealthy. It also increases cellulite (especially in the legs and glutes) for those lacking in type-2 muscle fibers.

Functional Alert: Too much cardio burns muscle for fuel, especially in the legs and glutes. This can cause a loss of muscle tone or roundness in the glutes, which can result in a noticeable increase in cellulite in some females. When muscle in the glutes is lost, there will be less muscle left to push up against the skin. This results in saggy skin, which reveals cellulite!

Now that you know too much cardio is bad, we want to clarify that a sedentary lifestyle and too much food (especially carbs and fats) are what is killing most people prematurely. The majority of people in the world need to exercise a lot more, but everything in moderation!

Cardio can help or hinder your immune system. Depending on your level of exercise, your immune system will become enhanced or it will suffer. The right level of exercise allows your body to produce more white blood cells to fight off infection, while too much exercise lowers your white blood cell count. After 45 combined years of experience in this field, we are convinced that too much cardio does more harm than overtraining with weights because it destroys your body composition and your motivation to stay committed to working out because of boredom, and it increases inflammation and free radical damage that accelerates the aging process.

Ronnie: *The energy we use for cardiovascular exercise is primarily made through aerobic metabolism, which, unfortunately, produces a significant amount of harmful free radicals.*[2-7] *On the other hand, the energy used for Functional Training is primarily made through anaerobic metabolism, which, if the heart rate is not allowed to remain too high, does not produce a significant amount of harmful free radicals.*[8,9] *Furthermore, both Functional Training and Functional Cardio performed on a consistent basis cause the body to become more resistant to oxidative damage. Exercising in moderation trains the body to activate increased concentrations of free radical scavengers (antioxidants), to destroy harmful free radicals, and to fight against oxidative stress.*[10] *However, in the case of Dysfunctional Cardio, the body cannot produce enough scavengers to both destroy the excessive harmful free radicals and to fight against oxidative stress.*[11] *The body is then put into a highly stressful state where hormonal imbalances throw it out of a fat-burning mode and into a fat-storing one.*[12] *This is also another reason to stay away from CrossFit® because it is based on maintaining an extremely elevated heart rate throughout the entire workout!*[13]

Kathy: *Cardio done in moderation is good for you, but a lot causes damage and premature aging. The damage from excess cardio is caused by the buildup of scar tissue around the heart and the body producing excess amounts of pro-inflammatory cytokines and free radicals.*[14]

You must listen to your body! When your legs feel tired, it's your body telling you it's time to back off the cardio. If you start feeling stale or chronically fatigued, then take off as much time as you need in order to get your energy levels back. You may find that you need a week off to get your energy levels back, and scale back when you start again. If you continue with the cardio even though your legs and body are tired, of course it's going to get worse because your legs and central nervous system are becoming more and more overtrained. It's very important to maintain leg strength in order to train with weights using enough intensity and load to maintain round glutes, help prevent cellulite, and maintain spine and hip stability.

Functional Alert: Performing cardio prior to Functional Training is counterproductive. You use energy that normally would be used to perform Functional Training more efficiently. In addition, cardio should be avoided altogether on the days you train legs with a lot of volume. Combining both on the same day usually results in overtraining!

If your primary focus is on losing body fat and muscle toning, but you are limited on time or energy, then skip Functional Cardio and focus solely on Functional Diet and Functional Training. Diet and weight training are more important than Functional Cardio in relation to looking good, being healthy, and being able to function during daily activities.

Moderate-intensity, steady-state cardio is heart healthy when used in moderation but can be bad for the heart when done in excess. Like other muscles, your heart responds in a healthy way to Functional Cardio. People who perform Dysfunctional Cardio can build up scar tissue in the heart just as people who overdo weight training can build up scar tissue in the joints, ligaments, tendons, fasciae, and nerves. When scar tissue builds up around them, it shrinks. When it shrinks, it pulls on those tendons, ligaments, fasciae, and nerves causing horrible pain, and the muscles lose their ability to contract in a functional manner. In other words, you get weaker! Likewise, when scar tissue builds up around the ventricles of the heart, it shrinks. When the scar tissue shrinks, it constricts the ventricles and cuts off blood delivery throughout the body. The heart muscle weakens because it can no longer contract in a functional manner. Dysfunctional Cardio is linked to the malfunction of the right ventricle, which is responsible for pumping deoxygenated blood through the lungs.[15-17]

Functional Alert: Endurance athletes can help prevent overstressing their hearts by systematically changing their training programs to give their bodies adequate rest. Some tend to massively overtrain!

FUNCTIONAL CARDIO

We are not saying you shouldn't engage in cardiovascular exercise—quite the contrary: Moderate-intensity, steady-state cardio helps your body function more efficiently on many levels. It's very unfortunate that many people's sedentary lifestyles result in unfavorable outcomes in terms of disease.

Functional Cardio:

- ☐ Changes the chemistry of the brain.[18-19]

- ☐ Causes the heart to pump blood and deliver oxygen to working muscles and all major organs, such as the brain. The cells in your brain start functioning at a higher level, making you feel more alert during Functional Cardio and more focused after you finish. Over time, you will experience a lower resting heart rate and your brain will function more efficiently.[20]

- ☐ Helps with the digestion after a meal.[21]

- ☐ Helps us cope with the stress we face in everyday life. Stress often becomes unmanageable, causing a Dysfunctional Immune System.

- ☐ Helps control anger, anxiety, and depression.[22,23]

- ☐ Lowers blood glucose (sugar) levels, which enhance the function of the pancreas.[24]

- ☐ Releases dopamine and testosterone, which increase sexual function and brain function.[25]

- ☐ Increases brain serotonin and dopamine, which are responsible for helping maintain mood balance.[26]

- ☐ Improves the functionality of the lungs, which helps prevent COPD.

- ☐ Improves kidney function by lowering blood pressure. High blood pressure is widely known for causing kidney failure, strokes, and heart attacks.[27]

- ☐ Improves the function of the liver by preventing the buildup of fats in liver tissue.[28]

- ☐ Decreases visceral fat (fat that lies deep inside the body that can compress vital organs, blood vessels, and lymphatic vessels) and subcutaneous fat (fat that lies just beneath the skin that can negatively affect one's overall appearance).[29]

- ☐ Purges Dysfunctional Toxins (through sweat, burning of calories, and speeding up the elimination of food through your digestive tract) and lowers body fat, which improves immune functions and lowers the risk of getting cancer and other life-threatening illnesses.[30]

- Stimulates the movement of lymph fluid by increasing the rate of blood that gets transported to the capillaries.[31]

- Reduces the risk of disease by improving the antioxidant system.[32]

- Helps prevent getting an enlarged heart.[33]

Some people (personal trainers included) can't stand cardio and won't do it. If we are training clients who get upset at the thought of doing cardio, we eliminate it altogether if that is what it takes to keep them moving forward with the Functional Diet and Functional Training. There are a lot more people dying from obesity and a lack of Functional Training than a lack of direct cardio exercise. As long as you are working fast enough between Functional Sets, you will still be getting a decent amount of cardio. Intense Functional Training, while taking minimal rest between sets, will lower your pulse rate. This means you don't have to do additional cardio on a treadmill, elliptical, etc., unless you need to burn some additional calories to offset your caloric intake. Also keep in mind that we believe most cardio equipment in the gym exaggerates the amount of calories burned during usage. It takes great effort and adjusting the machines to a high-resistance level, to try and burn as many calories as you would by hiking, running, swimming, and biking outdoors. If you can read a book or newspaper while attempting to do cardio on a stationary machine, you are not training with enough intensity for it to be considered Functional Cardio! However, low-intensity cardio will do one good thing: it keeps you occupied and relaxed so that you are not sitting around on the couch eating. Therefore, if you eat out of boredom, going outside and taking a walk is a good thing for you. Going for a walk on a flat surface is not an effective way to burn calories—it's just not intense enough. However, walking on a flat surface is a good way to help increase circulation.

Functional Alert: Performing Functional Cardio in the water can be great for people with bad joints. Most prefer swimming laps using various strokes and group classes such as Water Aerobics and Aqua Zumba®. Mainstream Zumba® is harder on the joints than exercising in the water, but a lot of people, especially women, love dancing in a group setting!

FUNCTIONAL CARDIO

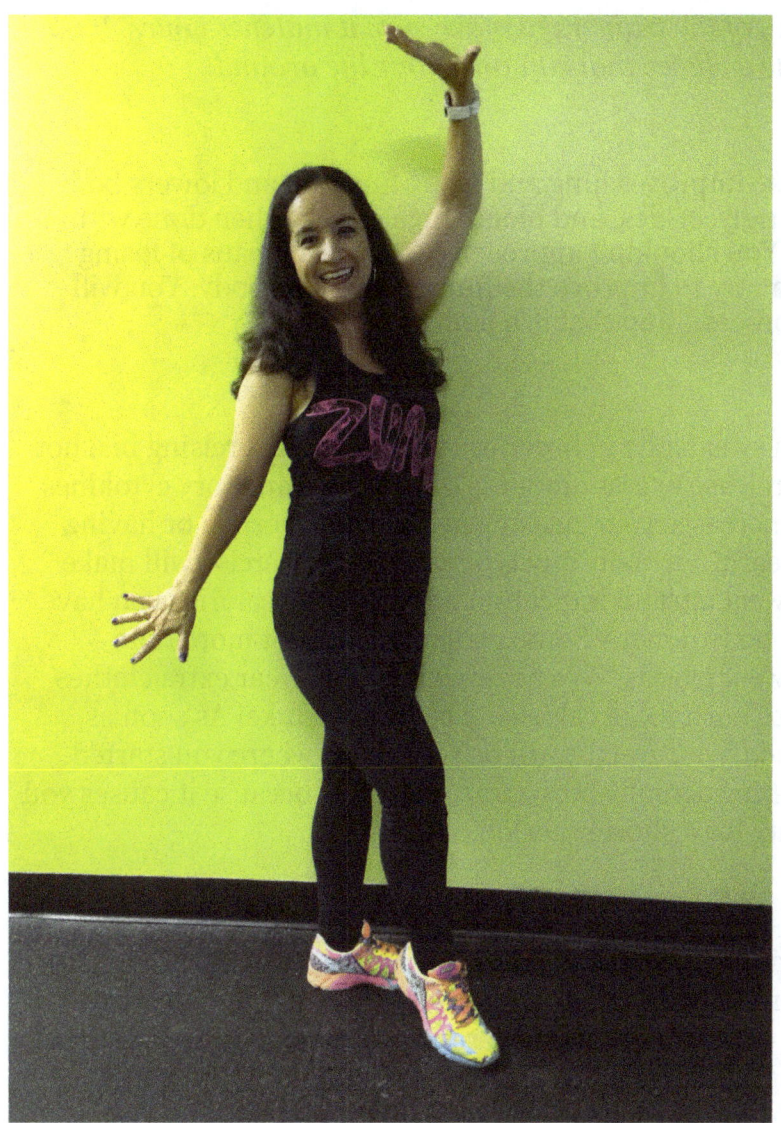

Diana Berry, Zumba Instructor

In 2010, I was obese and desperate to find guidance on how to motivate myself to exercise and keep the commitment to my health. I was a regular member of the gym, but could not maintain a consistent schedule of exercising three or four times a week. One of my coworkers mentioned the personal trainers at Gold's Gym and how getting set up with the right one could change your lifestyle and put you on the road to fitness success.

I finally decided to hire a personal trainer at that time. At the same time, I started taking Zumba. I called the gym requesting a woman trainer and asked for a professional and qualified person who could work with me and educate me through the process. I was assigned to Kathy Rowland as my new trainer. On the first day I met with Kathy, we went through my fitness needs and goals and she suggested a program to follow. She was and always has been very professional throughout the years. During my training with Kathy, and later on with Ronnie, I have been able not only to train but also to learn about the fitness industry, nutrition, and teaching. Since I started training with Kathy in 2011, I have lost a total of 32 lbs of body fat, I have shaped my body, and I have become a well-known Zumba instructor in the industry. Something that started as a training session has become a second job for me and has brought me invaluable fitness knowledge. Having excellent mentors like Kathy and Ronnie has brought me an experience and fitness knowledge that I could not have any other way. After good and bad experiences with personal trainers I strongly suggest for people before engaging in any mentoring or training relationship, to study the qualifications and personality of the trainers to make sure it matches yours. If you find the right one, you have made a choice that can turn your life around!

We believe the best cardio exercise improves lung and heart function and lowers body fat, blood pressure, cholesterol, triglycerides, and blood-sugar levels when done within the limits your body can handle. You shouldn't approach cardio as a means of losing weight at all costs, but rather as a way to improve the function of your body. You will burn away some body fat in the process, and that is a bonus.

Functional Alert: Don't wear a sweatshirt in order to sweat more. Exercising in a hot environment causes the body to release excess amounts of pro-inflammatory cytokines and free radicals. It also greatly increases your risk of getting hyperthermia or having a heat stroke which can lead to death! Virtually any type of intense exercise will make you sweat, but the amount you sweat isn't an indication of how many calories you have burned. Sweating just cools your body down.[34] Some people sweat a lot more than others because they have more sweat glands.[35] We have seen people wear extra clothes while performing cardio hoping to burn more calories. This is a mistake! As soon as you replenish your body with fluids, your weight will be right back where you started. Performing exercise in more clothing actually burns fewer calories because it causes you to train at a lower level of intensity for a shorter period of time!

A major problem we see with mainstream cardio is that it lacks enough intensity to make a noticeable improvement in body-fat loss. Short-to-moderate bursts of moderate-intensity, steady-state cardio helps build up reserve capacity in your heart and trigger the expansion of your lungs. This helps you train more intensely with weights, especially with compound leg movements such as squats, lunges, and leg presses.

High-intensity cardio and high-intensity interval cardio are more effective than moderate-intensity, steady-state cardio for improving your ability to play sports such as football, basketball, and sprinting. But high-intensity cardio and high-intensity-interval cardio and too intense for the average person looking to maintain a lifestyle of fitness because it runs down the central nervous system and the immune system. High-intensity cardio and high-intensity-interval cardio increases the production of pro-inflammatory cytokines and free radicals.

It's best to perform the absolute minimum amount of moderate-intensity, steady-state cardio required to maintain optimal health and body composition. This will help ensure you don't overtrain! For the person with an average metabolism, it only takes 20 minutes of moderate-intensity, steady-state cardio 3 times a week in addition to Slingshot Functional Training or Basic Functional Training sessions. With Advanced

Functional Training, there's a chance you might get all the moderate intensity cardio your body needs. Those who want to max out their fat loss can perform moderate-intensity, steady-state cardio 6 times per week. We can't hand out specific times for how long you should perform cardio because it's different for everyone. What we can tell you is that people with a slower metabolism will need more cardio than those with a faster metabolism. The absolute maximum amount of moderate-intensity, steady-state cardio anyone should perform is 3 hours total per week. This can be accomplished by performing 30 minutes of moderate-intensity, steady-state cardio 6 days a week, 45 minutes 4 times per week, or 60 minutes 3 times per week.

Functional Alert: Having some body fat and left-over energy after your workouts is a must for sexual function!

We recommend that you see your doctor before starting any form of exercise if you smoke, are morbidly obese, or have a chronic health condition. Pushing cardio and trying to get your heart rate up while using high blood pressure medication is dangerous. These medications were designed to slow your heart rate down. If you push it too much, you risk going into cardiac arrest—the electrical system of the heart will malfunction.[36] This is another reason to avoid CrossFit®!

Functional Alert: High-intensity cardio and high-intensity interval cardio is an advanced form of cardio only to be performed by certain athletes. High-Intensity cardio and high-intensity interval cardio is not recommended for the average person trying to lose body fat. It puts too much stress on the body which leads to over-training. These extreme forms of cardio can also lead to cardiac arrest in people who are obese, out of shape, or have an underlying heart condition. Over time the thyroid can react to the stress and decrease T3 production and slow down your metabolism! [37]

CHAPTER 8

How the Immune System Functions

Your immune system is the foundation of living a long and healthy life! In this book we show you how to build the best immune system possible for your genetic makeup so you can max out your life expectancy and stay as healthy as possible in the process. You might be surprised to find out that the immune system is involved in progressing or slowing down all life-threatening diseases. Every health condition is caused by a Dysfunctional Immune System and/or causes a Dysfunctional Immune System. Due to genetics, some people's immune system provides less protection than others'. Genetics accounts for approximately 25% and lifestyle accounts for 75%.[1] In most cases, your immune system does a great job of keeping you healthy until you pass middle age. When your immune system doesn't function properly due to old age, genetics, and/or Dysfunctional Toxin overload, health problems will arise and your life span will shorten!

Functional Alert: Some people's immune systems deal with events that cause stress better than others'. If you are one of the unlucky ones, there's a great chance you will develop a serious medical condition before reaching old age, if you don't apply the principles found in **Functional Training with a Fork** to improve immune deficiency and function!

Instead of posting thousands of complicated studies about all the different types of Dysfunctional Toxins (any foreign object the body does not recognize) and how they cause chronic inflammation and oxidation, we are going to save you time and effort by explaining the most important things you can do to manage chronic inflammation and oxidation, so your immune cells can perform the different functions they were intended to. You will need to read through this entire chapter to discover them!

Dysfunctional Toxin overload blocks communication between immune cells, preventing them from performing their job as a team. For instance, a Dysfunctional Immune System leads to medical problems such as dementia, cancer, heart disease, diabetes, autoimmune diseases, and organs that change in size and perform less efficiently due to hypo-function or hyper-function.

Functional Alert: The majority of people in the U.S. die from heart disease every year. The second leading cause is cancer. Chronic lower respiratory disease, stroke, Alzheimer's, diabetes, autoimmune diseases, and infections follow![2]

There's a long list of Dysfunctional Toxins. The external Dysfunctional Toxins that we consume in our diet are: pesticides, chemicals, food preservatives, heavy metals, hazardous waste, hormones, antibiotics, various medications, and food and water contaminated by pathogens, such as parasites. Microbes—such as viruses and bacteria—which enter the blood stream are also Dysfunctional Toxins. There are many hidden Dysfunctional Toxins in plastics, etc. There are also the Dysfunctional Toxins we can smell such as household cleaning agents, second-hand smoke, colognes, candles, air pollution, etc. We believe many over-the-counter and prescription medications are Dysfunctional Toxins. In order to avoid being poisoned, your body stores both ingested and inhaled Dysfunctional Toxins in fat cells. Research has shown that people with bad lifestyles can hold upwards of 800 Dysfunctional Toxins in their fat cells![3]

In addition, there are internal Dysfunctional Toxins that are released inside of our body, such as excess pro-inflammatory cytokines, excess free radicals, excess white blood cells, excess cortisol, excess blood sugar, excess insulin, excess triglycerides, and excess LDL cholesterol. Tumors also fall into the category of internal Dysfunctional Toxins. Unmanaged stress, combined with obesity, is one of the most destructive Dysfunctional Toxins of all.

Functional Alert: The excess of external Dysfunctional Toxins usually leads to the development of internal Dysfunctional Toxins!

In order to be as healthy as possible, you want to be exposed to the least amount of Dysfunctional Toxins. In order to do this, you must follow a Functional Diet to the best of your ability. A good way to minimize Dysfunctional Toxins from being stored in body fat is to stay relatively lean through Functional Diet, Functional Training, Functional Cardio, and Functional Hormone Replacement.[4,5] Immune system dysfunction caused by the accumulation of Dysfunctional Toxins in fat cells greatly increases your odds of getting cancer, heart disease, diabetes, Alzheimer's, etc., but you have a choice in doing something about it by implementing **Functional Training with a Fork**!

There's still a lot that researchers don't understand about the immune system. What they do know is extremely technical. Therefore, we are going to explain how the immune system functions in an oversimplified manner. Your immune system is composed of functional cells, organs, tissues and proteins that defend your bodies against Dysfunctional Toxins.[6] Think of Dysfunctional Toxins as anything that tries to damage the cells, tissues, and organs that activate your immune system. Your immune system is multifunctional: There is an innate immune system and an adaptive immune system that work together as one when Dysfunctional Toxins (external and internal Dysfunctional Toxins) are detected.[7, 8] First the innate response kicks in; the more powerful adaptive response comes later. These two systems communicate with each other through vast numbers of chemical mediators that allow them to coordinate a given response.

Our collective research shows that stem-cell function plays a key role in how long you will live in good health. Hematopoietic stem cells located in your bone marrow are involved in the production of red blood cells (hemoglobin) and white blood cells (b-cells and killer t-cells).[9] Red blood cells carry oxygen to tissues through blood. Your blood also delivers white blood cells to repair your body's tissues. Your immune system weakens as you age and when it has to deal with excess amounts of Dysfunctional Toxins (both internal and external Dysfunctional Toxins). [10] This weakens the stem cells ability to produce healthy new red blood cells and white blood cells. Both red blood cells and white blood cells have short life spans and must be constantly restocked in order for you to survive! Unfortunately, science has yet to figure out a way to make your stem cells produce new, healthy red blood cells and white blood cells as you get older and/or are exposed to excess amounts of Dysfunctional Toxins. The best solution for counterbalancing the problem is Functional Hormone Replacement along with the rest of the principles found in **Functional Training with a Fork**. Using testosterone therapy maintains the production of healthy red blood cells and following every principle found in **Functional Training with a Fork** helps prevent the need for an oversupply of white blood cells. This lowers the production of pro-inflammatory cytokines and free radicals. The immune system remains more functional because the body's cells are able to exchange oxygen more efficiently!

Functional Alert: Once you have permanently damaged your body and continually need more white blood cells for damage control, there will be no way to get them after you get older. This means the time to change over to a functional lifestyle is now!

In order for your immune system to function properly, two things must happen: First, the cells, tissues, and organs must recognize that they have been invaded by Dysfunctional Toxins. Second, your immune response must be activated quickly before the Dysfunctional Toxins can contaminate other cells, tissues, and organs. Cytokines (both anti-inflammatory and pro-inflammatory) have a built-in radar that locates both internal and external Dysfunctional Toxins. When Dysfunctional Toxins are located, your b-cells are signaled by cytokines. If the Dysfunctional Toxins appear to be a serious threat, your body releases more pro-inflammatory cytokines than anti-inflammatory cytokines. This results in chronic inflammation, chronic oxidation, and the release of excessive amounts of white blood cells (b-cells and killer t-cells). Your b-cells confront Dysfunctional Toxins and remember them. B-cells also signal killer t-cells to come and destroy the Dysfunctional Toxins. As time progresses, the b-cells produce antibodies. These antibodies remain in your body and more easily recognize Dysfunctional Toxins, which helps prevent the contamination from occurring a second time. Unfortunately, as you age and/or are exposed to excess amounts of Dysfunctional Toxins, your immune system can become underactive. When Dysfunctional Toxins are not terminated by killer t-cells because the immune system is in a weakened state, Dysfunctional Toxins eventually leads to the destruction of your body.[12]

Functional Alert: Did you know that type-1 diabetes is caused when the immune system mistakenly attacks the cells of the pancreas, resulting in chronic inflammation and oxidation?[13] Did you know that rheumatoid arthritis is caused by the immune system mistakenly attacking the joints, resulting in chronic inflammation and oxidation?[14] Did you know that chronic inflammation, chronic oxidation, and plaque buildup in the arteries is decided by the immune system?[15] Did you know that most women out live males by approximately five years because their immune system ages more slowly?[16]

Chronic inflammation and oxidation go hand in hand. In fact, they feed off one another! Chronic inflammation is like a "fire" inside the body. Chronic inflammation occurs when there's an increase of pro-inflammatory cytokines (destructive cell-signaling chemicals) that contribute to the progression of all diseases. Excess pro-inflammatory cytokines cause problems for healthy cells and accelerate the aging process. Smoking, excess alcohol, pesticides/herbicides, food preservatives, obesity, and unmanaged stress from a lack of Functional Exercise, and sugar/insulin and hormonal imbalances cause some of the most extreme forms of chronic inflammation!

Oxidation is a chemical reaction combined with oxygen that also creates a "fire" inside the body.[17] Oxidation is a natural process that happens during normal cellular functions. The body metabolizes oxygen very efficiently, but approximately 2% of cells will become damaged during oxidation and turn into free radicals.[18] Free radicals are damaged cells that cause problems for other healthy cells.[19] Free radicals injure other cells and damage their DNA, which creates the foundation for all diseases. Excess free radicals accelerate the aging process. Smoking, excess alcohol, pesticides/herbicides, food preservatives, obesity, unmanaged stress from a lack of Functional Exercise, and sugar/insulin and hormonal imbalances cause some of the most extreme forms of free radical damage!

HOW THE IMMUNE SYSTEM FUNCTIONS

Functional Alert: When the fire from chronic inflammation and the fire from chronic oxidation feed off one another, they become a firestorm! Allow us to illustrate: A big, wild land fire creates its own tornado. This is a result of a large amount of rising heat and air that sucks more air into the fire, creating a rising tornado that builds on itself, getting bigger and stronger. It can jump around and change direction just like a regular storm tornado. This is what happens inside your body when a firestorm (such as cancer) is ignited! [20]

In a healthy, young person, short periods of acute inflammation and oxidation build up immunity and are essential for fighting off diseases.[21] However, as people age, they tend to have lengthy periods of chronic inflammation/oxidation and thus have a harder time fighting off diseases. Once your immune system begins to malfunction from lengthy periods of chronic inflammation and oxidation, a viscous cycle is set in place. Inflammation just feeds off itself, causing further inflammation and oxidation.

There are no diagnostic tests for much of the inflammation and oxidation going on inside your body. You can't depend solely on doctor visits for a clean bill of health. Sometimes doctors are right and sometimes they are wrong! You can't place all the blame on doctors when something goes wrong because some of the interactions going on inside your body can't be detected with x-rays, blood tests, urine tests, hair samples, etc. We refer to these interactions as tiny fires that can't be seen with modern diagnostic tests. For example, signs and symptoms of liver cancer often don't show up until the later stages of the disease, but once it turns into a big fire, it creates its own weather—a destructive tornado inside the human body!

Functional Alert: Pro-inflammatory cytokines cause inflammation and free radicals cause oxidation. Excess inflammation and oxidation lowers cellular oxygen levels!

The #2 killer in the U.S. is cancer.[22] Lowering your risk of developing cancer starts with you! One thing you can do is to not smoke or be around others who do. Carbon monoxide (a Dysfunctional Toxin) caused from smoking, sticks to hemoglobin and decreases the blood's ability to transport oxygen.[23] This depletes cells of oxygen and they can no longer function properly. Smoking is linked to all cancers, not just lung cancer! [24]

Functional Alert: Dr. Otto Warburg won a Nobel Prize for proving cancer is caused by a lack of oxygen respiration (the set of metabolic reactions and processes that take place in the body's cells). Warburg discovered that the respiratory enzymes in cells become damaged or die when cellular oxygen levels get too low. Chronic inflammation and oxidation within and around cells restrict oxygen exchange of the cells and cause dysfunction![25]

Once a cell's DNA is damaged from pro-inflammatory cytokines and free radicals, it becomes precancerous. The more pro-inflammatory cytokines and free radicals present, the more cancer causing damage occurs! A Functional Immune System usually destroys precancerous cells before they turn into a tumor. If you have a Dysfunctional Immune System, your body is less capable of destroying these precancerous cells. If a cancerous tumor is formed then you are fighting for your life!

Every year, there are roughly 2 million new cases of cancer and many will die.[26,27] The survival rate for cancer has improved a little over the past 30 years due to the technological advances in screening, chemotherapy, radiation, and surgery. The medical community is giving it their all, but they are still not winning the war. We don't believe the medical community has been very successful in treating people who are in the later stages of cancer by prescribing drugs that cost billions of dollars. The cancerous cells become more immune to chemotherapy treatments over time. In addition, the immune system becomes drained from trying to kill off the cancer cells and dealing with more chemotherapy. Ironically, this would mean that the #1 side effect of long-term chemotherapy is helping the cancer live because it weakens your immune functions![28] The immune system will be stronger when first beginning chemotherapy than after extended treatments. This means we have a much better chance that our immune system, combined with the chemotherapy, will kill off the cancer cells before they can feed and grow.

Functional Alert: We believe our exposure to Dysfunctional Toxins, the explosion of obesity, hormonal imbalances, and unmanaged chronic stress from a lack of Functional Training are going to continue increasing the rates of cancer if people don't act to improve the functionality of their immune systems. Preventing cancer with **Functional Training with a Fork** is much easier than trying to cure cancer once it occurs!

Ronnie: *I spent several years reading various studies on cancer to try to make sense of it all. What I learned from reading is that there are a lot of highly intelligent people out there trying to figure out how to cure cancer. I think the reason no one has yet to figure it out is because we all have different immune systems and our bodies react differently to internal and external Dysfunctional Toxins. If our obesity epidemic, sedentary lifestyles, and poor dietary habits are not reversed in America, cancer may one day rival heart disease. Most chronic inflammation and oxidation comes from* *what we consume in our food, being overweight, sugar and hormonal imbalances and unmanaged stress from a lack of Functional Exercise. Everyone is vulnerable to chronic inflammation and oxidation in today's highly toxic and highly stressed society. Inflammation and oxidation is a reaction of the body's tissues from being exposed to any form of Dysfunctional Toxins. Some people think that since Dysfunctional Toxins are in all food, they are destined to get cancer and just eat whatever. They are totally missing out on the big picture, which is combining "conventional medicine" (being screened by doctors and preventing cancer-causing infections through vaccinations) with "functional medicine" (following **Functional Training with a Fork**).*

When being screened by doctors, instead of placing all your emphasis on a complete blood count, have your doctor check for vitamin and mineral deficiencies. Also, have them check your urine and blood for the accumulation of Dysfunctional Toxins such as mercury, lead, arsenic, pesticides, etc. Blood and urine will indicate exposures that are chronic and recent.[29]

It's not uncommon for personal trainers to have sickly, overweight clients who blame their doctors for not stressing how important proper exercise, nutrition, and healthy hormones are for disease control. You must keep in mind that most doctors are only trained to try to figure out what is wrong with you and some of them are not in the best of shape themselves. They go mostly by what you say and then they write out prescriptions and/or run diagnostic tests. This is called conventional medicine. Doctors often have a very difficult time trying to differentiate between what is causing imbalances and what is causing dysfunctions within the body. This often leads to poor management and further deterioration of the disease until the patients take matters in their own hands and begin applying the principles in this book.

Doctors' job descriptions don't require them to write out proper exercise and diet plans. Time is money and even the doctors who know about these things don't have the time to teach each individual patient how to eat and exercise properly. Keep in mind that the multi-billion dollar pharmaceutical and health care industries make capital gains off of your illnesses—illnesses that can often be better managed by applying **Functional Training with a Fork!**

GMO and the Immune System

As the world population continues to grow, food production must also grow if America wants to remain the agriculture leader of the world. It's estimated that about 80% of processed food contain genetically modified organisms (GMOs) in one form or another.[1] These foods include high- fructose corn syrup, canola oil, soybean bean oil, soy flour, etc.[2] GMO foods were introduced so everything could be grown faster and larger in order to keep everyone around the world fed. We have some concerns about the new generation of GMO foods on the market, but it appears to be too late now—we have allowed large corporations and our government to become the functional equivalent of God on earth! One of the things that concerns us the most is that the people behind GMO foods are fighting against labeling food that contain GMOs. If they are safe, then why would they be against it? No one knows how harmful they may be, but what we can tell you is that farmers on certified organic farms are prohibited from feeding GMO crops to their animals. If it's not good enough for these animals, then it really makes you wonder if it's good for us! Organic farmers are also prohibited from producing GMO foods, so this tells us even more.[3,] In the United States, most food companies are not required to tell you which food is GMO.[4] It seems to us that we have the right to know what kinds of food we are eating.

Functional Alert: We must never allow ourselves to confuse objective information with marketing efforts from large organizations. Our opinion is that some of the studies being performed by large corporations stop before problems with a product can occur, which is an advanced form of deception and half-truths by omission!

Unfortunately, it looks as if the conventional food we and our kids eat are never going to be normal. More pesticides and herbicides are being used now than ever before because bugs and weeds are becoming immune to the chemicals.[5] It's something we all need to face because looking the other way won't make this particular problem go away. We are of the opinion that our food industry deserves our suspicion until it decides to label food containing GMO and do away with all growth hormones; excess preservatives, refined sugar, salt, antibiotics, herbicides, pesticides, and heavy metals; and stop selling food that come from highly toxic countries such as China that lack regulation of food products![6] In order to get things changed, we need to find out who's allowing these things to happen and demand change in a peaceful manner! America is self-destructing by conforming to standards of behavior based on misguided principles. The causes of America's dysfunction are not a mystery. What is the remedy? Everyone needs to begin taking personal responsibility and accountability for their actions. Until this occurs, we can forget change in America!

Functional Alert: A lot of people ask, I wonder what's causing all these bizarre diseases if it's not genetics, obesity, and unmanaged stress? Our answer, Dysfunctional Toxins in our food supply are largely to blame! Take a look at the alarming number of deformities in sea creatures from the BP oil spill and it's easy to see that Dysfunctional Toxins are the blame for a large spectrum of diseases in both wildlife and humans![7]

All grass-fed livestock produces leaner beef void of GMO corn. Conventional grain-fed livestock produces meat that is lower in omega-3s and contains GMO corn.[8] GMO corn is the main ingredient in animal feed.[9, 10] We are convinced that the GMO diet fed to livestock is affecting not only their health (e.g., bloating, stomach ulcers, diarrhea, organ failure, reproductive disorder, etc.) but ours as well! [11-15] Most cows are fed grain composed of GMO corn; therefore, their meat contains GMO corn. We eat their meat, and the GMOs accumulate in our bodies.

Functional Alert: When GMO food is fed to livestock (e.g., pigs) it leads to dysfunction of their GI tract. This causes them to get sick more often and have to take more antibiotics.[16] The GMO and extra antibiotics they are given are passed on from livestock to humans.[17] This is very scary because the human digestive tract is very similar to animals such as pigs![18]

Many hidden ingredients in processed food are being made out of GMO corn (e.g., fructose corn syrup is used in just about everything).[19] Many Americans are clueless that their diets are high in GMO corn, which is contained in various food products. GMO shows up in our bodies in ways we could not even imagine. For instance, tests on human hair samples have shown a high concentration of GMO corn. Unfortunately, most Americans now have a larger percentage of carbon (our second-most abundant element) composed of GMOs in their bodies from eating hidden sources of GMO corn.[20, 21]

One of our concerns about GMO food is a built-in pesticide called Bt-toxin.[22] This gene is produced from Bacillus thuringiensis bacteria and is being added to most corn crops. Monsanto, a large agricultural company, has taken over a large portion of the farming industry.[23] There are plenty of farmers who are against Monsanto, but are being forced to use their products.[24, 25] Their products include Roundup Ready® seeds that contain Bt-toxins (built-in pesticides). In addition, these seeds are specifically altered to resist large amounts of Roundup®, an herbicide farmers use to kill weeds.[26] Guess who makes Roundup® for the farmer's crops? If you guessed Monsanto, you would be correct! [27]

Let us explain: The presence of weeds and pests leads to a measurable reduction in the average yield of crops. These Roundup Ready® seeds grow into plant-based food that can withstand massive amounts of the weed killer Roundup® and invading pests. Unfortunately, this means farmers can spray the living daylights out of their crops to keep the weeds from taking over while the built-in pesticides take care of the pests. Now, guess who consumes these Dysfunctional Toxins? We do!

Bt-toxins kill pests by causing holes to develop in their stomachs after they nibble on plant-based food. If they're putting holes in pests' stomachs, we can only imagine what they're doing to ours. Keep in mind, our stomachs are 75% of our immune system! We and others believe that the Bt-toxins alone cause irritable bowel syndrome from chronic inflammation and oxidation of the GI tract, along with many other diseases stemming from a Dysfunctional Immune System.[28-37]

Our organic farmlands are gradually being contaminated by GMO pollen.[38] Insects and winds often carry GMO pollen to other areas.[39] The pollen lands on organic crops and contaminates them by changing their DNA to GMO.[40] Then the organic farmers can be forced to buy GMO seeds and change over to conventional farming![41]

A recent study entitled "Pesticides in Mississippi air and rain: A comparison between 1995 and 2007," reveals that glyphosate (the main ingredient contained in Roundup®) was found in more than 75% of the air and rain samples tested from Mississippi in 2007 during growing season.[42] In other words, we are breathing Roundup®, drinking Roundup®, and eating Roundup®!

Functional Alert: A new study links GMOs to causing gluten intolerance! [43] Food allergies are also on the rise in the United States!

Europe and more than 60 other countries have set forth regulations against various GMO foods because of their potential dangers.[44, 45] We would like to point out that many studies are available about the potential dangers of GMO food and you can find them on the Internet. Thanks to the Internet and independent scientists, the public is gradually learning about the ability of glyphosate to cause birth defects as well as dysfunction of all major organs in the body.[46,47] We are of the opinion that the consumption of Roundup® in GMO food is causing devastating health problems for all age groups. The health problems could be immediate as well as long-term. Since no one can discredit the scientific studies that show Roundup® is harmful, we believe everyone needs to do their best to avoid these particular Dysfunctional Toxins as much as possible!

Functional Alert: The majority of the United States citizens that we have come in contact with believe it's time our country started looking out for its own citizens. We don't believe for one minute that the farming industry can't grow enough non-GMO food in the United States to keep its citizens and animals fed. Just think about all the food that is wasted daily in homes, restaurants, delis, etc. If we put an end to that, we wouldn't have to produce as much food!

A huge problem we as Americans face is special interest groups.[48, 49] We certainly can't place all the blame on them, but they are constantly lobbying Congress to void and/or modify its FDA/EPA rulings and guidelines to meet the needs of big business. Could it be that the FDA and USDA are run by the very people who used to work for these same food companies profiting from our food supply? As usual, most things have a way of getting back to money! The food industry, like the government, has lost a lot of its credibility with the American public. Government officials need to stop taking lobbyist money and do what is right, but it doesn't look like that's going to happen. We need to have as many Dysfunctional Toxins as possible removed from our food. We are not saying to get rid of the FDA, but rather make the agency more responsible for protecting our health.

The amount of money currently flowing into the system in the form of political contributions is playing the largest role in who gets what within the economy. The lobbyists always want something in return, such as financial support, tax changes, changes in regulations, etc. As a result, the people giving the money to the government officials and the government officials themselves get benefits from what happens to their stocks and campaign funds. The rest of Americans suffer because the deals being made behind closed doors hurt the health of the overall economy. The end result is multitudes of people without enough money to buy the healthiest food, lacking sufficient regulations on the safety of our food supply, and paying increased health care costs!

The majority of people living in the United States believe in a set of principles rooted in the ideas of fairness. Everyone in America should be proud to be living in the greatest country on earth. However, everyone reading this book, regardless of their political affiliation, wants major policies to be fixed that aren't being fixed. If we as a society don't work together and protect our great nation's food and water supply, it won't always be "the land of the free and the home of the brave." It will turn into the land of the dependent and home of the sick! Things would be so much better if politicians would actually work together and follow up on their promises. We've entrusted the government with too many of our services and we're beginning to pay for it as a nation (e.g., increased health and financial problems). We believe the solution to getting things back on track in the future begins with making politicians aware of our concerns. Politicians want to make us happy so we will elect them. If they're not willing to keep our food safe, we should send a strong signal that we're not going to elect or re-elect them. We have a choice to turn our backs on the politicians who have turned their backs on our and their own families' health.

Hormones, Antibiotics, and the Immune System

We believe children are reaching puberty earlier these days because of the hormones and other Dysfunctional Toxins, such as pesticides/herbicides, in our food supply. Hormones trick the body into thinking it's older than it actually is and Dysfunctional Toxins act as estrogens and endocrine disruptors inside the body.[1-4] We think obesity plays a role as well, but a lot of thin kids are hitting puberty early, which is a sign that obesity isn't the only culprit.

Certified organically grown meats, eggs, and dairy are prohibited from using hormones and antibiotics.[5] We don't think it's necessary to give animals all these hormones for weight gain and milk production when a better option is available. You can make animals gain weight using the same methods that cause people to put on pounds. Eating larger, more infrequent, meals throughout the day instead of several smaller ones causes weight gain. When hormone-free animals are allowed to eat smaller meals throughout the day, they will usually eat less. With a means to self-feed or always have food, the animals are never going to let themselves get real hungry. Therefore, they won't eat enough calories in one sitting to stretch out their stomachs, which would allow them to eat more food and gain more weight. As the animals gain weight, their hunger hormones change, which allows them to gain even more weight. If you hand-feed animals or give them access to food only three times a day, they will get very hungry before the next meal comes around and gorge, just as humans do. Think of going to a buffet and trying to get your money's worth!

Since the use of antibiotics and hormones in most farm animals may be here to stay, we would like to encourage the FDA to pass a law stating that conventional farmers who treat their animals with antibiotics and/or hormones must not sell any animals, eggs, or milk until the particular drug used has been flushed from the animals' systems. For example, separate the chickens and allow enough time for a particular antibiotic to leave their systems before going to market. Many people can't afford to eat organic foods, so we believe the right thing for the FDA to do is to put reasonable restrictions on conventional farmers. With today's advanced technology, no one should have to consume meat, eggs, and dairy that contains antibiotic or hormone residues! Unfortunately, 80% of antibiotics made in the U.S. are used on farm animals.[6] Long-term exposure to antibiotics weakens the immune system by decreasing good bacteria in the gut.[7] This is something everyone needs to be concerned about if they want to keep their immune systems functioning properly. The conventional food industry, as it stands now, is actually costing us more in the long run when you add up the cost of our health and environment. We hope the industry will begin to understand this and make some needed changes.

People need to shop smart when buying meat. We believe the most important meat to buy organic is chicken. Eating meat free of antibiotics and hormones will dramatically decrease your exposure to these Dysfunctional Toxins. We also encourage people to stay away from all forms of processed meats (e.g., most deli meats, bacon, and hot dog wieners that usually contain sodium nitrite, etc.) and farm-raised fish that contain antibiotics.[8] Eat only wild-caught fish on the bottom of the food chain, which contain no antibiotics and fewer quantities of Dysfunctional Toxins such as PCBs and mercury. Also, avoid fried fish, frozen fish sticks, and breaded fish.

Many people simply don't take enough time these days to shop smart! They are overbooked, overworked, stuck in traffic, etc. The U.S. is in desperate need of developing various fast-food chains that serve food lower in calories on the higher end of the Functional Food Spectrum as opposed to fried food on the lower end. Furthermore, it would be much more convenient if grocery stores had built-in farmers' markets that sold affordable products because everyone likes to buy local. This would greatly help the masses of people who have to eat on the run in today's busy society. Grocery stores and fast-food chains are in business to sell what the consumers want. If more Americans would let it be known they wanted to purchase organic, more farms will invest in organic farming and organic food would become more available and less expensive. As for now, we look to local farmers' markets for some of our produce, and we buy organic meats and both organic and conventionally grown produce at the grocery store. We also avoid restaurants because of the health risk, low nutritional value, and high-calorie content.[9]

Pesticides, Fertilizers, and the Immune System

More than 2,000 years ago, all the food that God provided for us to eat was clean. Today, that rule doesn't apply because we live in a polluted environment. The contamination of our food supply in America is a clear and present danger. Dysfunctional Toxins cause birth defects, illness, and death to all living creatures.

One of the best ways to make money farming produce is from a tree. We live in the South where conventional peach orchards are abundant. (Growing organic peaches in South Carolina where we live is very difficult due to higher humidity and more insects.) Farmers say they do their best to limit the amount of high-risk synthetic pesticides they apply. You might ask, How toxic are these pesticides to the immune system? Let's put it to you this way: We have been told they can strip the paint right off tractors! We have also been told by several people that their horses will stand up on their hind legs and bolt when they get a whiff of the high-risk pesticides being sprayed.

Functional Alert: High-risk pesticides used on conventional crops are more effective at killing crop invaders and they are more effective at killing you!

Organic farmers use more natural pesticides and conventional farmers use more synthetic pesticides.[1-2] We consider all pesticides, whether natural or synthetic to be Dysfunctional Toxins. Both versions get embedded into our food supply and can't be completely washed off.[3,4] Pesticide residue gets washed into local streams, poisoning wildlife and aquatic plants (which help keep the air clean).[5] It also ends up in our drinking water.[6] Pesticides have been found in drinking water sources at concentrations of potential concern to our health.[7] Make no mistake—it doesn't matter whether these pesticides are from natural plant-derived matter or from synthetic material, they are absorbed the same way when you eat them and can have a negative impact on the function of your immune system!

The term "organic" doesn't mean chemical- or synthetic-free as many have been led to believe. It simply means organic farmers are required to use natural pesticides and lower-risk synthetic pesticides.[8] Even though we believe organic is significantly safer, don't let the term "natural" fool you! Just because a pesticide is called natural doesn't mean it's safe. Organic farmers use chemicals that are derived from botanical and mineral-bearing sources.[9,10] There are a lot of Dysfunctional Toxins in natural things that can kill you. For example, fungi, bacteria, arsenic, cyanide, etc., are all naturally plant derived, but they are still toxic.[11]

Functional Alert: A certain percentage of Dysfunctional Toxins are here to stay. Instead of worrying about things we have very little control over, we must start worrying about the things we can control. We can apply **Functional Training with a Fork** to actually do something to help purge our bodies of these Dysfunctional Toxins!

If the same amount of pesticides are used repeatedly, an even greater proportion of pests survive the following year because their parents built up a resistance that they passed along to their offspring.[12] No one knows the full long-term effects with either form of pesticide application, but we believe there is enough evidence to prove that the pesticides used by organic farmers are much safer for consumption than those used by conventional farmers. For example, studies have shown much lower urinary pesticide levels among people consuming organic versus conventional food.[13] This means fewer pesticides are left on organic food during consumption, even though it usually takes more applications of the natural pesticides to do the job because they are weaker.

Functional Alert: Anything that can kill bugs and weeds can eventually kill humans if allowed to accumulate inside the body! The good news is your body becomes more efficient at eliminating all external Dysfunctional Toxins when following the principles found in **Functional Training with a Fork**. This is because your body-fat levels will be lower; you'll be eating more soluble fiber/prebiotics and probiotics; your immune system, circulatory system, and lymph system will be running smoother; and your metabolism will be revved up due to having more muscle tone, increased testosterone, and balanced sugar/insulin levels!

If the organic food (produce and meats) are coming from countries outside the U.S. (e.g., China), we believe most of it is contaminated and contains a lot more high-risk pesticides than conventionally grown produce in America.[14] Let's face it: China has turned into an environmental nightmare! Runoff from pesticides, fertilizers, and air pollution contaminates both land and water for the people who grow produce, causing immediate as well as long-term health problems. These Dysfunctional Toxins wipe out many species of plants and animals, not just insects! We can only imagine how contaminated the water is that is being used on both organic crops and conventional crops outside the U.S. Many foreign countries are motivated by high profits, and Dysfunctional Toxins are not as strictly regulated. Another concern is the partnerships we have with some of these other countries. Can we be assured that the FDA is really testing all the food coming from foreign countries such as China where there is already less regulation on Dysfunctional Toxins? We believe the answer is no! In fact, the FDA samples less than 1% of all regulated food products.[15] Is this leading to more Dysfunctional Toxins being shipped to America? We believe the answer is absolutely!

Functional Alert: It's foolish to consume anything coming out of China. The package might say "Pacific Salmon" in big print, but look for the small print on the bottom of every product you buy. If the label says "Made in China" or "PRC" (Hong Kong), choose a different product!

Eighty percent of seafood in America is imported.[16] There are approximately 4.5 million fish farms in China.[17] The fish are raised in contaminated ponds and fed raw sewage. Then they are shipped to America![18] Did you know that China is the largest producer of seafood in the world?[19] Did you know that 80% of America's tilapia comes from China?[20] Did you know that catfish shipped from China is one of America's top 10 most-consumed fish?[21] It's very disturbing that the FDA only has the ability to inspect approximately 1% of the fish and shrimp at the border coming from China and only 0.2% is tested in a lab.[22] It's even more disturbing that more than 60% of the 1% gets rejected![23,24] Unfortunately, the FDA doesn't have the authority to seize the fish and shrimp. If it gets rejected at one port they travel to other ports and sometimes find one that allows the contaminated species to enter the food markets in America.[25] We often wonder how much of the food being served in America's restaurants is coming from China? The U.S. requires labels on fish and seafood to mark their place of origin. However, it's extremely rare for restaurants to provide information on their menus regarding where their food comes from. That alone should be enough to keep you out of restaurants so you can lose weight and avoid some major causes of dysfunction and disease!

Functional Alert: Companies are not required to label where ingredients in most food come from, only where the food is processed.[26, 27] This means you are unknowingly consuming a lot of food ingredients made in China!

Air pollution in China and Mexico has become a huge health threat.[28] The pollution in China and Mexico is no longer just their problem; it's also ours! "What goes up must come down!" China and Mexico have some of the world's most polluted air, and it's absorbed by clouds before they leave those countries. The Dysfunctional Toxins contained within rain lands directly into the Pacific Ocean, polluting the fish we consume with heavy metals and other Dysfunctional Toxins. Moreover, as the polluted air from Mexico, and particularly China, enters California from the Pacific Ocean, it accumulates on the western end of the U.S. In other words, Californians, in particular, are breathing second-hand smoke from Mexico and China.[29] The remaining 49 states are also being affected by this air pollution because more than 50% of the United States' fruits, vegetables, and nuts are produced in the state of California.[30] The state is also our #1 dairy-producer![31] We believe the production of organic food in any contaminated environment still produces food containing a lot of harmful Dysfunctional Toxins. Air pollution is causing many deaths in the U.S. and has now become the single largest environmental health risk![32] There are Dysfunctional Toxins in air pollution that significantly aggravate allergies and asthma.[33] Nowadays when people go outside, the air often smells like the noxious fumes of a chemical plant or carbon monoxide from heavy traffic, even if they aren't in close proximity to either a plant or a highway. We believe the super-toxic air pollution entering the United States is one of the reasons inhaled allergies and food allergies are on the rise! [34]

Functional Alert: The extraordinary growth of trade between China and the U.S. and Mexico and the U.S. has had a negative impact on the U.S. economy due to job losses. Ironically, outsourcing jobs is still having a negative impact on the purity of the water, air, soil, and produce coming out of California, etc. The U.S. loses on both accounts!

We recommend buying locally grown fruits, vegetables, and meats when they are available because they reach the shelves faster and it helps support the local farmers. Get to know your source! Some people have turned into vegetarians and stopped eating meat, thinking that it would get them away from most Dysfunctional Toxins, but they were wrong! Most farmers don't like having to use Dysfunctional Toxins, but in order to stay in business, they have no choice. Neither farmers nor the FDA can tell you much about the countless numbers of harmful Dysfunctional Toxins being sprayed on crops every spring and summer. It's as much a mystery to them as the general public. Our opinion is that you can only tamper with Mother Nature so much before she becomes angry. We feel that there are safer paths conventional farmers could be taking, and the large food companies need to start doing everything in their power to help support them and to help our population become healthier, even if it means losing a few profits.

The accumulation of external Dysfunctional Toxins is difficult to monitor even though some have been directly linked to various medical conditions. For example, tobacco was on the market for decades before the link to COPD, cancer, heart disease, strokes, diabetes, sexual dysfunction, organ dysfunction, and Alzheimer's was confirmed! It wasn't very long ago that we learned second-hand smoke was also a killer. Right now, no one knows with certainty which external Dysfunctional Toxins are causing the most deaths.

Functional Alert: The America public should be outraged about how much cigarettes alone have caused the cost of healthcare to rise. According to an extensive report on smoking and health from the Department of Health and Human Services, the economic toll exceeds $157 billion each year in the United States.[35]

The best thing we can do now is take a rational look at fixing the problems we can control because at this point, it doesn't look as if America can ever go back to the days where food, water, and air didn't contain all these Dysfunctional Toxins. Avoiding all Dysfunctional Toxins isn't realistic for today. Our best option at this point is to avoid as many Dysfunctional Toxins as possible and purge the ones that are building up in our bodies. This can be accomplished by applying **Functional Training with a Fork**!

Any type of vegetable with roots, such as potatoes, celery, and carrots, will contain more pesticides (both natural and high-risk pesticides). This is because pesticides get absorbed into the roots and become more concentrated inside the vegetable.[36, 37] This makes French fries cooked in smoking, oxidized oil a deadly combination! Likewise, apples, grapes, blueberries, strawberries, peaches, cherries, and lettuce have soft skins that absorb more natural and high-risk pesticides.[38] In order to ingest fewer higher-risk synthetic pesticides, you should buy organic versions of these foods!

Functional Alert: The consumption of high-risk pesticides cause the body to produce excess amounts of pro-inflammatory cytokines and free radicals![39]

You will need to do your own research as time progresses and make personal decisions on whether or not a particular organic product is worth spending the extra cash. You parents out there shouldn't feel guilty about buying non-organic fruits and vegetables if you can't afford organic. The most important thing is to feed your kids fruits and vegetables instead of processed junk food. In addition, wash the produce vigorously with water. Unfortunately, washing the produce won't remove all pesticides from the skin, nor will peeling fruits and vegetables protect you from pesticides spread throughout its tissues.[40, 41] In the end, you are destined to consume some pesticide residue whether you go with organic or conventionally grown so be prepared to use **Functional Training with a Fork** to purge these Dysfunctional Toxins from your body!

Functional Alert: A healthy choice is not just whether it's organic or conventional. Your family needs to be eating some fruit and vegetables, healthy fats, plenty of non-starchy vegetables (Free Food), probiotics, and adequate amounts of lean protein!

Organic farmers use cow manure as a natural fertilizer and this is a good thing because it reduces heavy metal content in food and replenishes minerals in the soil.[42, 43] Doctor's Data Analytical Laboratories found higher amounts of heavy metals, such as lead and mercury, in food grown with synthetics compared to organic products.[44] The dumping of synthetic fertilizers partially composed of sewage sludge or biosolids on organic farmland is prohibited in the U.S., but it's allowed with conventional farming. This alone makes organic food more appealing! The best way to avoid produce grown in sewage sludge is to buy organic food. If you grow your own, avoid any fertilizer that says it contains biosolids. It's gross to think that all the things going down our toilets and drains in homes, hospitals, and industries are being indirectly dumped onto conventional farmland by way of synthetic fertilizers. It's estimated that sludge contains more than 60,000 Dysfunctional Toxins! [45-59]

The sludge is treated and turned into biosolids or fertilizer before being administered to the soil, but conventional methods are not able to eliminate all the Dysfunctional Toxins. The use of sludge as a fertilizer is being promoted by some as a good disposal option because incinerating it causes air pollution. On the other hand, some are labeling sludge as ground pollution!

Functional Alert: Bill Boyce won a $550,000 court judgment against Augusta Georgia on his claim that Dysfunctional Toxins in sludge caused more than 300 of his cows to die![60]

Conventional farmers use synthetic fertilizers and organic farmers don't. [61, 62] Heavy metals in synthetic fertilizers get absorbed into plant-based food.[63] When you consume the plant-based food your body produces more pro-inflammatory cytokines and free radicals.[64]

Dysfunctional Toxins from food is linked to organ damage. For instance, the epidemic of diabetes is related to diet and obesity and it can be accelerated by heavy metals. Type-1 diabetes is a result of the immune system destroying the cells of the pancreas responsible for producing insulin. Why are both type-1 and type-2 diabetes on the rise? Obesity and consuming too many carbs and fats are mostly to blame. However, Dysfunctional Toxins such as mercury are also to blame because once they accumulate in the body, they cause the immune system to attack the pancreas! Therefore, when Dysfunctional Toxins such as mercury are stored in the body, the internal organs often become dysfunctional.

There is a study showing that type-2 diabetics (people who generally have big bellies and less muscle tone) have a higher concentration of the heavy metal mercury in their bodies. Researchers have discovered that having high levels of heavy metals, such as mercury, in our bodies has an accumulative effect on our risk for developing life-threatening diseases. In 1987, researchers tested the toenail clippings of 3,875 diabetes-free adults. By 2005, 288 people in the study were diagnosed with diabetes. It's no surprise to us that those with the highest mercury levels in their toenails were 65% more likely to develop diabetes than those with the lowest levels. This correlates with other laboratory studies we have read that suggest that mercury is toxic to the insulin-producing beta cells in the pancreas.[65]

We believe a lot of people have health problems that are being caused or accelerated by Dysfunctional Toxins. Doctors simply don't know enough about preventing most diseases because they can't control the Dysfunctional Toxins in our food supply. Doctors can diagnose many health problems, but they can't always pinpoint the causes; for example, an escalating number of children are being born with ADHD and autism due to having low levels of oxygen in their cells from exposure to Dysfunctional Toxins while in their mother's womb and/or complications during birth, but no one can prove which Dysfunctional Toxin or combination thereof is the cause because everyone has a different immune system.[66, 67] For example, smoking cigarettes causes greater damage to some people than others, but it eventually damages everyone. Some may get COPD, some may get lung cancer, and some may get heart disease. Others may get all three!

Functional Alert: It's of the utmost importance for pregnant females to keep as many Dysfunctional Toxins from reaching the fetus as possible. This is best accomplished by consuming food on the higher end of the Functional Food Spectrum, keeping a little muscle tone, performing a little low-intensity cardio, not allowing body-fat levels to skyrocket, staying away from all medications and drugs, and staying well hydrated. They need to get plenty of sleep and take a multivitamin and mineral supplement. In addition, they should always check with their doctors before starting an exercise program and diet and before taking dietary supplements!

Body-Fat Levels and the Immune System

Dysfunctional Toxins get stored in body fat. Keeping body-fat levels in the lower ranges will help prevent the accumulation of Dysfunctional Toxins because there will be less space in fat cells in which they can take refuge.[1] If fat cells become enlarged, more Dysfunctional Toxins can be stored. This disrupts the body's immune system and decreases the production of key fat-burning and muscle-building hormones, such as t3/t4, testosterone, and growth hormone.[2-5] Moreover, excess body fat lowers mood and sexual-enhancing hormones, such as testosterone, dopamine, and serotonin.[6-8] When Dysfunctional Toxins are stored in body fat, they also increase fat-storage hormones, such as insulin[9], leptin[10], cortisol[11], and estrogen.[12] As you can see, obesity causes your hormones to become out of balance, setting you up for future weight gain and an array of health problems.[13] When you lose body fat (decrease the size of your fat cells), Dysfunctional Toxins are released into the bloodstream and the body disposes of them. Once you get rid of Dysfunctional Toxins, your metabolism increases!

Functional Alert: Body fat functions like an organ and releases pro-inflammatory cytokines, free radicals, and white blood cells.[14-16] The larger your fat cells become, the more of these it releases![17]

Anti-inflammatory cytokines and white blood cells are discharged by your immune cells to manage excess amounts of pro-inflammatory cytokines and excess free radicals caused by obesity.[18] This scenario gets much worse when your body is also dealing with external Dysfunctional Toxins entering your GI tract, accumulating in your fat cells, or being discharged from fat cells. Sometimes, this discharge of inflammatory mediators (anti-inflammatory cytokines, pro-inflammatory cytokines, and free radicals) is kept in check by the immune system. However, other times the reaction becomes uncontrollable because too many white cells are activated in one area. This results in the release of excess amounts of pro-inflammatory cytokines and free radicals that damage various cells, tissues, and organs.[19-21]

Our definition of a Dysfunctional Toxin Firestorm is a lethal immune system reaction consisting of pro-inflammatory cytokines and free radicals stimulating the release of white blood cells, and white blood cells further stimulating pro-inflammatory cytokines and free radicals, and so on. The cycle continues causing excessive amounts of pro-inflammatory cytokines, free radicals, and white blood cells to be released, resulting in chronic inflammation and oxidation. This results in lower cellular oxygenation and a Dysfunctional Immune System.

Obesity often causes a Dysfunctional Toxin Firestorm. [22, 23] The primary symptoms are swelling and fatigue. In some instances, the immune system malfunctions to the point of causing death. The liver is no longer able to do its job, the kidneys begin to fail, and the lungs start filling with fluid. The heart will slow down because of increased pressure from fluid in the lungs. The brain will realize that the other organs have shut down and will stop sending messages to the heart to continue beating. In some cases, the weakened response from the immune system allows a Dysfunctional Toxin, such as a virus, to cause cancer.

Functional Alert: Obese people who are under repeated stress release increasing amounts of pro-inflammatory cytokines, free radicals, and white blood cells. People who aren't obese also experience this problem, but to a much-lesser degree![24] The good news is that even moderate body-fat loss can cause a significant reduction in pro-inflammatory cytokines, free radicals, and white blood cells. This results in increased cellular oxygenation and a better-functioning immune system!

Dysfunction Junction

Dysfunction junction occurs when body fat disrupts the function of the organs, arteries, lymphatic vessels, and immune system. Subcutaneous fat (fat lying just beneath the skin) can negatively affect one's overall appearance and increases pro-inflammatory cytokines and free radicals. Have you noticed that when you gain weight in your stomach, your intestines have more trouble digesting your food? This is a result of accumulating more visceral fat when you gain more subcutaneous fat.

Visceral fat (fat lying deep inside the body), squeezes on your organs like a boa constrictor. It also compresses blood vessels, which constricts the flow of oxygenated blood throughout the entire body and causes an increase in blood pressure.[1] This is one of the primary reasons you get out of breath more easily and can't think as clearly when you have a bulging belly! Not only does visceral fat squeeze on organs compressing blood vessels and slowing down blood flow, it also constricts lymph vessels, which slows down the flow of lymph fluid throughout the entire body.[2] Consequently, as Dysfunctional Toxins accumulate, cells are unable to function properly, resulting in various metabolic and medical problems.

Functional Alert: Your blood pressure lowers when you lose body fat!

Increased fat around your mid-section is linked to having more health problems than if the fat gets stored elsewhere, because it intersects with many major organs, blood vessels, and lymphatic vessels. Central obesity increases the risk of clots in the arteries.[3] It also increases leaks and ruptures in blood vessels and lymphatic vessels. Visceral fat causes the body to release more pro-inflammatory cytokines and free radicals that damage the inner lining of the arteries, etc.[4] Functional Diet, Functional Training, Functional Cardio, and Functional Hormone Replacement are effective at eliminating both visceral fat and subcutaneous fat.[5-9]

Obesity (coming from subcutaneous and visceral fat) creates an oxygen deficiency in our cells.[10, 11] The water in our cells is capable of holding a lot of oxygen. When these cells become chronically inflamed from obesity they are only capable of holding a little water, which lowers our oxygen and changes the structure of the cells. When this occurs, our once-dominant aerobic metabolism is overpowered by our anaerobic metabolism and our immune system begins to malfunction.[12] This allows bacteria and viruses to flourish, which can cause numerous types of cancer, etc.[13]

Consuming excess calories generates chronic inflammation and oxidation in the form of excess pro-inflammatory cytokines and free radicals.[14] Many studies have shown this promotes the growth of cancer cells.[15] This is why not allowing yourself to become overweight is one of the most important things you can do to increase your life-span!

Functional Alert: Body weight can be deceptive because it doesn't indicate how much is from muscle and how much is from fat. There's no accurate standard for ideal body fat regardless of age, sex, and genetics. However, excess fat in the abdominal area is the most dangerous. We don't believe bioelectrical impedance devices such as body-fat scales and hand held devices are accurate. In fact, we believe they underestimate body fat in people with high body-fat levels and overestimate it in people who are lean. We believe they also overestimate body-fat levels in older people who lift weights, take testosterone, and have a lot of muscle tone. We also believe bioelectrical impedance devices underestimate body-fat levels in older people who are lacking muscle tone. As you get older, it's perfectly normal not to be able to eat as much food without gaining body fat as you did when you were younger. You don't want to go overboard with body-fat loss for your genetics or you'll lose your sex drive and not have any energy. Some people can become anemic or chronically cold from a lack of body fat needed for insulation!

When our cells become chronically inflamed from obesity and/or Dysfunctional Toxin overload, our bodies will pull vital minerals, such as calcium, from organs, bones, and fat cells and shuttle them into the bloodstream to help neutralize the chronic inflammation and oxidation.[16] If the bloodstream remains chronically inflamed, your arteries and organs will gradually become impaired.[17] The body will try to counteract the inflammation and oxidation by latching onto calcium, which it will place on the walls of the arteries, causing a calcium deposit. The calcium deposits provide a double whammy by working as a team along with plaque buildup to scar the inside of your arteries![18] Eventually, there will not be enough space left for the blood to flow through the arteries, which lowers oxygen even more, causing a stroke or heart attack. If part of the scar breaks lose, it can cause pulmonary embolism and an even more severe stroke or heart attack than a blockage alone.[19]

Obese people who eat on the higher end of the Functional Food Spectrum will have fewer Dysfunctional Toxins stored in their fat cells than obese people who eat at the lower end of the Spectrum. This same rule applies to thin people. In addition, you can also be skinny, but still be considered clinically obese if you have a poor lean muscle mass-to-fat ratio.[20] In other words, you are skinny fat! A marathon runner who has an abundance of type-1 muscle fibers is a prime example. Some of them run in excess, which causes them to lose what few type-2 muscle fibers they have.[21] They end up with poor muscle tone, which decreases hydration and increases the buildup of Dysfunctional Toxins. If you are considered clinically obese and are eating food on the lower end of the Functional Food Spectrum, you are like a walking toxic factory, full of inflammation/oxidation and ready to explode! Your immune system becomes like a battery that is slowly losing its charge. Having a Functional Immune System is a must if you want to live a healthy, long life.

Some people are naturally lucky and have a fast metabolism. They eat as if their stomachs were bottomless pits, but never gain weight. On the other hand, they are unlucky in the sense that they have no gauge to let them know that their bodies are becoming chronically inflamed and oxidized on the inside because they are eating food on the lower end of the Functional Food Spectrum. This same rule applies to those who can eat a lot of food on the lower end of the Functional Food Spectrum and not gain weight because they burn off a lot of calories performing excess amounts of cardio; for example, marathon runners. They may think they are getting by because their waistlines are staying small, but, on the inside, their bodies are staying inflamed and oxidized. Using dangerous drugs, such as cigarettes and diet pills, to stay thinner further compounds the inflammation and oxidation.

Functional Alert: Regardless of your metabolism or age, no one can escape the harmful effects of a Dysfunctional Diet. Heart surgeons commonly run into trouble with plaque buildup in thin people. In addition, pointing the finger at body fat as the sole contributor to contracting type-2 diabetes is misleading. Thin people also get cancer and autoimmune diseases!

Yo-Yo Dieting and the Immune System

Yo-yo dieting is worse for your immune system and overall health than staying obese! People who never learn to change their behavior usually fall into the trap of yo-yo dieting. We have seen people who do great on a weight-loss diet for a little while, but eventually they go back to their old ways of eating. The problem is that they never learned the skills needed for long-term behavioral changes—skills that are required for a Functional Diet. Out of desperation, they usually go on some form of crash diet that is too restrictive in calories to be maintained long-term. Looking for rapid body-fat loss is a sure sign they have never learned to motivate themselves every day to eat sensibly. In addition, it shows they have yet to learn how to control perceived stress and negative emotions and recognize that when they make a mistake, it's time to move on and do better the next time.

One of the most devastating effects of yo-yo dieting can be seen in the immune system. It depletes white blood cells that fight off infections and prevent cancer.[1,2] Why does this occur? When you begin losing body fat (shrinking fat cells), the Dysfunctional Toxins stored in your fat cells are released back into the bloodstream and have to be eliminated, causing the immune system to work overtime.[3] That is a side effect of losing body fat!

When you first begin losing body fat, it's not uncommon to experience headaches, acne, fatigue, bad breath, stinky sweat, and irritable bowel syndrome. Once these Dysfunctional Toxins are eliminated from the body, you will feel better than ever! However, if you get into a cycle of yo-yo dieting (losing weight rapidly, regaining it back rapidly, then losing it rapidly, etc.), you set yourself up for chronic diseases because your body is continually having to try to eliminate the accumulation of excessive amounts of Dysfunctional Toxins.

While yo-yo dieting promotes fat loss in the short-term, you will regain that fat, and more. In addition, low-calorie diets without Functional Training lead to severe muscle wasting. This means that once you get back to your normal eating habits, you'll be left with a body that has less muscle than before, and even more body fat. The increase in body fat, coupled with the loss in muscle tone, causes your metabolism to burn off fewer calories, which means it's going to be much harder to lose weight in the future. Many people are under the false impression that if they decrease their body weight by 20% with diet alone, their metabolic rate will also decrease by only 20%. In reality, their metabolism would decrease by around 30%![4] This excessive body fat leads to dysfunction of major organs and vessels, which further destabilizes the immune system.

HOW THE IMMUNE SYSTEM FUNCTIONS

Functional Alert: It is imperative that you lose body fat and keep it off so that, in the future, your body does not have to deal with the massive amounts of Dysfunctional Toxins that are released from fat cells during a significant body-fat loss!

Yo-yo dieting also slows down your metabolism by causing the thyroid to work less efficiently, leading to future weight gain.[5] The thyroid gland is like a tentacled squid. It branches out and controls many functions of the body. Once the thyroid becomes dysfunctional, it decreases production of t-3 and t-4, which are hormones responsible for regulating your metabolism. When t-3 and t-4 get low, your metabolism slows down and you gain body fat. This condition is called "hypothyroidism" and it often diminishes your sex drive. In addition, hypothyroidism can cause heart problems, such as an enlarged heart and heart failure. Hypothyroidism decreases the heart's ability to pump and increases bad cholesterol, blood pressure, and water retention.[6] This results in more inflammation and oxidation, which further weakens the immune system.

Diabetes is common in yo-yo dieting.[7] People who have deprived themselves end up rebounding and overloading on carbs and fats. This causes sugar levels to skyrocket and the pancreas to become overworked. You will feel hungry and tired and can experience dizziness, thirst, frequent urination, and blurred vision. This results in chronic inflammation and oxidation which weakens the immune system.

Impaired kidney function often occurs when people rapidly gain back all the body fat they once lost. The Dysfunctional Toxin overload from the excess food puts a lot of strain on the kidneys. It's common to experience edema in the lower legs and feet because the kidneys cannot work fast enough to filter and expel the excessive Dysfunctional Toxins and sodium that are building up in the body. Rapid weight gain usually causes drastic increases in blood pressure, which can result in kidney failure and stroke! Even people with seemingly normal kidney function during a rapid gain in body fat can be leaking albumin (the main protein of human blood plasma) from their kidneys into their urine.[8] The loss of albumin thickens the blood, resulting in a decreased blood volume in the blood vessels.[9] This causes wear and tear on major organs and vessels. It also causes the body to release excess amounts of pro-inflammatory cytokines and free radicals.

Functional Alert: Yo-yo dieting is not only dangerous for the general population, it's also dangerous for bodybuilders, figure and bikini competitors, etc., who enter multiple competitions a year and experience a rebound effect after each. If you compete, it's very important to remain relatively lean year round in order to avoid having health problems. We have witnessed competitors getting swollen ankles, kidney dysfunction, heart dysfunction, high blood sugar, high blood pressure, and infections immediately following a show due to the rapid change in body fat. The changes in one's diet after a competition must be gradual and small in order to prevent rebound weight gain, and organ and immune system dysfunction!

Yo-yo dieting weakens your cardiac output because you are losing heart muscle. The constant gaining and losing of body fat causes shrinking and swelling of the blood vessels. These abrupt changes over time can create small tears in the blood vessels, which can cause heart palpitations, plaque buildup, and hardening of the arteries.[10] In addition, levels of electrolytes (electrically charged minerals) in your body can become too low during rapid weight loss and too high during rapid weight gain. This can short-circuit the function of the entire body and cause permanent damage to all organs, especially the heart!

Yo-yo dieting also causes fatty liver disease. This not only causes the liver to malfunction, but also the kidneys, heart, thyroid, brain, pancreas, etc. All organs are interrelated and when one becomes dysfunctional, it creates a domino effect!

Fatty acids are released by visceral fat and travel to the liver where they increase the production of bad cholesterol and sugar in the blood. When the liver is unable to break down fats, they build up in liver tissue.[11] This causes chronic inflammation and oxidation, which scars the liver. If the scarring is severe, it can cause liver failure. If your liver cannot handle the excess fat and sugar when rapidly regaining body fat, the fat and sugar will accumulate throughout the body, causing all your arteries to harden and accelerating aging across the entire spectrum, especially your brain, heart, and genitals. Moreover, when blood sugar is unable to be stored fast enough, the liver becomes clogged and slows down your metabolism.[12]

The liver is one of the most important of all our vital organs. It is responsible for filtering and removing Dysfunctional Toxins. Obesity and/or exposure to excess amounts of Dysfunctional Toxins can cause Dysfunctional Toxins to accumulate in the liver as it tries to detoxify them. This sets up the stage for chronic inflammation and oxidation, depleted glutathione levels, and an immune system that malfunctions.

Functional Alert: Functional Training with a Fork gets rid of yo-yo dieting once and for all by creating a permanent lifestyle change!

Fiber and the Immune System

A large percentage of food contains both soluble fiber and insoluble fiber. Soluble fibers tend to provide better results for reducing appetite and blood sugar and for improving cardiovascular health. Insoluble fibers tend to provide more benefits in the area of preventing constipation and increasing the rate of food moving through the digestive tract.[1] Both types of fiber are essential for eliminating Dysfunctional Toxins in the body so the immune system can function properly. The extra fiber from eating on the higher end of the Functional Food Spectrum aids in the elimination of Dysfunctional Toxins—fewer will have to undergo metabolism in the body.[2] Any Dysfunctional Toxins that remain outside the fat cells are primarily managed by the amino acids and the probiotics/prebiotics that help your immune system suppress an invasion of these toxins.[3]

Functional Alert: Larger amounts of fiber are needed in today's society because we are exposed to more Dysfunctional Toxins. Fiber latches onto a modest portion of Dysfunctional Toxins in the digestive system and gets rid of them before they can be metabolized and stored in fat cells. Fiber also reduces LDL cholesterol, which sticks to the arterial wall![4]

Fruits, starchy vegetables, oats, beans, barley, nuts, seeds, and whole grains are good sources of fiber, but don't overdo them or you will gain weight. A one-cup serving of kidney beans contains approximately 15 grams of fiber. They contain both soluble (prebiotics) and insoluble fiber. Oat bran has about as much soluble fiber per serving as navy or black beans. Whole rolled oats is another good source. One small apple has 5 grams, one small banana has 3 grams, and a half cup of blueberries has 3 grams of fiber. Many herbs and spices also contain some fiber. People who struggle to eat enough fiber can get it through juicing fruits, vegetables, and even oats in a blender. Go easy on them because they contain carbs/sugar! The best way to increase your fiber intake while keeping calories low is by using fiber supplements. They have almost no digestible carbs. With the help of a psyllium husk fiber supplement (composed of about 70% soluble fiber and 30% insoluble fiber), along with your dinner and some oats for breakfast, it's easy to reach target fiber levels! Ground flax seed is another option for increasing fiber. But flax seeds contain about twice as much insoluble fiber as it does soluble fiber (prebiotics).

Functional Alert: Most people can't get enough daily fiber through food without overshooting their carb intake. This makes taking fiber supplements very important!

When using a fiber supplement such as psyllium husk, it's best to start with a low dose (e.g., 3-5 grams) and gradually increase to the needed amount. You can take 5-15 grams at dinner to reach target goals. Your target goal should be 20-40 grams of fiber per day. The amount of fiber you need is connected to the number of calories you eat in a day. We recommend approximately 15 grams of fiber for every 1,000 calories consumed. So if you are consuming 2,000 calories a day, aim to get around 30 grams of fiber. If you are consuming only 1,200-1,500 calories a day aim for 20-25 grams. For those who consume 3,000 calories or more per day, we have found that it's best not to go above 40 grams of fiber per day in order to prevent stomach upset. Always consume at least 8 ounces of fluid with your fiber supplement to prevent an upset stomach.

Functional Alert: Taking a fiber supplement before going to bed allows the body to trap Dysfunctional Toxins while you are asleep so they can be eliminated the following day. It also significantly lowers your appetite and the desire to eat anything else after your last meal!

Food ranging on the upper end of the Functional Food Spectrum also provide more antioxidants and phytonutrients (4,000 phytochemicals) to help combat free-radical damage, inflammation, and immune system dysfunction.[5] If you neglect to consume enough fiber throughout the day, you open the door for more Dysfunctional Toxins to be stored in fat cells, causing a vast array of symptoms: some immediate, some showing up later. Some effects are direct and some are indirect. Most people don't eat enough fiber throughout the day to help them stay full and eliminate enough Dysfunctional Toxins to keep their blood clean!

Functional Alert: The more food you consume from the lower end of the Functional Food Spectrum, the faster you progress from inflammation and oxidation to chronic inflammation and oxidation!

When Dysfunctional Toxins are ingested, they have to go through the GI tract and then the liver before they get stored as body fat. Eating too much food and/or the wrong kinds of food assaults the digestive system, liver, and fat cells, causing the immune system to become dysfunctional. The rich Dysfunctional Diet, as we refer to it, combined with a sedentary lifestyle, is making people sick and overweight.

Highly processed junk food and fast food are cheap and plenty tasty, but they are loaded with calories and Dysfunctional Toxins and lacking in fiber, protein, probiotics, nutrients (vitamins and minerals), phytonutrients, carotenoids, and antioxidants. These kinds of food are ranked on the lower end of the Functional Food Spectrum. Don't be fooled by labels on highly processed food that say "contains added fiber" because it's usually not the same kind of fiber found in real food such as oats, fruits, and vegetables.[6]

Functional Alert: There are different types of fiber that function differently and provide us with distinct health benefits. It has never been proven that added isolated fiber in many food products is effective at latching onto Dysfunctional Toxins for elimination. Therefore, stick to real food or products that contain intact natural fiber!

Fiber causes the body to release fewer pro-inflammatory cytokines and free radicals.[7] Therefore, the cells, tissue, and organs become less inflamed and the immune system doesn't have to work as hard to heal those areas. This leaves your body with more white blood cells to help prevent the growth of pathogens, kill infections, and export Dysfunctional Toxins from the body through feces. Fiber helps get rid of obesity by making you feel full, lowering blood sugar, and decreasing the workload on the pancreas.[8] When you consume carbs they turn into blood sugar. The pancreas has to release insulin to deal with the excess blood sugar that isn't used for fuel or taken up by the muscles and liver. When too much blood sugar is left in the body, it acts like a poison causing chronic inflammation and oxidation inside the body, especially the arteries, and puts a strain on the immune system. The excess sugar is shuttled to the liver and turned into triglycerides to be stored as body fat. The more body fat you accumulate, the less efficient the pancreas becomes at making insulin to deal with the excess blood sugar. This is referred to as insulin resistance. The pancreas eventually begins to malfunction to the point that insulin shots are needed to control blood sugar in order to prevent it from poisoning the body. This condition is called diabetes, which leads to dysfunction of all major organs. Now you see why obesity, a Dysfunctional Diet, and organ dysfunction go hand in hand!

Functional Alert: Fiber promotes the burning of fat for fuel and gut microbe metabolism.[9] The average American consumes only 10-15 grams of fiber per day.[10] You should be consuming around 20-40 grams of fiber daily!

Probiotics, Prebiotics, and the Immune System

Probiotics and prebiotics help maintain healthy levels of good bacteria in your GI tract which determine immune functions![1] In this age of the overconsumption of antibiotics, medications, food preservatives, pesticides, herbicides, and heavy metals, there is a greater need for prebiotics and probiotics to prevent intestinal and immune system dysfunction. If your digestive tract is incapable of digesting your food, your cells won't get the nutrients and oxygen they need to function optimally. Therefore, healthy intestinal functions play a major role in staying well. People who are malnourished are more vulnerable to infectious diseases.

Functional Alert: Chronic inflammation of the GI tract, unmanaged stress, and low testosterone are linked to autoimmune disease!

Prebiotic food simply are soluble fiber that the good bacteria (probiotics) feed on in your digestive system.[2] Probiotic food contain live bacteria, and they help your body maintain healthy PH levels in the blood, thus reducing the risk of external Dysfunctional Toxins invading the body.[3,4] Probiotics also destroy Dysfunctional Toxins released by other Dysfunctional Toxins, such as pesticides and bacteria.[5] They enhance GI tract immune function so that the GI tract and the immune system are compatible and work together.[6] Probiotics are living organisms inside your body and can sustain themselves unless something, such as antibiotics, comes along and destroys them. Bifidobacterium and lactobacillus are the most highly studied good bacteria. These good bacteria called "probiotics" require prebiotics such as inulins and fructooligosaccharides for growth and survival.[7] In a sense, this makes prebiotics just as important as probiotics!

Functional Alert: In a recent study, researchers were able to make mice obese or lean by altering their gut bacteria.[8] This is why taking prescription antibiotics or consuming them in your diet causes you to gain body fat!

We believe that conventional probiotic supplements end up delivering a very small percentage of what is claimed on the label—or nothing at all—because they don't contain any real probiotic strains.[9] Probiotics are living bacteria, thus making them highly sensitive to changes in environmental conditions. The acid in your stomach destroys a large percentage of the probiotics before they can reach the stomach.[10] Therefore, it takes an ample supply of probiotics and prebiotics stemming from fibrous plant-based food to allow probiotics to multiply and grow. Yogurt is the most popular source of probiotics because it contains viable probiotic organisms that reach the colon alive! If you decide to take a probiotics supplement, we highly recommend that you ask your doctor to write you a prescription for a pharmaceutical-grade one.[11]

By consuming probiotics, you reduce the risk of antibiotic-associated diarrhea. Lactobacillus acidophilus is a probiotic, or good bacteria, that lives inside your digestive tract.[12] It lowers cholesterol levels! [13] This good bacteria also lives inside every female's vagina. It also helps prevent yeast infections.[14] Antibiotics are notorious for causing yeast infections because they deplete lactobacillus acidophilus. Eating food such as yogurt and supplements containing effective strains of lactobacillus acidophilus can help females prevent yeast infections while they are taking antibiotics. However, they have to consume enough prebiotics (non-digestible/soluble fibers) so the probiotics can eat and survive. Having a healthy balance of bacteria fights life-threatening fungal infections, which are on the rise! [15]

Functional Alert: Lactobacillus acidophilus can often be consumed by individuals who suffer from lactose intolerance!

Most brands of yogurt contain two common probiotics: lactobacillus acidophilus and bifidobacterium bifidum.[16] These two probiotics have been intentionally added to improve the health of the GI tract, which improves the health of the immune system. This means your body will produce fewer pro-inflammatory cytokines and free radicals!

We highly recommend ingesting probiotics through food, especially shakes made of organic yogurt (low in sugar/carbs and fat) and liquid egg whites. Our preferred choice of yogurt is CARBmaster® yogurt because it contains very low carbs, sugar, and fat. It's also inexpensive and taste great!

Adding yogurt to the liquid egg whites increases probiotics in your digestive tract. The additional probiotics work in conjunction with amino acids derived from the liquid egg whites, helping to improve the function of your immune system and preventing cellular damage! In addition to the yogurt with live and active cultures, some other food that contain probiotics are soft cheese, low-fat kefir, sauerkraut, and effective probiotic supplements, if needed. Unfortunately, a lot of the food that contain probiotics also contain a high amount of carbs, sugar, or fat.

We also recommend ingesting large amounts of prebiotics (fiber) to improve GI tract health. These are the types of food that make gut flora grow well, which aids in digestive system function and improves immune function.

Some people have problems with gas when they first begin a high-fiber, high-protein diet, but over time, they will build up a tolerance, and the good bacteria in their stomachs generated from the yogurt will help neutralize excess gas in the stomach and intestines. If not, they need to reduce the amount of protein and fiber they are consuming in one sitting.

Ronnie: *I developed a condition called geographic tongue. The medications I have to take for my chronic lower-back pain caused a bacterial imbalance and acid reflux in my GI tract. Certain food would cause me to develop painful blisters on my tongue. I visited several doctors and dentists who told me the condition was untreatable and not to eat food that made the condition worse. It got so bad that just about everything I ate made my tongue burn. After hours of exhausting research, I finally came to the conclusion that a lot of inflammation throughout the entire body starts in the GI tract, and that my inflamed tongue was due to bacterial imbalances. So, I began consuming more probiotics through CARBmaster® yogurt and increased prebiotic consumption through psyllium husk. My geographic tongue was cured after about six months. In addition, during the time I was experiencing this condition, I was also noticing a considerable amount of plaque buildup on my teeth between my regular dental teeth cleaning appointments. After the geographic tongue was cured, the plaque buildup on my teeth left. This is proof that an imbalance of good and bad bacteria in the GI tract causes chronic inflammation and oxidation throughout the body. My experience has made me suspect that bacterial imbalances play a role in causing cancer, heart disease, diabetes, autoimmune disease, etc. I also recommend flossing and/or using a water pick every day. Certain bacteria live in your teeth and can cause inflammation and oxidation in the body. This also leads to swelling of the arteries, etc.*[17]

Functional Alert: Excess exercise can lower your immune system. This is particularly true in elite athletes who often overtrain and/or don't get enough sleep. Consuming more probiotics and prebiotics is clearly more important for people who implement vigorous Functional Exercise as a lifestyle, so they don't risk running their immune systems down and then suffer from colds, viruses, etc.!

Heavy Metals, Antibiotics, and the Immune System

Avoid heavy metals and antibiotics for a stronger immune system. Heavy metals and antibiotics weaken the immune system and cause it to produce more pro-inflammatory cytokines and free radicals.[1, 2] In order to avoid ingesting excess heavy metals, stay away from larger fish at the top of the food chain. Eat organic meats and produce, which contain fewer heavy metals and nitrogen than non-organic because organic farms use natural fertilizers, not synthetic.[3]

You don't have to worry about ingesting excess antibiotics when eating wild-caught fish, organic lean red meat, organic lean chicken, organic lean pork, and organic lean turkey. We believe that conventional chicken, turkey, pork, red meat, and farm-raised fish are full of antibiotics and should be avoided.[4]

HOW THE IMMUNE SYSTEM FUNCTIONS

Kathy: *Years ago, I worked for a company packaging penicillin. Over time, my immune system reacted to the penicillin as a harmful substance. I constantly ran a low grade fever and experienced both chronic fatigue and irritable bowel syndrome. I went to several different doctors who wanted to put me on an antidepressant even though I kept telling them I wasn't depressed! I continued to have these symptoms until I no longer worked around the penicillin. During that time, I didn't know about the importance of probiotics and prebiotics to increase good bacteria in the GI tract. Now I stay away from foods containing antibiotics and consume plenty of probiotics and prebiotics in my diet. All the health issues I once experienced are gone. So no one can convince me that long-term exposure to small amounts of antibiotics in our diet are not harmful to one's health!*

Eating meats containing appreciable amounts of antibiotics can result in heavy metals, pesticides, food preservatives, etc., building up in your organs and tissues.[1] The gastrointestinal (GI tract) or gut makes up approximately 75% of your immune system.[6] This is because good bacteria, especially those located in your colon (part of the large intestines), live next to the immune system's lymphatic system, which is mostly composed of the GI tract. The lymphatic system is one of the most overlooked systems because it is vital to the circulation and production of white blood cells.[7] The GI tract contains approximately 400 types of probiotic bacteria.[8] These good bacteria reduce the growth of harmful bacteria, promote a healthy GI tract, and enhance the function of your immune system. Most of the heavy metals in your GI tract are eliminated by good bacteria![9] Antibiotics, other Dysfunctional Toxins, and chronic stress can interfere with this process because they destroy excessive amounts of good bacteria in the gut which allows the bad bacteria to overpower the good. When antibiotics are consumed through your diet or through prescription medications, it often prevents good bacteria from dominating bad bacteria. The bad bacteria overpowers the good and shuttles Dysfunctional Toxins such as heavy metals to various organs and tissues throughout the body. This increases the chance of carcinogenetic mutations and/or organ dysfunction because chronically inflamed organs and tissues become the targets of bacteria, viruses, and fungus. When this occurs, the organs and tissues begin to malfunction and the chronic inflammation/oxidation over an extended period prevents your immune system from making enough white blood cells to repair all the damage.

Functional Alert: According to the Center for Disease Control, more than 2 million Americans get sick from antibiotic-resistant bacteria each year, more than 23,000 of them die![10]

Antibiotics can cause leaky gut syndrome: Partially digested food enters the blood stream and the immune system has to work overtime to try to clean the blood, in addition to everything else going on inside your body.[11] A low white blood cell count is a sign that there is a decrease in disease-fighting cells circulating in your blood. Swollen lymph nodes are a sign of viruses, bacterial infections, and cancer.

Functional Alert: The Journal of the American Medical Association has linked antibiotic use to an increased risk of cancer.[12] The New England Journal of Medicine has linked antibiotic use to an increased risk of heart disease![13]

When there aren't enough good bacteria in the gut to prevent heavy metals and other Dysfunctional Toxins from entering the blood stream, killer-t cell production decreases, setting you up for an enormous spectrum of diseases.[14-16] In order to have good health, our good bacteria must dominate bad bacteria to properly digest food, absorb vitamins, and protect us from Dysfunctional Toxins, such as antibiotics and heavy metals that promote disease.

Functional Alert: Removal of heavy metals from the body is known as chelation.[17] Amino acids derived from protein-based food, such as liquid egg whites, help remove heavy metals from the body once they enter the blood stream![18]

Amino Acids and the Immune System

Amino acids bind together to form protein.[1] They are used in every cell of your body to build protein you need for survival. People working in the cancer field tell their patients on chemotherapy to eat more protein because the variety of amino acids contained in protein has healing properties.[2] Proteins perform a vast array of functions within our bodies, including reacting positively to events that stimulate a specific functional change in cells, tissue, and organs. In order to maintain proper immune function, you must continually restore amino acids in every meal because your body doesn't have a long-term storage system for protein like it does for carbs and fats. A high-protein diet, coupled with good insulin sensitivity, provides the amino acids needed for cells and molecules to make additional protein to help suppress Dysfunctional Toxins that can cause disease.[3] This becomes even more critical as you get older in order to prevent immune system malfunction. A high-protein diet, combined with Functional Training and Functional Hormone Replacement, becomes even more vital for proper immune system functions as we age because it helps preserve muscle tissue and blood-protein levels.

Functional Alert: Nitric oxide is synthesized from the amino acid arginine. A protein-rich diet, such as liquid egg whites, increases nitric- oxide levels. Nitric oxide penetrates the underlying smooth muscles and makes the arteries expand, lowering blood pressure and decreasing inflammation and oxidation. It also helps lower the production of excess white blood cells that would otherwise thicken the blood and cause further inflammation and oxidation. Amino Acids help put a stop to heart disease, sexual dysfunction, and brain neurodegeneration by improving blood flow and preventing damage to the endothelium (inner lining of the arteries)![4]

Amino acids have the healing power to help you feel good, look better, think clearer, and stay healthier. Your brain and body can't function properly without an adequate supply of amino acids. The primary reasons are because your dopamine, epinephrine, and norepinephrine levels decrease.[5, 6] A low-protein diet produces inflammation and oxidation in the brain that impairs learning ability, memory, and attention span. A high-protein diet improves learning, memory, focus, and alertness. Even dogs and cats look, feel, and perform better if they are fed a high-protein, meat-based diet instead of a wheat-, soy-, rice-, or corn-based one.

We get lazy and feel fatigued after a large meal composed predominately of high carbs and fats. A high-carb and/or high-fat diet greatly increases our chances for getting Alzheimer's, which accounts for approximately half of all dementia cases. Severe brain dysfunction isn't a normal part of aging. In fact, older people who have good vascular health continue learning as time moves forward.

One thing is for certain, diets low in protein in both animals and humans depress normal growth, increase susceptibility to many Dysfunctional Toxins, and kill exposed Dysfunctional Toxins later instead of earlier, which increases the development of pre-cancerous lesions. Low-protein diets also promote fatty liver disease; decrease muscle tone, strength, metabolism, glutathione levels, and immune function; increase blood pressure and water retention; and lead to plaque buildup, which, in turn, leads to decreased cognitive, sexual, and cardio function!

Functional Alert: A lack of amino acids causes the body to produce more pro-inflammatory cytokines and struggle with preventing free radical damage![7]

Protein-based food supply our bodies with a master antioxidant called glutathione.[8] Glutathione is synthesized in the body from three amino acids—L-glutamic acid, glycine, and L-cysteine—which are derived from protein-based food.[9] This highly potent antioxidant is more effective at preventing free-radical damage to cells than any other antioxidants in the human body because it's produced inside the cells.[10]

Glutathione is one of the body's most potent shields for defending against Dysfunctional Toxins once they enter the bloodstream or get stored in body fat. Furthermore, your body can't excrete Dysfunctional Toxins, such as the heavy metal mercury, until they bind with glutathione after immediately being ingested into your bloodstream or until they are being released back into your bloodstream as you lose body fat.[11] This binding process helps prevent Dysfunctional Toxins from continuing to circulate through the liver and blood vessels and eventually poisoning your system.

Functional Alert: You can use 100% whey isolate protein powder to boost glutathione levels if you are allergic to dairy (yogurt) and/or liquid egg whites. You should not see the word "concentrate" listed in the ingredients.[12] Use a protein powder that has the least amount of sugar, cholesterol, and saturated fat!

A high-protein diet is a must for everyone because our bodies are always fighting some form of imbalance. Adequate levels of glutathione are necessary so that other important antioxidants (such as vitamin A, C, E, and selenium) can be properly used within our bodies. Basically, glutathione recycles other antioxidants so fewer are needed to prevent diseases that are caused by excess inflammation and oxidation.[13] Glutathione is the most important antioxidant for maintaining a Functional Immune System and preventing cellular damage. A Functional Diet alone will help improve your antioxidant system, but combining Functional Training and Functional Cardio with a high-protein diet produces a synergistic effect.

Functional Alert: A diet containing plenty of antioxidants decreases the rate at which cells become inflamed and oxidized, thus preventing all types of diseases![14]

Your body's response to stress, hormones, diet, lifestyle, or environment can result in a Dysfunctional Immune System that no longer protects you from diseases. Dysfunctional Immune Systems kill multitudes of people per day in America! Your immune system is a highly complex network of white blood cells and protein made of amino acids that recognize and attack foreign invaders or Dysfunctional Toxins.[15] If the immune system becomes overworked from trying to simultaneously heal and protect multiple damaged organs, such as the brain, heart, liver, kidneys, and pancreas, it won't have enough antibodies left to extinguish all the inflammation/oxidation inside the body. This leaves you vulnerable for many short-term and long-term illnesses.

Globulin and albumin make up your total blood-protein level and help preserve antibodies as we age and help them function more efficiently. Approximately 38% of your protein blood plasma is made up of globulin. It's the main ingredient used to build antibodies and carry hormones.[16]

Approximately 55% of your protein content of blood plasma is made up of albumin. Albumin is a protein manufactured by the liver. It keeps fluid within the vessels and transports vitamins/mineral, electrolytes, etc. by way of the bloodstream.[17] If you develop chronic inflammation, the body requires additional albumin to try to repair the damaged tissues.[18] When albumin levels get low, edema (swelling due to excess fluid trapped in the body's tissues) can develop.[17] Edema can be caused by a blockage in blood vessels and leads to vein and valve damage, causing even more swelling. When the valves of the blood vessel become damaged, blood leaks back down the vessels, and fluid is retained in the soft tissue of the ankles and feet. The most immediate danger of edema in the lower legs is the increased risk of developing a blood clot that can travel to the lungs (pulmonary embolism). Edema in the lower legs is often a sign that the whole body has hidden edema and is causing dysfunction in multiple organs such as the brain, heart, and lungs.[18] Edema can also slowly poison the body, causing the immune system to work overtime on that particular problem, while leaving less total blood proteins to handle other problems.

Functional Alert: A Functional Diet high in protein, moderate in fats, and low in carbs and salt helps alleviate edema, and decreases body fat. Liquid egg whites (cooked or drunk) are known to contain an abundance of albumin to help fight against edema!

Protein, Bone Density, and Kidney Function

The same macronutrient that builds muscle, connective tissue, and cartilage builds up the bones. This macronutrient is protein! Scientific studies have shown that long-term, high-protein intake increases bone mineral density and reduces bone fracture incidence.[1] Protein uses calcium to improve bone health, especially in the elderly. A large proportion of deaths from falling are due to complications following a hip fracture. One out of five hip-fracture patients dies within a year of their injury.[2]

Research shows that a high-protein diet can impair kidney function for people who already have chronic kidney disease, but just the opposite is true in healthy individuals. In fact, the best way to prevent the decline in kidney function as we age is to keep protein intake higher and carbs and fats lower![3] Replacing carbs and fats with protein lowers blood sugar and blood pressure. A high-protein diet in normal people enables the kidneys to filter Dysfunctional Toxins at an accelerated rate.[4] On the other hand, high levels of blood sugar from a diet composed of too many carbs and fats impairs the kidneys' filtration system and causes Dysfunctional Toxins to build up in the blood.[4]

    A high-protein diet and phosphorous are both needed to maintain strong bones, help healthy kidneys get rid of waste, and regulate nerve impulses and heart rate. A lack of protein and phosphate can result in an irregular heart rhythm and even death. Phosphorous is the second most abundant mineral in the body; calcium is first.[5] If a healthy individual takes in too much phosphorus through protein sources, such as chicken, their kidneys will remove the excess phosphorous from the body through urine. When high blood sugar and/or high blood pressure prevent the kidneys from functioning well enough to remove excess phosphorous, bones can become brittle and heart disease can occur.[6] The kidneys may be unable to efficiently eliminate phosphorous if you allow yourself to become obese and/or you consume junk food ranked on the lower end of the Functional Food Spectrum (e.g., fast-food and soft drinks).[7] This leads to kidney disease! [8]

Functional Alert: High blood pressure or hypertension is referred to as the silent killer. It leads to chronic kidney disease. A lot of people with mild, elevated blood pressure (e.g., 140/90) are being prescribed drugs such as beta-blockers. These drugs often have serious side effects that include decreased sexual performance, dry mouth, insomnia, and fatigue! **Functional Training with a Fork** is a much healthier way of lowering a moderately elevated blood pressure. A high-protein diet and drinking plenty of fluids help lower blood pressure and blood sugar, reducing wear and tear of the kidneys over the long haul!

    We believe all colas are dangerous and can cause chronic kidney disease because they contain phosphoric acid. We believe dark colas are even worse because they contain a carcinogen called 4-methylimidazole (4-Mel). This carcinogen forms when ammonia is used to make the caramel coloring that gives them their dark brown color.[9,10] After looking at the research done on dark brown-colored sodas, we believe caramel coloring should be banned. It's absurd to put consumers at risk from an ingredient that is being added to make it look more appealing. This same rule applies to pancake syrups that use caramel coloring.

    Eating a low-protein diet reduces levels of albumin (the most abundant protein found in the blood needed to repair damaged tissues from excess inflammation).[11] Albumin is important for everyone because this particular kind of protein helps extract excess fluid from swollen tissues and puts it back into the blood where it can then be removed by the body.[12] The key to enhancing the filtering of your blood without excessively reducing albumin levels or excessively increasing phosphorus levels is to replace some of the other protein sources (e.g., meats and beans) with pasteurized liquid egg whites that are low in phosphorous.[13,14] Liquid egg whites are the healthiest protein for people with kidney problems and without. However, if you have kidney problems always consult with a physician about your diet.

Blood Sugar, Insulin, and the Immune System

Blood sugar and insulin imbalances lead to a malfunction of the immune system because excessive amounts of pro-inflammatory cytokines and free radicals are released.[1-3] Blood sugar and insulin imbalances are caused by consuming too many carbs from any source and/or too many refined sugars or by combining too many carbs and fats in the same meal. All carbs eventually turn into blood sugar. Fats slow down the burning of sugar derived from carbs for fuel when combined in the same meal. Less blood sugar is then being used for fuel and more insulin is being produced over a longer period of time to deal with the excess sugar remaining in the blood stream. Other factors leading to blood sugar and insulin imbalances include not exercising enough, obesity, and hormonal imbalances. Blood sugar and insulin imbalances cause the immune system to malfunction through four different pathways: hyperglycemia, hypoglycemia, hyperinsulinemia, and insulin resistance.

1. Hyperglycemia occurs when you have more blood sugar in your blood stream than your insulin (a hormone secreted by the pancreas that helps to regulate the level of sugar in the body) can manage. Drastic increases in blood sugar stimulate one's appetite. This problem is common with diabetics. Hyperglycemia leads to hypoglycemia, which causes sugar crashes.[4]

2. Hypoglycemia occurs when your insulin removes blood sugar too quickly, causing blood sugar to drop too low, making you feel tired, faint, irritable, and extremely hungry.[5]

3. Hyperinsulinemia occurs when the pancreas has to continually produce too much insulin to deal with blood sugar that remains chronically elevated after a meal. It's caused from constantly consuming too many carbs from any source and/or too many refined sugars or by combining too many carbs and fats in the same meal. Hyperinsulinemia causes the beta-cells in the pancreas to produce excessive amounts of insulin. When the pancreas becomes exhausted to the point of damage, a person becomes insulin resistant.[6]

4. Insulin resistance is a condition in which your body tissues have a lowered level of response to insulin. When you are insulin resistant, your brain craves carbohydrates because your pancreas can no longer produce sufficient amounts of insulin for the body's demands, then blood sugar rises.[7]

Functional Alert: Your goal should be to keep blood sugar and insulin levels as close to the desired range as possible. Blood sugar/insulin imbalances are a leading cause of rapid biological aging in today's society!

Unstable blood sugar and insulin levels damage the blood vessels that supply blood to vital tissues and organs.[8] Anytime you experience excess or unstable blood-sugar levels, oxygen is cut off to the entire body, including the brain and heart.[9] This is why you feel so sluggish during a sugar crash! The inner lining of blood vessels, known as the endothelium becomes damaged, decreasing the ability of the blood vessels to dilate.[10] This restricts the flow of oxygenated blood to vital cells, tissues, and organs. A lack of oxygen also damages the nerve endings that surround blood vessels. Over time nerve damage occurs and weakens electrical impulses throughout the entire body, including the brain and heart.[11] A great many of Americans with unstable blood sugar and insulin levels face cancer, strokes, heart attacks, amputations, dementia, sexual dysfunction (damaging blood vessels and nerve endings in the genitals, leading to a loss of feeling and sexual performance, and making orgasm difficult), vision loss, peripheral neuropathy (pain, numbness, and weakness in hands and feet), and autonomic neuropathy (damaging of the nerves that control the genitals, GI tract, bladder, and other organs).[12,13]

Functional Alert: Unstable blood sugar and insulin levels can demolish glutathione, our most important antioxidant for combating free radical damage to blood cells, blood vessels, and organs. In addition, when glutathione levels get low the body releases more pro-inflammatory cytokines and free radicals that damage the endothelium.[14, 15] Excessive amounts of pro-inflammatory cytokines and free radicals are bad because they cause cell mutations and damage immune function. Please take this under consideration the next time a friend or family member gets sick and you want to make them something sweet, such as cookies, cakes, and casseroles. The sugar and fats in these foods will cause unstable blood sugar and insulin levels and will further lower their immunity!

Your brain is your personality! Eating in a manner that controls blood sugar will improve brain function and bring out your best character. Eating right makes you smarter, more likeable, interesting, and pleasant to be around. It also helps you succeed academically and improves your ability to rationalize and make quicker and wiser decisions. There is a strong connection between brain function, sexual function, heart function, and immune function.

If you want to be smarter and prevent cognitive dysfunction, then you have to improve the blood flow to your brain and keep electrical impulses flowing. A diet high in carbs and/or high in fats has serious ramifications to brain health because clogged arteries are related to a person's mental health. Arteries determine blood flow to your brain, which is the main cause for developing dementia. What is good for the brain is good for every organ in the body. A new major study from researchers from the University of Washington suggests that high blood-sugar levels, even without the presence of diabetes, can increase the risk of dementia. They found that as blood-sugar levels increase, so does the risk for dementia![16] The bottom line is, you need to eat more protein and fiber and fewer carbs and fats in order to control your blood-sugar levels. This will help prevent damage to the brain's cells and tissues over time by reducing their exposure to pro-inflammatory cytokines and free radicals!

Everyone (even endurance athletes who are not overweight) who consumes a diet composed of too many carbs from any source and/or too many refined sugars, or who combines too many carbs/sugars and fats in the same meal is at risk of developing plaque and pits on the inner lining of their arteries. Furthermore, mixing carbs and/or sugar with saturated fats is worse than mixing them with unsaturated fats, because saturated fats alone cause insulin resistance.[17] When a diet causes chronic blood sugar and/or insulin imbalances, it damages the endothelium (the inner lining of the arteries). The inflammation signals the immune system to release pro-inflammatory cytokines and free radicals to help regulate the function of the endothelium.[18] Pro-inflammatory cytokines and free radicals act as messengers that form a communication link between your body's tissues and immune system.[19, 20] Having very high levels or long-lasting levels of either lead to disease! The continued release of pro-inflammatory cytokines and free radicals leads to further inflammation and oxidation, resulting in the release of excessive amounts of both from activated white blood cells.[21] This can cause multi-organ failure, cell and tissue damage, plaque buildup, and tumor growth.[22] As you can see, eating fewer carbs and fats prevent elevations in pro-inflammatory cytokines and free radicals. This helps maintain normal cellular oxygenation!

Functional Alert: Blood sugar and/or insulin imbalances provokes the release of excessive amounts of pro-inflammatory cytokines to overpower anti-inflammatory cytokines. Over time, this runs down the immune system by depleting white blood cells. The excessive release of pro-inflammatory cytokines and free radicals is linked to all diseases: diabetes, heart disease, cancer, autoimmune disease, stroke, Alzheimers, etc.!

High blood sugar is also causing an epidemic of type-2 diabetics and it's driving up the cost of everyone's health care! Diabetes is the most common disease of the endocrine system (consists of glands that produce and secrete chemical messengers called hormones that regulate the activity of cells and organs).[23,24] Excess blood sugar has a negative impact on the building blocks of our immune systems, leaving the white blood cells unprepared to fight off deadly bacteria and viruses. If you put a little sugar into your vehicle's gas tank, it won't run smoothly, and it may not run at all. Excess blood sugar has a similar effect on your immune system! Just because your blood-sugar levels are normal doesn't mean your body isn't releasing a lot of insulin at times from eating the wrong kinds of foods or combinations of foods. High-insulin levels are linked to chronic inflammation and oxidation, which cause your immune system to misfire! Ingesting moderate amounts of sugar (even fruit juice) in a meal, regardless of the form, impairs the function of white blood cells to destroy Dysfunctional Toxins by 50% for more than 5 hours.[25]

Some diabetics are finally starting to learn that insulin dosing for meals shouldn't focus only on counting carbohydrates, but also on dietary fat intake. It has been proven that combining an appreciable amount of carbs and fats in the same meal promotes weight gain in the form of body fat. Researchers found that type-1 diabetics who chose to eat a high-fat meal instead of a low-fat one need to use an average of 42% more insulin, even though both meals were equal in protein and carbohydrates. In spite of the additional insulin being added along with the higher-fat meal, sugar levels remained higher for up to 10 hours in the people who ate the high-fat meal along with their usual amount of carbs and protein for dinner versus the meals low in fat.[26]

Functional Alert: Fats dramatically increase blood sugar and insulin levels when combined with carbs!

Insulin is a storage hormone. It affects carbohydrate, protein, and fat metabolism.[27] Your body breaks these nutrients down into sugar, mostly from carbs, and very little from protein and fats. When you have low body-fat levels, coupled with an abundance of muscle tone, amino acids from ingested dietary proteins easily enter into the muscle cells for growth and repair. On the other hand, when you become insulin resistant from a lack of muscle tone and/or accumulating too much body fat, the body blocks amino acids from entering the muscle cells, making it very difficult to build muscle tone. The more lean muscle you build, the more calories from carbs you can eat without gaining body fat. The more body fat you accumulate, the more insulin resistant you will become, and the easier it will be to keep gaining body fat!

Functional Alert: Actively training your type-2 muscle fibers with the proper type of Functional Training help prevent insulin resistance, obesity, and premature death!

When insulin levels fall, you release body fat and burn it for fuel. When insulin levels rise, you accumulate triglycerides (fats) in body-fat cells.[28] When too much insulin is produced over a period of time, the body has trouble maintaining stable blood-sugar levels, causing you to stay hungry and tired. This is because your body does not allow blood sugar (fuel) to gain entry into your cells and provide you with the energy you need to remain fully functional. As a result, your activity levels will decrease, you will burn fewer calories, and you will consume more food.

Cholesterol and the Immune System

Optimize your immune system with healthy cholesterol levels. The single most important factor involved in optimizing your cholesterol levels is consuming more protein and fiber, and fewer carbs and fats! It's the same protocol needed to prevent becoming diabetic. The injury to our blood vessels is caused by high-carb diets, high-fat diets, and, especially, diets that are high in both carbs and fats!

Saturated fats are known to increase LDL (bad) cholesterol more than dietary cholesterol alone.[1] No one knows exactly why saturated fats cause LDL levels to elevate more than unsaturated fats do. We believe the answer to the question may lie with insulin resistance. Our cells can differentiate between saturated fats and unsaturated fats, and become more insulin resistant when we consume saturated fats versus unsaturated.[2]

You need a little saturated fat for optimal immune system functions. Therefore, it's okay to have limited amounts in your diet as long as you emphasize unsaturated fats, especially omega-3s and monounsaturated fats, which have some anti-inflammatory effects. High levels of LDL cholesterol in the blood from excess saturated fats are prone to inflammation and oxidation. Oxidized LDL cholesterol is a free radical generator! Once oxidation occurs, the immune system sends excessive amounts of white blood cells to the rescue and they often get converted into plaque when there is endothelium (inner lining of the arteries) damage. The plaque buildup in the arteries is irreversible![3-5]

It should be noted that having an excessively high white blood cell count is a bad sign![6] Over time, the plaque begins to build up inside blood vessels throughout the entire body. The continual buildup of inflammatory plaque over time can confuse the immune system causing it to attack its own healthy cells, tissues, and organs instead of attacking Dysfunctional Toxins or foreign substances.[7] The dysfunctional response from the immune system can also allow a Dysfunctional Toxin, such as a virus, to cause cancer because the body can no longer distinguish the virus from healthy cells, tissues, and organs.

The key to having healthy cholesterol levels is to optimize your cholesterol profile in order to lower inflammation and lower oxidation, improve the delivery of oxygenated blood to cells, and prevent the immune system from having to work overtime. Higher levels of HDL (good) cholesterol help reduce plaque buildup.[8] HDL particles help fight against inflammation and oxidation caused by elevated LDL levels that weakens the immune system.[9,10] Healthy HDL levels retrieve LDL (bad cholesterol that clogs arteries) from your blood stream before it can cause a scar or blockage.[11] The scar or plaque buildup is considered worse than a blockage because if a piece of hardened plaque breaks off, it can travel to the brain and cause a stroke. This scenario causes more permanent damage than an almost fully blocked artery that requires a stent. You want to get your LDL as low as possible and HDL levels high.

Functional Alert: The side effects of high LDL cholesterol is chronic inflammation and oxidation. The side effects of chronic inflammation and oxidation is immune system dysfunction!

The role fats play in causing clogged arteries is confusing to many people because they hear about the dangers of saturated fats, excess omega-6 fats, etc. Allow us to simplify things: Plaque buildup on the inside of the arterial walls is caused by embedded lipids from consuming too many dietary fats from any source. These lipids are composed of cholesterol and triglycerides.[12] All forms of excess dietary fats, whether saturated or unsaturated (monounsaturated or polyunsaturated) eventually turn into triglycerides and cholesterol inside the body causing plaque buildup over time.[13,14] Any dietary fat that isn't immediately used for fuel either gets stored inside body-fat cells to be used as a reserve backup for fuel, or accumulates in the blood stream as bad lipids (triglycerides and LDL cholesterol).[15] The bad lipids that are left in the blood stream clog arteries over time, which restricts blood flow to your cells, tissues, and organs![16]

Saturated fats produce larger amounts of triglycerides and LDL cholesterol than unsaturated fats. Saturated fats, omega-6 fats, and trans fats cause the most inflammation, oxidation, and plaque buildup over time. Omega-3 fats and monounsaturated fats create the least amount of inflammation, oxidation, and plaque buildup over time.[17,18] Replacing saturated fats and omega-6 fats with Omega-3 fats and monounsaturated fats is one of the healthiest changes you can make, besides eliminating refined sugar and eating more lean protein, fiber, and probiotics.

Functional Alert: A steady supply of protein in the diet increases Nitric oxide, which is made from an amino acid called L-arginine. Nitric oxide suppresses oxidation of LDL cholesterol, which prevents inflammation, plaque buildup, and further free radical damage![19]

The only fats you need to avoid altogether are trans fats or all hydrogenated oils because they dramatically increase inflammation and free radical damage to cell membranes. Trans fats increase LDL levels and lower HDL, which causes further chronic inflammation and oxidation inside the arteries.[20] A food label may say "Contains no trans fats," but still contains partially hydrogenated or hydrogenated oils.[21] If a food has fewer than 0.5 grams of trans fat per serving, the label will show zero grams trans fats even if partially hydrogenated oil is in the product.[22] You must read those labels carefully! The theory that you need to consume specific ratios of each type of fat has never been proven, but we believe you need to limit saturated and omega-6 fats (polyunsaturated), stay completely away from trans fats, and place more emphasis on omega-3s fats (polyunsaturated) and monounsaturated fats.

Functional Alert: Cutting back on saturated fats and eliminating trans fats will have no benefit if you replace them with refined carbohydrates (sugar)!

The idea of carbs in the diet causing plaque buildup also confuses many people because they hear about the dangers of sugar and that all carbs (whether they have a low, medium, or high insulin production) eventually turn into sugar. The glycemic index scale does not measure insulin production in relation to rises in blood sugar.[23] You may be surprised to learn that refined sugar has only a moderate glycemic index rating comparable to potatoes. However, potatoes are a lot more satisfying than refined sugar, and the sugar contained in potatoes acts differently inside the body. Allow us to simplify things: Processed sugars are derived from sugar cane or sugar beets and need to be avoided as much as possible.[24] Processed sugar has added chemicals and raises blood-sugar levels faster than natural sugar derived from plant-based food (e.g., apples, oatmeal, and potatoes).[25]

Any sugar from carbohydrates that is not used for fuel due to low activity levels or consistently high blood-sugar levels turns into triglycerides. Some of the left-over triglycerides that aren't immediately used for fuel get stored inside body-fat cells to be used as a reserve backup for fuel, while others accumulate in the blood stream as bad lipids (triglycerides and LDL cholesterol).[26] The bad lipids that are left in the blood stream clog arteries over time, which restrict blood flow to your cells, tissues, and organs!

Functional Alert: Excess carbs in your diet increase triglycerides, LDL cholesterol, inflammation, and oxidation just like excess dietary fats. Both macronutrients when consumed in excess make you fat and sick and keep you that way!

The ratios of your triglycerides and HDL cholesterol are also highly important. It's common for people with low HDL (good) cholesterol levels to have high triglycerides, which further encourages thickening of the blood. As triglyceride levels rise, HDL levels will usually fall, putting a strain on the function of one's immune system and the body's ability to retrieve LDL cholesterol before it oxidizes. When you lower triglycerides and/or increase your HDL, your immune system and health improves.

Sugar beets are exclusively made from GMO.[27] Plant-based foods are made up of natural sugar. They are broken down in the GI tract into a more usable form of sugar and provide steady control of insulin, energy, mood, and hunger.[28] This means less insulin production! On the other hand, refined sugars are incomplete foods because they aren't broken down into a sugar that is very usable. Refined sugars cause swings in insulin, energy, mood, and hunger. This means more insulin production! Think about how bad you feel after consuming a candy bar, ice cream, cookie, desserts, crackers, chips, white table sugar, sugar-laden cereals, and sugar in juice, soda, or alcohol. These foods and beverages cause the most chronic oxidation and inflammation inside the body's cells, tissues, and organs! The carbohydrates that cause the body to produce the most insulin, also cause the most damage to the inner lining of the arteries, creating larger pits in the inner lining of the arteries, which allow LDL cholesterol to oxidize and build up as plaque!

Functional Alert: Today high-fructose corn syrup is in most processed foods and sweetened drinks because it's cheaper to manufacture than sucrose (refined sugar from sugar beets and sugar cane).[29] However, high- fructose corn syrup and sucrose are not significantly different.[30] Both high- fructose and sucrose are bad for your health because they cause a lot of insulin production, which causes chronic inflammation and oxidation. However, high-fructose corn syrup is even worse than sucrose because it causes the body to produce even more pro-inflammatory cytokines and free radicals.[31,32]

Replacing processed sugar with natural sugar reduces your appetite and allows body fat to be more readily used for fuel because insulin is better managed. In addition, blood-sugar levels depend on how much fat or protein is eaten with the carbohydrates. When combined with carbs, fats increase blood sugar whereas protein lowers blood sugar.[33] Carbs, other than the ones listed as Free Foods, shouldn't be consumed without protein because they will increase hunger. In other words, neither natural sugars nor refined sugars should be consumed without protein! Not only does protein help stabilize blood-sugar levels, it helps counterbalance the effects sugar has on the pleasure center of the brain (the part of the brain that tells you, I want more food) by stimulating the reward center of the brain (the part of the brain that tells you, I've had enough food)! However, carb sources on our Free Food list can be consumed without protein if desired. In addition, fruits and vegetables have various nutrients and contain fiber to slow down the digestion of their natural sugars, which leads to more stable blood-sugar levels!

Cholesterol

There's only one type of cholesterol. It's a waxy substance that occurs in our tissues and is called a "sterol" because it's made out of an alcohol and a steroid.[1] Your total cholesterol count is made up of HDL cholesterol and LDL cholesterol along with one-fifth of your triglyceride level.[2] Cholesterol has three primary functions: First, it's used to manufacture bile acids, which help with the digestion of fats in our diet. Second, it's needed to make Vitamin D and steroid hormones. Third, it's also a structural component of all cell membranes, making it extremely important for overall functionality.[3] Your body is capable of producing all the cholesterol it needs without any help from the diet![4]

Bad cholesterol (LDL) and triglyceride levels become elevated from the following:

1. Your body makes too much on its own naturally due to your genetics.

2. You consume too much cholesterol.

3. You consume too many fats in any form (saturated, monounsaturated, and polyunsaturated), especially saturated fats.

4. You consume too many carbs (fast burning and slow burning), especially refined sugar.

5. You don't eat enough lean protein and fiber.

6. Your body doesn't get rid of LDL cholesterol efficiently due to a lack of prebiotics and probiotics, a sluggish metabolism from a lack of muscle tone, and low-thyroid hormones.

7. Your liver begins to malfunction from obesity and/or Dysfunctional Toxin overload.

8. You allow yourself to become overweight and have high blood sugar and/or insulin levels.

9. You drink alcohol in excess and/or mix alcohol with fats, which delays the effect of chylomicrons being broken down during digestion.[5,6]

10. You smoke.

Cholesterol has a lot in common with the baggage carousel at the airport. A single-level baggage carousel at an airport delivers checked luggage to passengers so they can pick up their personal belongings. This is how cholesterol works in your body!

Allow us to illustrate:

- Circulatory system (carousel)
- Cholesterol (one's personal belongings)
- Lipoproteins (luggage)
- Blood (conveyor belt)
- Liver (airport personnel)
- Excess LDL cholesterol (illegal drugs)
- Arterial plaque buildup (lost luggage)
- Bowels (baggage claim area)

Luggage containing one's personal belongings is loaded onto a conveyor belt by a baggage handler and moves around on a carousel until it's picked up in the baggage claim area. Likewise, lipoproteins (luggage) containing cholesterol (one's personal belongings) are sent into the blood stream (conveyer belt) by the liver (airport personnel) and travels through the circulatory system (carousel) until the bowels (baggage claim area) take it away.

Lipoproteins (luggage) carrying excess LDL cholesterol (illegal drugs) are brought back to the liver (airport personnel), which determines where it goes. Sometimes, your luggage gets lost and doesn't make its way back to airport personnel to determine its final destination. Likewise, sometimes lipoproteins (luggage) get embedded in the arteries causing arterial plaque buildup (lost luggage) and never makes its way back to be examined by the liver to determine its final destination: whether it will be either recycled or sent to your bowels where it is excreted in your feces.

Lipoproteins are made from a mixture of protein and lipids (triglycerides and cholesterol). The medical community puts lipoproteins into different (transportation) categories because cholesterol consists of three parts and two of the parts can't dissolve in water/blood. This means that cholesterol needs something to transport it throughout the body. Cholesterol is transported by various lipoproteins and the transportation methods determine what the cholesterol is called. In other words, there are various types of lipoproteins that transport cholesterol, but lipoproteins are not part of cholesterol. [7-11]

LDL and HDL Cholesterol

LDL and HDL cholesterol have different functions. Both HDL cholesterol and LDL cholesterol are required for good health. Both can be broken into subtypes by reclassifying their density, but it starts getting very technical from that point on. In fact, there are some lipoproteins that doctors have yet to figure out how to measure in blood tests. Therefore, we feel it's best to keep it simple and focus on what matters most: your ratio between HDL (good cholesterol) and total cholesterol!

Even though HDL and LDL are not actually cholesterol, we use the terms HDL cholesterol and LDL cholesterol throughout this book to simplify things. LDL is low-density lipoprotein that delivers cholesterol throughout your body. HDL is high-density lipoprotein that transports any leftover LDL back to the liver where it can be metabolized efficiently. The function of your liver helps determine how much cholesterol is in your body. Next, your liver makes a decision on whether or not to recycle or eliminate the LDL from your body. If your liver decides to produce more lipoproteins to carry extra cholesterol around the body you end up with a higher number of LDL cholesterol.[1]

Functional Alert: When following a diet higher in protein, probiotics, and soluble fiber/prebiotics and lower in carbs and fats, you end up with fewer lipids and more protein, which forms the HDL (good) version of lipoprotein. Likewise, when following a diet lower in protein, probiotics, and soluble fiber/prebiotics and higher in carbs and fats, you end up with more lipids and less protein, which forms the LDL (bad) version of lipoprotein! Therefore, you want to eat a high-protein, high-probiotic, high-soluble fiber/high-prebiotic diet, with fewer carbs and fats in order to boost HDL cholesterol and decrease the amount of LDL cholesterol made in your liver![2-4]

If your total cholesterol and/or triglycerides is too high, this may be an indication that your body has persistent high blood sugar or is insulin resistant, thus triggering the liver to produce excessive LDL cholesterol and triglycerides. However, it can also mean that the liver is clogged with too much fat and can't effectively filter the cholesterol out of the blood. Once your liver begins to malfunction, your immune system is compromised.

The Causes of Heart Disease

There's are many factors that play a role in heart disease. Excess cholesterol and chronically elevated or imbalanced sugar and/or insulin levels play a major role. Cholesterol comes from your diet in the form of all dietary fats to some degree and saturated fats and trans fats to a large degree. Dietary fats increase LDL cholesterol and play a role in the buildup of plaque and blockages of your arteries. However, plaque buildup becomes much more pronounced when carbohydrates (especially those with a high insulin production) are included.[1] Consuming carbohydrates, especially refined carbohydrates also increases your LDL cholesterol levels.[2] Cholesterol, which is being produced naturally in the liver, can be significantly lowered through Functional Diet, Functional Training, and Functional Cardio. Any extra cholesterol comes from your diet. (About 25% of the cholesterol produced resides in your brain to help it function properly, but too much, causes plaque deposits in the brain.[3]) Due to genetics, some people can eat foods that produce more cholesterol and still have low or healthy blood cholesterol levels. Likewise, some people can eat foods that produce less cholesterol and have a high blood cholesterol level.

Here are the facts: About 75% of heart attack victims have normal to low LDL cholesterol levels.[4] You're probably asking yourself, How could this be, if cholesterol causes heart disease? Research tells us that total levels of LDL cholesterol alone aren't the only cause of heart disease. In fact, endothelium dysfunction is the #1 cause of heart disease![5] The endothelium is the inner lining of the arteries. The endothelium lines the entire circulatory system, which delivers oxygen and vital nutrients to cells in all parts of the body and eliminates waste.[6] The primary cause of endothelium dysfunction is chronically elevated or unstable blood sugar/insulin levels.[7,8] This is why diabetics have more heart disease! Allow us to give a simplified explanation of how plaque buildup occurs:

1. A diet composed of too many carbs or too many carbs and fats is the primary factor that causes excess or unstable blood sugar/insulin levels.

2. Excess or unstable blood sugar/insulin damages the endothelium. Once the endothelium becomes damaged, it forms pits and becomes jagged. As a result both large- and small-sized LDL is trapped inside the pits where it becomes oxidized and turns into OxLDL. Excess blood-sugar levels are suspect for causing LDL cholesterol to shrink and become more easily trapped. Smaller LDL oxidizes faster than larger LDL because it's harder for HDL to remove from the endothelium.[9-30]

3. OxLDL causes chronic inflammation inside the arteries. This signals the immune system to send out white blood cells to engulf the OxLDL. The white blood cells then turn into foam cells. HDL cholesterol comes to the rescue and pulls the foam

cells off the arterial wall and takes them to the liver where they are disposed of through the bile.[31-32]

4. When there's an excess of foam cells, a shortage of HDL occurs, and they can't get all the foam cells off before they turn into plaque. Consuming moderate to excessive amounts of refined sugar compounds the problem by significantly lowering HDL levels.[33]

Functional Alert: As we age, it's inevitable that we will accumulate some plaque buildup in our arteries. **Functional Training with a Fork** will significantly delay arterial plaque buildup regardless of your genetics!

It's important to note that chronic inflammation and oxidation causes damage to the endothelium. (The human body requires some inflammation and oxidation to maintain good health because the tissues and organs are in a constant state of repair.) As previously stated, the pits inside the arteries are primarily caused by excess or unstable blood sugar/insulin levels that cause chronic inflammation and oxidation. Other factors that cause damage to the endothelium and increase inflammation and oxidation are a lack of Functional Exercise and Internal and External Dysfunctional Toxins such as high blood pressure, excess LDL and triglycerides, obesity, excess cortisol release from chronic stress, hormonal imbalances, bacteria imbalances in the GI tract, smoking, and excess amounts of alcohol. It's important to note that the possibility of getting heart disease is 300% more likely to occur when C-reactive protein levels become chronically elevated from excess amounts of pro-inflammatory cytokines and free radicals.[34, 35]

Functional Alert: Heart disease, Alzheimer's, and erectile dysfunction share common risk factors!

Plaque that forms on damaged areas of the endothelium is built on a less stable foundation. As plaque continues to form on a damaged area, it becomes less stable and is more likely to rupture. This is the most dangerous kind of plaque because once it ruptures, it turns into a blood clot. It can block off blood flow or travel to another area of the body. If the blood clot blocks off blood flow to the heart it causes a heart attack. If it blocks a blood vessel that feeds the brain, it causes a stroke.

Functional Alert: An aneurysm is abnormal swelling of a blood vessel (artery) due to chronic inflammation and oxidation. An aneurysm can occur in any part of the body. The most common type of aneurysm is an abdominal aortic aneurysm. Aneurysms of the brain are also quite common. Aneurysms can leak causing severe headaches or stroke-like symptoms. Many aneurysm rupture and kill within seconds! [36]

The most common causes of heart disease in today's society are from chronically elevated or unstable blood sugar/insulin levels from consuming too many carbs or too many fats, and especially from combining too many carbs and fats in the same meal. Combining refined sugar with saturated fat and/or tran fat is the worst! Think of carbs or fats as a fire and mixing carbs and fats in the same meal as pouring gas on the flames! For example, combining a baked potato with a fatty steak in the same meal is a recipe for disaster. However, you can take out the baked potato (starchy carb) to help stabilize blood sugar and insulin levels that would otherwise be increased and/or become unstable. In other words, now you are helping control the fire! In addition, you can add Free Foods (non-starchy carbs) to the fatty steak and still keep the fire under control because mixing them with fats doesn't cause excess or unstable blood sugar and/or insulin levels in the way starchy carbs would if they were eaten with the steak.

It's important to separate your carbs and fats in each meal to the best of your ability to keep the fire under control. You can have a lean chicken breast, with a salad using non-fat dressing (e.g., mustard mixed with artificial sweetener and a little water) or fat-free cheese, and a dry, baked potato. On the other hand, if you decide to eat a fatty steak, you can eat a salad with a tiny amount of olive oil or shredded cheese, but no baked potato. Adding the baked potato full of carbs that secrete insulin along with the steak full of dietary fats will chronically elevate blood sugar and insulin levels!

Functional Alert: After consuming a steak and a salad without a potato, there will be less blood sugar/insulin around; therefore, our bodies can more readily use the fats from the steak for energy. Furthermore, adding Free Foods to a meal composed of carbs, fats, or carbs and fats does little to lower insulin secretion. It boils down to the fact that Free Foods, such as a green, leafy salad, don't increase insulin levels in the same way starchy carbs would!

Blood-sugar levels and insulin production from mixing carbs and fats in the same meal is different from one person to another due to body-fat levels and genetics. Keep in mind that your lab work can show that your blood sugar is normal, but your body still may be producing too much insulin because of your diet or body fat. This means that you can still be damaging the inner lining of your arteries, which allows LDL cholesterol to more readily build up as plaque.

Once body-fat levels are reduced and more muscle tone is built, less insulin will be secreted in relation to food consumption. This makes maintaining desirable body-fat levels easier. Even people with fast metabolisms who are not overweight should avoid mixing a lot of carbs and fats in the same meal. They may appear slim on the outside, but damage will still be occurring on the inside of the body. This is what makes highly processed and fast food so harmful!

We also know from personal experience that when people are eating a lot of carbs or mix a lot of carbs and fats together in the same meal, they are actually hungrier and have less energy. They get lazy and want more food, more often! That is just the way our bodies work. A lot of people don't start getting concerned until they begin developing problems such as high blood pressure, high blood sugar, high cholesterol, or high triglycerides. For most people, the decision to limit their carb and fat intake was as much about reducing their cholesterol, blood pressure, and sugar levels as it was about losing body fat.

Topping carbs such as pasta, potatoes, and breads with fats such as butter, extra virgin olive oil, cheese, and sour cream leads to hyperinsulinemia and serious weight gain. Moreover, saturated fats, such as butter, are even worse than unsaturated fats, such as extra virgin olive oil, because they cause more insulin resistance without any carbohydrates being present. When you consume high amounts of saturated fats from processed meats, such as sausage, bacon, etc., along with high glycemic carbs, such as white flour and refined sugar, your body secretes more insulin for a longer period of time. It becomes worse than a fire. It's more like a wildfire that causes a lot of damage and takes much longer to get under control.

Numerous people are doing themselves a great disservice. We have seen a lot of people go on a diet and lose weight before their doctor appointment. The reasons they do this is so their doctors won't fuss or so they can avoid being put on prescription medications or taking larger doses when their lab results come back. It's not uncommon for their lab results to come back in the normal range. However, a week later their lab results would be anything but normal! They go back to eating incorrectly and gain all the weight back. Some doctors don't realize that many of their patients are pre-diabetic. The only people who can benefit from such reckless behavior are their potential beneficiaries. Millions of Americans are pre-diabetic and don't even know it. The A1C testing method can help detect pre-diabetic conditions in some, which would otherwise go undetected using standard methods. We believe that testing for A1C values provides a more accurate measurement of sugar levels than the fasting blood-sugar test. This is because your A1C shows your average blood-sugar level over a three-month period. However, A1C testing can't detect all the blood sugar spikes people are having after eating meals composed of too many carbs and/or fats. When their blood-sugar levels spike, significant thickening of the blood occurs, which causes a reduction of oxygen. These spikes in blood sugar are causing a lot of people to take medications to thin their blood, lower blood pressure, and reduce cholesterol. These medications have potentially dangerous side effects. There is a good chance you can get off these medications. **Functional Training with a Fork** is the prescription you need for preventing spikes in blood sugar and insulin and the terrible side effects that go along with them!

Functional Alert: Cholesterol medications help lower LDL cholesterol, but they don't prevent the endothelium from becoming damaged by chronically elevated or unstable blood sugar/insulin levels![16]

We also think it would be wise for you to ask your physician to order a C-reactive protein (CRP) test to check for severe inflammation and oxidation, in addition to the other cardiovascular tests, such as cholesterol and blood sugar, in order to try to detect other forms of consistent inflammation and oxidation. Unfortunately, there is no diagnostic test that shows all inflammation and oxidation inside the body. This means you have to take responsibly for your own actions and choose between an anti-inflammatory/oxidative lifestyle and a pro-inflammatory/oxidative lifestyle. Pro-inflammatory/oxidative choices add up over time and one day chronic inflammation and oxidation will kill you!

Hormones and Cholesterol

Functional Hormone Replacement improves liver function to optimize cholesterol levels. Functional Hormone Replacement is defined as treatment by a well-trained physician based on your symptoms, not by a scale that supposedly predicts what is considered to be normal hormone levels for your age. There are numerous studies showing the positive effects of healthy levels of testosterone and estrogen on male and female cholesterol levels. A lack of testosterone causes a lack of estrogen. Testosterone converts to estrogen which lowers LDL (bad) cholesterol and increases HDL (good) cholesterol.[1] When estrogen levels get low near menopause (women) or andropause (men), the bad cholesterol goes up and the good cholesterol goes down![2] Your cholesterol gets out of whack from this lack of testosterone and estrogen. In addition, the diminishing supply of estrogen causes a diminishing supply of nitric oxide![3] Estrogen stimulates the release of nitric oxide. Nitric oxide penetrates the underlying smooth muscles and makes the arteries expand, lowering blood pressure and decreasing inflammation and oxidation. It also helps lower the production of excess white blood cells that would otherwise thicken the blood and cause further inflammation and oxidation. Adequate amounts of estrogen help put a stop to heart disease, sexual dysfunction, and brain neurodegeneration by improving blood flow and preventing damage to the endothelium (inner lining of the arteries).

Functional Alert: It's important to note that a small amount of testosterone gets converted into estrogen, which is also important for maintaining healthy cholesterol levels, especially in men because they don't take estrogen replacement. Healthy progesterone levels in females stimulate lipoprotein lipase that the cells use to break down triglycerides, resulting in lower triglyceride levels.[4, 5] Low thyroid levels and excess cortisol also increase LDL cholesterol![6]

The liver is the body's largest organ and it plays a key role in maintaining healthy immune functions. The liver recruits and circulates white blood cells that play critical roles in first-line immune defense against invading Dysfunctional Toxins.[7] If fat forms around the liver due to not having enough testosterone to prevent insulin resistance, it will begin to malfunction and be unable to handle the excess LDL and triglycerides coming in. The LDL and triglycerides will then congregate in the arteries, causing inflammation/oxidation and plaque buildup. A recent study by Bayer Schering Pharma in Berlin found that testosterone therapy significantly improved liver disease.[8, 9]

Functional Alert: Healthy testosterone levels regulate pro-inflammatory cytokine expression, specifically TNF-a and IL-1B. Inappropriate expression can create an immune response that damages the endothelium.[10, 11] Testosterone helps prevents damage to the endothelium by improving the communication link between the endothelium and the immune system!

We understand that there are some people who need cardiovascular drugs such as statins, blood thinners, high blood pressure meds, etc. However, we believe most people would be a lot healthier and look and feel better using a Functional Diet, Functional Hormone Replacement, Functional Training, and Functional Cardio, while leaving all those other medicines alone. For the people who are at an average risk with only modestly raised LDL cholesterol levels, statins are probably a bad idea. You have to look at the overall picture and realize we live in a capitalist society. Highly priced cardiovascular drugs generate a considerable amount of profits for some pharmaceutical companies.[12-14] When taken as a whole, the vast number of studies in regard to Functional Hormone Replacement show a reduction in obesity, diabetes, heart disease, stroke, cancer, and autoimmune disease when hematocrit levels are kept in normal ranges and estrogen dominance is avoided. Functional Hormone Replacement is available to Americans at a very affordable price. Some pharmaceutical companies would face huge economic losses if a lot of people used the inexpensive hormone testosterone to reduce their reliance on a vast array of expensive prescription drugs. On the other hand, insurance companies would save a ton of money in the long run. We'll let them fight that one out!

Functional Alert: We believe that some doctors are too quick to say medical problems, such as high cholesterol, are due to genetics as opposed to one's lifestyle. If you have high blood sugar, high cholesterol, and high blood pressure, ask your doctor about **Functional Training with a Fork**!

With the new era of socialized medicine coming into effect, there is an increased demand for many drugs, especially drugs to help control high blood sugar, high cholesterol, and high blood pressure. Now, more than ever, it becomes highly important to use affordable hormones, exercise, and nutrition to remain healthy because a lot of the other drugs are silently doubling and, in some instances, tripling in price![15] In addition, **Functional Training with a Fork** is the healthy route.

Some people have to use a statin to reduce the amount of LDL cholesterol in their blood streams, but these drugs often cause a host of side effects, such as memory loss, immune system dysfunction, sexual dysfunction, muscle pain/weakness, and CoQ10 deficiency that in and of itself can lead to heart failure or the need for a pacemaker.[16-24] We feel it's best to stay away from statins unless you fall into the category of having excess amounts of LDL cholesterol that cannot be controlled solely with a Functional Diet, Functional Hormone Replacement, Functional Training, and Functional Cardio.

Functional Alert: Low testosterone and estrogen is a common trait in men and women suffering from heart failure. People who experience chronic heart failure have high rates of depression and sexual dysfunction. Proper Hormone Replacement for men and women leads to major improvements in moods and sexual function after having had a heart attack. Using antidepressants to combat depression usually causes sexual side effects and more heart problems![25]

Functional Training, Muscle Tone, and the Immune System

Functional Training amplifies the immune system by increasing muscle tone! Our blood is composed of approximately 60% water.[1] The muscular system is composed of approximately 75% water.[2] Muscles attract water like a magnet. They share water with other parts of the body, allowing them to stay more efficiently hydrated.[3] Functional Training is needed to build muscle tissue, especially the type-2 muscle fibers. These larger muscle fibers are highly responsible for hydrating the body and increasing the blood's ability to supply cells with oxygen, which improves immune system and organ functions. Functional Cardio, which mostly focuses on training the type-1 fibers, doesn't help improve hydration of the body to any appreciable degree. In fact, too much cardio can cause a decrease in the type-2 muscle fibers and cause dehydration.

If you want to prevent your cells from becoming damaged or mutating, give them plenty of oxygen with Functional Training and muscle tone! A lack of oxygen is linked to all forms of diseases. Oxygen helps keep inflammation/oxidation under control; however, low oxygen causes chronic inflammation/oxidation and damages the body, forcing the immune system to work overtime. For example, kidneys need oxygen-rich blood cells to do their job. When the kidneys don't get enough oxygen, they develop fibrous tissue that causes them to malfunction.[4] When your kidneys begin to malfunction, you no longer have a functional filtration system to remove Dysfunctional Toxins from your body. This poisons the body and over-works the immune system. Oxygen is needed in each cell in your body if you are to remain alive. Your blood supplies the body with the nutrients it needs for good health. It does little good to eat a diet rich in nutrients if it's not being delivered to the cells through oxygenated blood. A lack of nutrients is linked to all forms of chronic diseases.

Functional Alert: Functional Training-induced muscle tone reduces the production of pro-inflammatory cytokines and free radicals![5]

The amazing thing about the muscles is they act as a reservoir to fuel the immune system. An optimal functioning immune system requires an abundance of muscle tone, which is made up of amino acids. The muscles and immune system need a constant blood supply of amino acids, derived from protein-based foods, to remain intact. When the body gets low on amino acids it produces more pro-inflammatory cytokines and free radicals.[6] Muscle tissue is made up of mostly amino acids derived from protein we consume in our diet. Glutamine makes up approximately 50% of amino acids located in the blood stream and muscles.[7] Approximately 60% of intracellular muscle is composed of glutamine.[8] All cells require glutamine as an energy source for cell-specific functions. Glutamine lowers inflammation and oxidation and boost the body's ability to increase its level of growth hormone.[9-11] The body doesn't have a long-term storage supply of amino acids other than muscle tissue. It's very common for cancer victims to lose most of their muscle tissue because their over-worked immune system revs up protein metabolism.[12] As a result, their bodies eat into muscle tissue once they devour all the dietary protein. Muscle loss causes a decline in white blood cells because they are using up their reserve of amino acids! These white blood cells make up a large portion of the immune system and help destroy cells infected with viruses, various cancers, etc. The function of the immune system relies on glutamine as one of its main fuel sources.[13-15] This vital amino acid can be reduced by as much as 50% in your muscles during times of chronic inflammation and oxidation, with accompanying tiredness, weakness, and fatigue.[16]

Functional Alert: Glutamine has a vital role in removing the waste product ammonia from the body.[17] Elevated blood ammonia can affect brain tissue, leading to symptoms such as confusion. Immune system function and brain function decline as we age. However, we can help compensate by maintaining muscle tone and consuming adequate protein!

Another amazing thing your muscles do is supply your body with the master antioxidant glutathione. This is the most important antioxidant for preventing free radical damage! Some of the glutamine in your body gets converted into glutathione.[18] The glutathione is shipped to inflamed tissues and organs as needed for the removal of Dysfunctional Toxins, such as heavy metals. Your immune system is functionally divided into tissues and organs.[19] These two locations are where immune functions begin and where balance is preserved in the body. This means that maintaining muscle tone results in higher glutathione levels, which keeps excess Dysfunctional Toxins out of organs and tissues and improves immune functions!

It has been reported that critically ill patients with chronic inflammation and oxidation have a significantly increased need for glutamine.[20] Low levels of glutamine have been proven to be an independent factor for causing death. Glutamine helps repair and replace stomach lining in order to enhance nutrient absorption. There have been a number of research studies that show that having an adequate blood supply of glutamine is associated with intestinal health.[21] A lack of glutamine weakens the functions of your immune system and causes problems with absorbing nutrients. This leaves you susceptible to a wide array of infections and vitamins and mineral deficiencies. People with various forms of irritable bowel syndrome (IBS) find that a high-protein diet has a soothing effect. There are also people who find it necessary to add L-glutamine in supplement form in addition to their daily diet to assist in controlling IBS. When nutrients are better absorbed, your immune system functions more efficiently to help fight off various diseases. The health of your digestive system is very important in establishing long-term, health-related goals.

Dehydration and the Immune System

Without water you would die. Your immune system works better when your muscles and organs are functioning properly. Water helps immune system functions by:

- Delivering nutrients and oxygen to the cells of the body.
- Carrying white blood cells from the bone marrow throughout the entire body.

HOW THE IMMUNE SYSTEM FUNCTIONS

- ☐ Improving the function of the digestive system so food can properly digest and deliver vitamins and minerals to specific areas.

- ☐ Removing Dysfunctional Toxins from the blood stream through urination (kidneys) and the bowels (liver).

    Stay well-hydrated on a daily basis—even if you have to force yourself to drink sufficient amounts of water! Start hydrating before you feel thirsty. Water works directly with your kidneys and indirectly with your liver to filter out Dysfunctional Toxins.[1] That empty-pit feeling in your belly is often not hunger for food, but rather your body telling you it's hungry for fluids. Hunger is often a sign your body is dehydrated.[2] If you don't get enough to drink, you will feel tired and hungry because your body thinks it needs food for energy. These signals begin before you even feel thirsty.

    Staying well-hydrated helps keep your blood thinner, making it a natural way to help the heart pump blood more efficiently. Thinner blood is less likely to form clots![3] Staying well-hydrated increases your metabolism and causes less wear and tear on the internal organs.[4] Water also helps keep your connective tissues and joints well-hydrated, which helps deter degeneration. Water is also needed for muscle repair and nutrient absorption of foods during digestion. A lack of water causes mild constipation that slowly poisons your body. Dehydration results in the body producing more histamine, which make any allergies you might have inherited become worse.[5]

    Dehydration leads to headaches, lack of libido, dizziness, low or high blood pressure, and a rapid heartbeat because the heart needs to pump faster to make up for having less oxygenated blood being delivered to cells. When blood begins to thicken, your heart rate stays elevated for longer periods of time. Hematocrit levels rise, which thicken blood and increase your chances of having a heart attack or stroke. Thick blood causes wear and tear on your organs in the same way a car engine low on oil can damage parts.

Functional Alert: Dehydration causes the body to produce excess amounts of pro-inflammatory cytokines and free radicals![6]

When you become dehydrated, your ability to breathe is greatly affected. Your lungs need fluid to decrease mucous.[7] The main function of your respiratory system is to provide oxygen for the body's cells and remove the carbon dioxide they produce.[8] Carbon dioxide is formed when the body uses oxygen as part of the process of converting sugar to energy.[9] If you allow yourself to become dehydrated, lung function decreases and the removal of carbon dioxide will be inferior.[10] Your blood cells will become inflamed and oxidized and they will irritate the inner lining of the arteries, encouraging plaque buildup and an overactive immune system! When you become dehydrated, carbon dioxide takes the place of the oxygen you need to remain alive. You must remain hydrated so carbon dioxide can be removed from the cells, transported through the blood, and eliminated from the body through the lungs or you will die!

Functional Alert: The human brain is composed of 95% water.[11] Headaches, the most common health complaint, are usually caused from dehydration, electrolyte imbalances, high blood pressure, neck pain, unmanaged stress, and hormonal imbalances, such as low testosterone and/or estrogen levels![12]

Unlike muscle tissue, fat tissue holds very little usable water. Water makes up roughly 55% of your blood that circulates and provides nutrients and oxygen to the body.[13] Around 65% of the non-obese human body is made of water whereas obese people's bodies are made up of only 45% water.[14] This is a key reason why obese people are more prone to dehydration and blood clots! It's even worse for those lacking muscle tone. Your bones are composed of about 50% of water and your muscles, approximately 75%.[15]

When the body as a whole begins getting low on water, the muscles will share water with other surrounding tissues and organs to keep balance. Having more muscle throughout the body means having more water on reserve for vital organs, tissues, and cells during times of need! We are often unaware of the fact that our body as a whole is becoming dehydrated until we begin to get a headache or feel fatigued. Different parts of the body are like warehouses that hold water. It's a concept similar to how the body stores glutamine in the muscles and shares with other organs, tissues, and cells when needed.

Functional Alert: It's a myth that drinking plenty of water helps flush fat from your system. However, staying well-hydrated allows the kidneys to function optimally, which prevents the liver from having to work overtime. The end result is the liver metabolizes more fat and your thyroid functions better! [16]

Loss of type-2 muscle fibers encourages dehydration! In the elderly, body water content begins to decline because their type-2 muscles decline in number. Most of this can be reversed with Functional Training and Functional Hormone Replacement! Less muscle tone coming from type-2 fibers means less water circulating around the body, which also means less blood, oxygen, and nutrients circulating. This is one reason a lot of elderly people stay cold.

Functional Alert: There is a dehydration epidemic among elderly people all across the world![17]

Water and the Immune System

Water is nature's best diuretic. The more water you drink, the more water you will eliminate, up to a point, when consumed with a high-protein, lower-carb diet in addition to the proper amounts of sodium. If you drink more water, you will end up needing to go to the restroom more often for a while. It might seem like an inconvenience at first, but it's worth it in order to remain fully hydrated and eliminate any excess water retention and Dysfunctional Toxins that may be lingering in your blood stream outside the cells. Drinking more water helps prevent kidney strain and aids the immune system in fighting off infection.

Various tissues, organs, etc., are made up of cells.[1] Water exists both inside and outside our body's cells. You need water in both areas for good health. It's very important to know the locations inside the body of excess water you are trying to eliminate, as well as the location of water you want to retain.

Extracellular space means "outside the cell."[2] You want to get rid of any excess water in the extracellular space because it causes edema and fluid retention in the organs, which is linked to breathing problems, high blood pressure, increased pulse rate, cirrhosis of the liver, kidney failure, heart failure, and dementia! Excess water retention outside the cells becomes exaggerated when you have high blood pressure, kidney dysfunction, or heart dysfunction, which cause the volume of extracellular fluid surrounding the cells to be greater than normal. Edema or swelling can appear throughout the entire body or be localized in certain parts. The buildup of excess fluid gets stored in the circulatory system and body tissues beneath the skin.

Excess water can often be seen around the face, feet, ankles, and stomach. Water retention makes you feel sluggish, gives you a puffy look, and hides muscle tone. Excess water retention causes the body to produce excess amounts of pro-inflammatory cytokines and free radicals.[3] Failing to drink enough fluids ironically causes water retention because without sufficient water in the extracellular space, fluid continues to shift out of the cells into that space.[4] This causes the cells to shrink and impairs cellular function and the immune system![5-7] However, adequate amounts of extracellular water (fluid outside the cell) are necessary because the water hydrates your organs, such as your brain, which are constantly monitoring and repairing your body for daily functions. Extracellular water also oxygenates your blood and keeps your muscles looking toned, since muscle is mostly composed of this water. Therefore, the lack of extracellular hydration and excess water retention is detrimental to your health!

Functional Alert: It is quite common for people to think they are holding water, when in reality they are holding body fat! Body fat makes you look as if you are holding water. When you are lean, you look as if you are holding very little water. When you are super lean, you appear as if you are holding no water at all!

Water retention (excess extracellular water) can also be caused by the thyroid not functioning properly. Having low-thyroid hormones impairs the kidneys' filtering abilities, causing fluid imbalances throughout the entire body.[8] A lack of iodine (generally obtained from table salt) and/or sugar/insulin imbalances, are known culprits for causing thyroid dysfunction.[9,10] Thyroid dysfunction occurs when the immune system produces excessive amounts of antibodies that attack the thyroid gland.[11]

Intracellular space means "inside the cell."[12] This is the water you want to retain because it increases overall oxygenation and improves cellular and immune function! Allow us to illustrate: Putting water in your body is like putting fuel in your car. Until the water (oxygenated fuel) gets into your cell (the engine) it won't run.

While drinking adequate amounts of water helps eliminate excess water retention outside the cells, it actually increases water inside the cells. Drinking adequate amounts of water helps with the removal of Dysfunctional Toxins from the GI tract, blood, tissues, and organs, which prevents immune system malfunction. The lack of intracellular water is strongly linked to the onset of many life-threatening illnesses and a lack of vital nutrients being metabolized inside the cell.

Having adequate water inside the cells prevents your body temperature from changing rapidly. If your body temperatures gets too hot or too cold from a lack of water, they often prevent water from getting inside the cells.[13,14] It's extremely important that you drink enough water so that oxygen can get into the cells and the lungs can eliminate carbon dioxide. When there is a combination of high carbon dioxide levels and low oxygen levels, cells, tissues, organs, and the immune system can no longer work in sequence and together as a multifunctional system.[15]

Functional Alert: Staying well-hydrated helps prevent the formation of kidney stones. A water hardness above 5 mmol/L is linked to a higher incidence of kidney stones for those who are genetically prone to this ailment.[16] Adding a little lemon juice to your water aids in preventing calcium stones by increasing citrate levels to deter formation. However, you can't use other juices to get the same effect because they don't lower calcium levels, and some juices increase oxalate levels that can actually lead to the formation of more kidney stones![17] Supplementing with magnesium also reduces the recurrence rate of calcium oxalate kidney stones!

Excess Water Consumption

Too much water consumption can lead to overhydration, causing hyponatremia. This condition causes you to have low sodium, potassium, magnesium, and calcium levels and is harmful to your overall health.[1] It leads to the overproduction of pro-inflammatory cytokines and free radicals. It also causes cells to swell, resulting in muscle cramps, nausea, and even death. Under normal circumstances, hyponatremia doesn't usually occur unless your water intake exceeds approximately 2 gallons or 256 ounces (32 glasses of water per day). Obviously, people who sweat a lot due to exercising or working in hot and/or humid weather need to replenish their fluids. They will also need to consume more sodium, potassium, magnesium, and calcium. Most people who exercise under normal circumstances who consume a high-protein diet can remain fully hydrated drinking half a gallon (64 ounces, 8 glasses of water) to 1 gallon (128 ounces, 16 glasses of water) per day. In general, people who weigh more and/or have more muscle require more water. You also get water from some foods (e.g., drinking liquid egg whites mixed with one yogurt) and fruits and vegetables.

Functional Alert: The use of serotonin-specific reuptake inhibitors (a class of drugs typically used as antidepressants) can cause hyponatremia.[2] Drugs that help control high blood pressure can do the same. This helps explain why dry mouth is a common side effect of these drugs.

Drinking caffeinated beverages causes some dehydration. Therefore, if you drink a cup of coffee or unsweetened tea, only half of that cup should count toward your daily fluid intake. Contrary to popular belief, carbonated beverages are still moderately effective at hydrating the body even though they are not healthy. Carbonated drinks contain phosphoric acid, which is associated with kidney dysfunction, bone loss, and an increased risk of developing kidney stones.[3,4] Fortunately, more people are drinking fewer carbonated drinks and more noncarbonated drinks, such as bottled water, artificially sweetened bottled water, and sugar-free sports drinks containing electrolytes.

Functional Alert: Intake of sports drinks containing sugar are bad for your health and will cause you to gain body fat!

Alcoholic beverages don't count toward your daily fluid intake because they lower the body's production of antidiuretic hormone which causes severe dehydration.[5] Drinking plain water all day can be a little hard to stomach for some people. Therefore, you may need to drink something artificially sweetened. It's important to drink enough fluids to stay hydrated. Dehydration can actually cause stomach upset!

Coffee and tea are full of antioxidants that provide numerous health benefits![6] Organic coffee and tea are the healthier choice because most conventional coffee and tea are heavily sprayed with high-risk synthetic pesticides.[7] It's important to remember that they come from all over the world. Some of these places spray their coffee and tea with Endosulfan and Carbofuran. The Environmental Protection Agency and World Health Organization believe both of these high-risk pesticides are cancer-causing agents.[8,9] Some of the coffee and tea coming from outside the United States have tested positive for the high-risk pesticide DDT.[10] This pesticide was banned many years ago because of its ability to cause a 5-fold increased risk in cancer![11]

Functional Alert: Don't wait until you are recovering from cancer to get away from normal store-bought coffee and tea with all the high-risk pesticides!

A moderate amount of sugar-free, caffeinated coffee will help boost metabolism and suppress your appetite. Decaffeinated coffee will also suppress your appetite. Don't rely on excessive amounts of caffeinated coffee to boost your metabolism because it's not healthy and it can cause anxiety, headaches, dehydration, and an energy crash. A good plan is to drink some caffeinated coffee or tea in the morning with breakfast and thirty minutes before workouts to boost metabolism and energy, and to relax air passages so you breathe more freely.[12] Drink a little decaffeinated coffee at other times of the day to help suppress appetite. People who are sensitive to caffeine need to drink only decaffeinated coffee.

Water Sources

There is no perfect water source! An abundant supply of clean, safe drinking water is essential for good health. The lifespans of humans have increased due to improvements in modern-day plumbing and the quarantine of toxic waste dumps, which can infiltrate our water sources. But we live in a society where Dysfunctional Toxins are constantly leeching from spills in factories and running off farmland into water sources where we obtain our drinking water. The constant recycling of water from our homes, businesses, hospitals, etc., prevents it from being 100% free of Dysfunctional Toxins.

Functional Alert: The majority of bacteria found in drinking water comes from the filters of water treatment plants.[1] We believe their filters need to be changed with greater frequency to prevent the buildup of dangerous bacteria. This same rule applies to house water filters!

Tap water, like all drinking water produced in the United States, is continuously tested and monitored.[2] No water-purification device can remove every Dysfunctional Toxin. Even after being purified at a water treatment plant, our drinking water often contains extremely low levels of Dysfunctional Toxins (e.g., antidepressants, antibiotics, the sex hormone estrogen, pesticides, lead, arsenic, fluoride, and chlorine).[3] Every water source available (city tap water, well water, bottled water/spring water, filtered water, softened water, and distilled water) has its pros and cons, and it's up to you as an individual to figure out which water source or sources you choose to drink. The truth is, all water sources are usually fine to drink and the idea that certain types of water are superior at promoting cellular hydration and eliminating Dysfunctional Toxins from the body has no scientific basis.

We recommend that you check your annual Water Quality Report, which provides testing results and a list of possible Dysfunctional Toxins in your water.[4] You can usually find testing results on your water provider's website or have them mailed to you. This will help determine if there are Dysfunctional Toxins present in your water that need to be dealt with more aggressively in order to prevent the weakening of your immune system. Every city is required to publish reports about the safety and quality of their drinking water system. If your local water source is below standard, then you have other options (e.g., use a carbon filter, install a reverse osmosis system with a carbon filter, drink distilled water, or purchase bottled drinking water from a reputable water bottling company). If you do decide you want to install an in-home filtration system, you should have your water tested by a certified independent laboratory first to find out what's in your water. Beware of companies that try to sell water-treatment devices by offering to test tap water at no cost. Free offers to test your water are usually part of a sales promotion.[5]

Functional Alert: Water is water in terms of hydrating the body! Don't fall for all these marketing scams about structure-altered waters that make false claims and use scare tactics to try to sell you their products. There are a lot of myths surrounding these products!

Electrolytes and the Immune System

Salt intake for normal, healthy people should be around 1,500-2,500 mgs per day, depending on their needs. Excess salt consumption is a huge problem in today's society. It causes high blood pressure, which injures the blood vessel walls and invites plaque buildup. As a rule, people who consume more carbs need to consume less salt. This is because carbs cause more water retention and adding too much salt with them can make you swell. Salt is mostly composed of sodium chloride and, to a lesser degree, potassium iodine.[1] Sodium is a mineral required by your body for many critical processes, such as controlling blood pressure and fluid balance in your body. Sodium is needed for sufficient nerve impulses (e.g., brain and heart function), muscle contractions, and sexual function.[2] Without sodium, your muscles won't move. The electrical system of your heart begins to short-circuit without sufficient amounts of electrolytes (sodium, potassium, calcium, and magnesium). In fact, the underlying cause of cardiac muscle dysfunction that often kills a person is due to a lack of electrolytes. A sign of electrolyte imbalances is blood pressure changes![3] Consuming adequate amounts of sodium, calcium, potassium, and magnesium from fresh produce and/or supplements is important in keeping your blood pressure normal. Sodium, in conjunction with potassium, calcium, and magnesium, functions to properly adjust the amount of fluids inside and outside the cells.[4] When your sodium levels are extremely low or high, your blood becomes acidic, which leads to chronic inflammation/oxidation and immune system dysfunction![5-7]

Functional Alert: Sea salt and table salt have the same nutritional value.[8] Salt is your friend when used properly, but it can be an enemy and cause chronic inflammation/oxidation when abused. Everyone's requirements are a little different when it comes to water and salt. Athletes can suffer just as much from low-salt levels and other electrolytes as from low-water levels!

People with high blood pressure often need to slightly reduce salt intake in order to reduce water retention, whereas people with low blood pressure may need to slightly increase it to enhance water retention. Body-fat levels play a much larger role in reducing blood pressure than reducing sodium intake. If at all possible, we believe it's wise to lose edema around your ankles, feet, and abdomen through losing body fat, exercising, increasing water consumption, and reducing carbs and sodium, instead of taking potentially hazardous diuretics such as Lasix that often lower sodium, potassium, and magnesium levels too much. We believe the long-term use of some diuretics often leads to needing a pacemaker and other heart problems.[9] Side effects of losing excess sodium, potassium, and magnesium along with water are confusion, dizziness, headache, fatigue, muscle weakness, cramps, nausea, and sexual dysfunction.

Functional Alert: A lot of elderly people die from dehydration due to a lack of muscle tone, water, and electrolytes. It's also causing a lot of younger people to suffer from abnormal function of their cells, tissues, organs, nerves, muscles, and immune systems. People who have ADD/ADHD can often improve their concentration by taking a daily magnesium supplement!

Your sodium levels should remain moderate unless your doctor suggests otherwise due to a life-threatening condition such as kidney dysfunction or congestive heart failure. Sodium causes you to retain fluid and a healthy person needs to retain some fluid. Sodium prevents muscle and strength loss by maintaining a sodium-potassium muscle pump, and if your heart muscle stops, you die! Low sodium intake decreases blood pressure because it decreases water volume, which, in turn, lowers blood volume. Lowering sodium too much can cause the blood to thicken! Remember, blood is composed of around 55% water. Therefore, due to its dehydration effects, a lack of salt makes blood thicker in the areas of the body that need thinner blood to remain functional!

Functional Alert: A lot of people experience heart attacks early in the morning. It's often due to dehydration and/or sleep apnea. People tend to lose a lot of water through urination at night because their legs are level with their kidneys while lying down. This makes the kidneys remove more water than normal. To help counteract this, you'll want to make sure there will be plenty of water left in your system in the early morning hours before waking up. Make sure to drink some fluids before going to bed, but not in excess because you'll be up all night going to the bathroom. Also, eat some salt for dinner or during your pre-bedtime snack so that your body will retain more water. You'll find this helps prevent night-time dehydration, which can help prevent heart attacks, muscle cramps, joint pain, headaches, allergies/asthma, dry mouth, etc. Furthermore, your brain needs adequate water, some healthy fats, and protein before going to bed in order to produce melatonin for a good night's sleep.[10] Melatonin helps protect the brain tissue from chronic inflammation and oxidation, which helps protect against Alzheimer's and boosts cognitive function![11]

Ronnie and Kathy: *When following the protocol above, we need to empty our bladders less frequently at night which helps us get a better night's sleep. It also helps prevent morning headaches and brain fog because your brain is functioning on a full reserve of water. We usually get our sodium from various spices, mustard, or salt we put on our lean meat for dinner.*

Unknowingly allowing yourself to become dehydrated always results in a soft, smooth, flat appearance to the muscles. The fastest way to lose muscle tone is to drop sodium levels too low while trying to shed water weight. This is why getting into a hot tub will actually cause you to lose muscle tone unless water and electrolytes are quickly replenished. When salt content is reduced in your muscles, so is water content. Sodium attracts water, so less salt equals reduced water content in your cells, including your muscle cells. You need water in your cells for them to remain healthy, but you don't want too much. Potassium flows inside the cells and pushes excess sodium out to eliminate any excess water inside cells. This is referred to as the "sodium pump!"[10] There is more potassium inside the cells and more salt residing outside the cells. This is how it must be to have good health and prevent the release of excess pro-inflammatory cytokines and free radicals.

Functional Alert: Joint problems are one of the major causes of disability around the world. Pain and swelling increase when the cells inside the tissue have too much sodium and not enough potassium. Consuming excessive amounts of sodium and not enough potassium increases joint pain!

It's important to note that a high-carb, high-salt diet will cause your body to retain excess water in bad areas and your blood pressure to rise. Blood pressure rises because the heart has to pump harder to keep it moving through your veins and arteries. A high-protein (40% of daily calories), moderate-salt diet will help your body eliminate excess water in bad areas, causing blood pressure to go down. When consuming a high-protein diet, you should increase your fluid intake to prevent intracellular dehydration. Some may find the need to supplement with potassium and magnesium to avoid muscle cramps, nausea, abnormal weakness, anxiety, and irregular heartbeats. Most people get enough calcium in their daily diet if they consume yogurt on a daily basis. High levels of magnesium are rare because the body is very efficient at eliminating what is not needed. A potassium level that is too high or too low can be serious. When sodium levels go up, potassium levels go down, and vice versa.

Functional Alert: Adequate fluids and electrolytes are very important for processing protein and proper organ function. The immune system is a collection of cells that travel through the bloodstream. Every cell in your body is interrelated and requires electrical signals to function properly! It's recommended to consult your doctor as needed to have your electrolyte levels checked!

Functional Sex Improves Immune Functions

Functional Sex is the only kind of sex proven to dramatically enhance your overall feeling of well-being and the function of your immune system. Engaging in Functional Sex on a frequent basis is one of the most underrated things you can do to live a longer, happier life! The more Functional Sex you have with the one you love, the more your body secretes feel-good chemicals such as oxytocin and dopamine.[1] During orgasm, your body releases chemicals that boost immune functions and alleviate stress.[2] A Functional Sex life helps keep the immune system functioning properly by increasing immunoglobulin A (IgA) proteins and dramatically lowering stress. These proteins are the body's first line of defense against Dysfunctional Toxins. Researchers suggest that couples who have a Functional Sex life can live up to 8 years longer, whereas people who are indifferent to Functional Sex often die earlier.[3,4] People who engage in regular Functional Sex experience less prostate and breast cancer, prostate enlargement, urinary incontinence, risk of heart disease, and stroke.[5-7] They also enjoy exercise more than those who don't engage in Functional Sex, eat a healthier diet, watch their body fat, sleep better, have more youthful enthusiasm, obtain more relief from chronic pain, suffer from less depression, and have a greater appreciation for life! Functional Sex improves immune functions by producing more IgA.[8] IgA is an important antibody that compiles up to 15% of the total immunoglobulin produced in the entire body.[9] Functional sex decreases pro-inflammatory cytokines and free radicals.

Functional Alert: You must feel desirable before you can truly get in touch with your sexual desires!

The truth is that sexuality is based first on looks and second on personality traits. You need both traits to experience Functional Sex! Functional Sex is defined as having a strong physical attraction combined with the deepest emotional connection during sexual intercourse. This cannot be obtained through one-night stands. Regular Functional Sex plays a huge role in maintaining a happy status in relationships. For sex to be considered functional, both partners must be equally involved. This requires knowing your partner's deepest psychological thoughts in an intimate way. It also requires revealing yourself to them with your guard down in a way that shows your true emotions and sexual desires; for example, shared fantasies and role playing that offer you as a couple the most sexual pleasure and satisfaction. Functional Sex falls under a large spectrum. Emotional connections during sex can range from nothing exotic to bondage-discipline. Since the emotional connection made during sex is vital to a healthy relationship, it's very important to find someone with the same interest in order to have what's considered Functional Sex!

Functional Alert: Relationships are often the most meaningful part of people's lives. A high-frequency Functional Sex life plays an enormous role in maintaining a happy marriage and preventing the other person from cheating!

Regardless of life's circumstances, make time for each other and stay connected emotionally and physically. Without one, it's hard to have the other. A healthy relationship requires the emotional side as much as the physical side. Trust is the foundation for Functional Sex because it creates a safe environment for Functional Sex to grow. The term "soulmate" is defined as a person who strongly resembles another in attitudes and beliefs. We would take it a step further by saying there's a very specific look that two people in love share with one another both inside and outside the bedroom. This particular look of sharing one's soul with one another brings about a whole new meaning of soulmates!

Functional Alert: Your brain is the most important sex organ on your body!

Oxytocin is called the love hormone because it causes you to feel more connected to your lover.[10] It also greatly increases the intensity of your orgasm. For those of you who have nonfunctioning sex organs, you don't have to have an orgasm to get the body to secrete oxytocin. Kissing, touching, and cuddling causes this hormone to be secreted from the brain. If you are not in a sexual relationship, you can still get a spike in oxytocin. Cuddling with your pet also causes oxytocin to be secreted, creating a strong bond between you and the animal. Oxytocin reduces stress hormones in the body, thereby helping the functions of the immune system.[11] The hormone also has anti-inflammatory properties, which helps chronic pain sufferers.

High-frequency Functional Sex encourages people to want to look good naked. It's true! This is what motivates many to build sexy bodies. The most effective natural aphrodisiac for boosting long-term libido in both men and women is Functional Training to build muscle tone, along with a Functional Diet, to reduce narrowing of the blood vessels in the genitalia, resulting in better overall sexual function.

Functional Alert: Reducing stress through Functional Training or Functional Exercise (Functional Training and Functional Cardio) has a surprising payoff: It makes your sex life better!

The ultimate trait both males and females desire is a thing called sexual chemistry! Both males and females are turned on sexually by the way the opposite looks and reacts. Since both males and females are stimulated visually to a very large degree, it's imperative to stay fit to keep your better half's libido and passion in high gear. David Buss is considered a specialist in the field of sexual researchers. He performed a widespread survey of 37 various cultures. He found that on a scale of 0.0 to 3.0, looks were only 0.5 less important for women than men![12]

Functional Training causes the natural release of testosterone and dopamine, which increase your libido. Both hormones rise in correlation with one another. Functional Cardio also plays a role, and sex is actually considered Functional Cardio because it strengthens your cardiac muscles. Testosterone functions as an aphrodisiac hormone in brain cells and dopamine dramatically intensifies these effects.[13] Dopamine is one of the most important neurotransmitters for enhancing sexual desire![14] It also plays a role in signaling killer t-cells to eliminate Dysfunctional Toxins in the body.[15] When your dopamine levels are high, you are happy and more motivated. However, if your dopamine levels are low, you feel unmotivated and become depressed and irritable.

Whenever you lift weights using intensity, you create a spike in dopamine and testosterone that lasts for hours. Functional Sex itself also boosts dopamine levels. High levels of dopamine can be very beneficial for getting you addicted to Functional Sex and Functional Training. Both men and women have an increased interest in Functional Sex and a better sex life when they regularly engage in Functional Training! This is a result of tearing down and rebuilding muscle fibers, which stimulates the production of dopamine and testosterone. An increase in sex drive can be noticed immediately after a good workout. Leg training produces the most profound effect on releasing dopamine and testosterone because it requires the most effort. This makes regular Functional Training very important for improving your libido. Working out together is a stimulating experience that gets couples in the mood. Combining Functional Training with Functional Sex is a win-win situation if you want to be in a better mood, have more intimacy in your relationship, and have better overall health!

Functional Alert: Most people are surprised to find that sexual activity makes them smarter by promoting nerve growth in the brain. This has been proven through Magnetic Resonance Imaging (MRI). If you want to max out your brain's full genetic potential, have lots of Functional Sex! [16]

Obesity rates have advanced from epidemic to pandemic, and this has had a major impact on Functional Sex and divorce rates. Even though you are the same person your spouse dated years ago, your appearance may have changed so dramatically from gaining so much body fat that they may no longer feel attracted to you and/or you no longer feel desirable. A lot of people don't understand that the root cause of marital problems often stems from a lack of Functional Sex! Functional Sex requires showing very strong feelings of enthusiasm toward another person. Without passion, there is a very good chance your marriage will fail.

We express our passion in many ways. One of those ways is building a great body for our significant other. Show them that you have passion for them by developing the best body you can for your body type! We ask that you stop this lack of concern before it's too late. We have seen struggling couples fall back in love with one another after they decided to lose weight and get a toned body. The lifestyle change caused them to feel good about themselves and it changed their attitude and hormones. Many had to get Functional Hormone Replacement as well. Quite often, it's the added body fat, accompanied by low testosterone levels/dopamine, that started all the negativity and disinterest toward one another. The weight gain and low testosterone/dopamine happen so gradually that most people are not even aware of it. It's very common for couples to blame their marital problems on money disputes. Ironically, many of these same people were once perfectly happy with one another without having a lot of money. We believe obesity, low testosterone, and a lack of Functional Training limit one's ability to have a Functional Sex life to its fullest. We urge you to lose the body fat, get toned, fix your hormones, if needed, and try to keep the mate you once fell in love with and could not live without. We believe a lack of Functional Sex is more responsible for today's high divorce rates than financial difficulties! Why? Well, think about it. What is the first thing people do when they get divorced? Is it to try and make more money? No! They try to lose weight and get in shape! Why? Because they want to attract someone who shows strong feelings of enthusiasm toward them, and vice versa, so they can have Functional Sex and a relationship with that person!

Functional Alert: The passion of yesterday isn't good enough for the passion of today!

> **Ronnie:** *Ladies, your man wants you to tell him how proud you are of him on a daily basis. Sincerely acknowledge what he has done as the greatest thing in the world. He likes to be put first! Make him his favorite healthy meals. He loves it when you sincerely thank him for his efforts. Males find femininity, personality, showing physical affection, having common interests, spending money wisely, being kind yet willing to speak your mind when necessary, and looking sexy with class to be incredibly seductive. There is no getting around it because it's true.*

> *The vast majority of men notice the same thing. We are visual creatures and appearance is what first catches our eye. Men love a nice body and a good personality to go along with it. As a woman, you want to have the best version of your body type and make sure to show off your body with class. If you avoid Functional Training and/or have low testosterone, you can't expect to make the most of your body. I have never understood why all these attractive people (both male and female) allow themselves to remain obese. I want you to know you don't have to remain that way! I have had a lot of people tell me they were unhappy in their relationships or marriages. I ask them, "Do you still love them?" They often say, "Yeah, I do, but they are unwilling to do*

anything about their weight or lack of muscle tone. It seems they are always starting their diet, hormones, and exercise program next week!" In other words, they have become unhappy in their relationship and the other person is either clueless or doesn't care. This kind of dysfunctional behavior destroys passion in marriages. If you are withholding Functional Sex for any reason, your marriage will be on the rocks!

Don't let hormonal imbalances, obesity, or even your kids, ruin your relationship by causing you to neglect Functional Sex. Don't allow anything to destroy your emotional connection. Divorce can be a life-changing event that causes severe stress! I have seen this happen enough times in my career that I feel the need to speak out on this very important subject. Admit it, there are some things you may never be able to take back, such as allowing yourself to remain extremely moody, obese, or sexually dysfunctional, or to cheat on your mate. As many people painfully find out later, you can spend the rest of your life apologizing for these situations. This is why I always suggest that couples take action now so that they don't have to face a life-altering situation!

Kathy: *Men, your woman wants to know how beautiful she is on a daily basis! You can relay the message through words and/or actions; for example, giving her a hug and telling her how beautiful she looks or holding her hand during a movie. Guys, females find masculinity, honesty, confidence, humor, and your ability to consciously connect to the here-and-now with purpose and direction to be incredibly attractive. Your woman also prefers you to be well-built and nicely groomed. Staying in shape puts you at an advantage because so many guys are out of shape nowadays. You can't get into shape if you neglect Functional Training and a Functional Diet and if your testosterone levels are too low. A lot of women indirectly encourage their men to get into shape when they say they want them to lose weight for their health. While health is a concern, it's not their only concern. What many women are not telling men directly is that when they gain a bunch of body fat, they are not as physically appealing to them. You should praise your woman every day and show her respect. One of the main ways you can praise each other is by staying fit for one another to maintain a Functional Sex life. It shows you care enough about each other to look your best!*

FUNCTIONAL TRAINING WITH A FORK

There is no such thing as a perfect marriage. People give up on one another too fast, especially after the infatuation period ends or obstacles in life appear. Our marriage and sex life continue to improve after 20 years. Here are some secrets we have used to keep our marriage Functional:

- We both know what we want out of life and are going in the same direction with the same mind-set. We have a lot in common and spend most of our time together. We work together, eat together, watch television together, work out together, sleep together, and go to church together. The more time we spend together, the closer we become, and the better we get along. We work together as a team and know when to give each other some needed space. We both have a strong work ethic and we love our jobs as Personal Trainers!

- We have sexual intercourse at least once a day. The passion and sex are there!

- We use creativity to keep romance alive. We can't expect passion to keep soaring if we're not trying.

- We both remain happy as long as we have Functional Sex frequently, remain consistent with our Functional Training and Functional Hormone Replacement, have healthy food that tastes good, and remain emotionally connected. The combination of these things keep us in a good mood.

- We love each other for what the other one does and how we make each other feel. We tell each other we love and appreciate each other on a daily basis, then back it up with action, not just words.

- During a disagreement we turn directly to each other for a resolution. Getting others involved in our personal business would usually do more harm than good. When you allow others to get involved in your personal lives, you can expect things such as biased opinions or a person being neutral instead of speaking up for what's right. All this does is stir up more drama, creating more disconnection and distrust.

- We don't talk bad about one another.

- We have open communication and are willing to compromise. We hold the eye rolls when we get frustrated at one another, but we do have some healthy arguments occasionally. We realize they are sometimes needed to accomplish something useful as a couple. Sometimes it's the only way to

HOW THE IMMUNE SYSTEM FUNCTIONS

get to the root of the problem in such a way that both of us can be content with the outcome. We have learned that one party can't always be the winner in healthy arguments. This would break down our level of trust and closeness. We never make the other one feel like a loser when the argument is finished. We stay connected and make each other feel sexy and desired. There is no loneliness or disconnection in our marriage.

- We stay in shape for one another through Functional Training, a Functional Diet, and Functional Hormone Replacement. We don't allow ourselves to get out of shape, eat a Dysfunctional Diet, or get low hormone levels. We realize these could destroy our relationship.

- We admire each other's physical appearance and abilities every day. We both feel secure about ourselves and our self-worth.

- We don't test or play games with each other, nor do we have trust issues. We aren't on the Internet (e.g., Facebook) causing marital discord. We don't try to make each other jealous. God put us together for a reason and we are very grateful for that.

- We encourage one another to follow our personal goals. Luckily for us, we both have the same goals in mind. We are more interested in spending quality time with each other than in materialism.

- We always support each other financially, physically, and mentally. For example, Kathy has supported Ronnie through his back surgeries, chronic pain, and limitations. Likewise, Ronnie has supported Kathy through her ankle surgeries, chronic pain, and limitations. We do our best to not allow negative circumstances to affect our marriage. We will always be there for each other regardless of what happens in the future.

- We are never dishonest with each other or hide secrets in our marriage. We trust one another!

- We are both highly dependable people. If we tell one another we are going to do something, we always follow through.

- We both allow one another to have opinions. Luckily for us, we have so much in common it makes it easy because we rarely have to agree to disagree. We both put God first and have the same spiritual mind-set and moral values. We also have the same interest when it comes to sex, politics, music, and entertainment.

- We don't try to change one another. We have grown together much stronger and wiser than either one of us would have by ourselves.

- We know better than to hold a grudge or try to get revenge.

- We realize our relationship is the most important thing in our lives because it's what makes our marriage strong and helps us be the best parents possible. Our son, Austin, means the world to us!

- We take ourselves lightly and joke with one another a lot.

- We realize we still have a lot to accomplish together as a couple. When times get tough, we don't run away, but draw even closer. We focus on the present and don't let bad things that could happen in the future control us.

- We both have learned to accept one another's faults and deal with the things we can't change. Why would we want to change one another since we have a functional marriage?

Sleep and the Immune System

Sleep is needed for proper immune function. A good night's sleep lowers inflammation and oxidation, and keeps the immune system functioning properly.[1] Sleep deprivation causes your white cell count to get too low, which leaves you vulnerable to a host of deadly diseases![2] A lack of sleep increases cortisol, a hormone that increases body fat by causing blood sugar and insulin imbalances and it decreases muscle tone by stripping amino acids from muscle tissue. Sleep deprivation also lowers testosterone and growth hormone, which increases body fat and decreases muscle tone. Not sleeping well causes sugar cravings, weight gain, diabetes, blood thickening, strokes, heart problems, diabetes, cancer, poor brain function, depression, anxiety, lack of sex drive, headaches, tunnel vision, nausea, and a Dysfunctional Immune System. When you don't get enough sleep, you increase your risk of being in an accident, especially a traffic accident. Neglecting to get enough sleep impairs comprehension and decision making. This becomes a huge problem in professions where it's important to be able to judge your level of functioning (e.g., a truck driver, surgeon, or police officer). Sleep is a very individualistic thing. Your body will let you know whether or not you are getting the sleep you need.

If you snore, you probably have sleep apnea and need a BIPAP or CPAP. Our choice is the BIPAP because it mimics normal breathing patterns by providing a high level of pressure when you inhale and a low level of pressure when you exhale. The CPAP provides continuous positive airway pressure that is hard for many to tolerate. Sleep apnea is very serious business because oxygen levels in the body drop, which causes premature death. Sometimes sleep apnea is caused from obesity and can be cured by losing body fat. Sleep apnea also poses a major risk to pregnant women and their unborn child.

Functional Alert: Intense Functional Training and Functional Sex helps turn your mind off at night by reducing anxiety that can cause insomnia. They greatly improve your chances of achieving REM (rapid eye movement) sleep. During REM, the mind releases stress that builds up during waking hours, decreasing the body's production of pro-inflammatory cytokines and free radicals while you sleep.[3] Replacing carbs with a little dietary fat and protein before going to bed also helps prevent insomnia. Fats and protein help prevent blood-sugar levels from bottoming out while you sleep. This deters the adrenal glands from having to secrete insomnia hormones (epinephrine and norepinephrine) to call up stored sugar.[4] It also helps lower the production of pro-inflammatory cytokines and free radicals while you sleep!

Drugs and the Immune System

A lot of drugs are Dysfunctional Toxins![1] Take as few prescription and over-the-counter medications as possible. Some prescription drugs slow the heart rate (e.g., blood pressure medication), causing the metabolism to slow.[2] As your metabolism slows, your circulatory system provides less force to your lymphatic system. When fewer Dysfunctional Toxins are being filtered through the lymph nodes, they are more apt to back up in your system, poisoning your body. The effect is further compounded if the drugs cause constipation, which allows even more Dysfunctional Toxins to accumulate and further poison your body. The bottom line is, some drugs can cause immune system dysfunction by producing excess amounts of pro-inflammatory cytokines and free radicals.

Functional Alert: It's very common to experience a loss of libido when taking drugs such as anti-inflammatories for pain, beta blockers for high blood pressure, statins for high cholesterol, over-the-counter allergy medications, and medications to control diabetes![3-7]

Drugs used to control blood sugar and some birth control pills are notorious for causing individuals to store more fat without any changes in diet or activity levels. There are a lot of drugs that tend to increase one's appetite, which slowly leads to weight gain over a period of time (e.g., prednisone, antihistamines, allergy medications, antibiotics, antidepressants, drugs for seizure disorder, migraines, mood stabilizers, etc.) and should be avoided if at all possible.[8] Some drugs make people gain weight from fatigue and lower levels of activity. Others contribute to insulin resistance. All drugs, whether they be prescription or over-the-counter, can have an adverse effect on your sexual function.

Functional Alert: A lack of muscle tone, accompanied by excess body fat, hinders the kidneys and liver from processing and clearing medications. Building muscle tone and losing body fat makes you less prone to drug toxicity!

Vitamins, Minerals, and the Immune System

Adequate amounts of vitamins and minerals improve immune function, resulting in fewer pro-inflammatory cytokines and free radicals. Your immune system won't function properly if you are deficient in nutrients. Vitamins and minerals help your immune system recognize all forms of disease in order to defend against them.[1] These diseases can be overlooked by a Dysfunctional Immune System that is low on crucial vitamins and minerals. Many of you will need to take a one-a-day multivitamin and mineral supplement to ensure you are getting plenty of nutrients.[2] Older people and those who exercise often require more vitamins and minerals. Most nutrients work together, so being deficient in one or more often leads to a deficiency in another.

Functional Alert: Prescription and over-the-counter medications are notorious for causing vitamin and mineral deficiencies for all age groups because they decrease absorption!

When it comes to multivitamins and mineral supplements, you won't overdose if you take one suggested serving every day. Taking large dosages of multivitamin and mineral supplements or single supplements could cause you to over dose. Your biggest concern should be fat-soluble vitamins, not water-soluble ones because they are not eliminated from the body as quickly. Fat-soluble vitamins are A, D, E, and K.[3]

Stay away from supplements that contain potentially dangerous stimulates and herbs. We recommend buying only multivitamin and mineral supplements containing the USP logo on the label. The USP logo means that the dietary supplement must meet certain standards.[4] Another option is to have your doctor write out a prescription for certain pharmaceutical-grade supplements. Some of you will find the need for additional supplements, such as Vitamin D3. Some of you will need iron, zinc, magnesium, potassium, etc. Everyone's body chemistry and diet is different and so are their nutritional requirements. Don't let other people persuade you that vitamin and mineral supplements are a waste of time or unsafe when used properly. On the other hand, don't let deceptive marketing tactics persuade you to buy these so-called miracle supplements that have no proven track record and cost a fortune. I am sure that, like us, after reading some of these supplement ads, your jaw drops and you ask yourself, Is there anything this "wonder drug" can't cure? We must stop this nonsense of miracle cures through mega-doses of supplements and start protecting ourselves from Dysfunctional Toxins that increase inflammation and oxidation. Excessive levels of anything have never been proven to have a positive effect on disease prevention or life expectancy; quite the contrary, they can make you sick and shorten your lifespan!

Getting your antioxidants from food provides many more benefits than the vitamin supplements because you get fiber, carotenoids, phytochemicals, polyphenols, quercetin (flavonoid antioxidant found in pigmented fruits and vegetables), etc. (A supplement has yet to be made that will give you the same benefits as eating an apple and blueberries, but that isn't to say they are of no benefit.) Carotenoids, which provide the bright coloration of many vegetables, serve as antioxidants. There are more than 600 known natural carotenoids, all of them synthesized in plants.[5]

Refined carbohydrates and fatty foods are lacking in phytochemicals (chemical compounds that occur naturally in plants). Scientists estimate that there may be as many as 4,000 different phytochemicals, that affect the outcome of disease conditions due to their ability to prevent chronic inflammation and free radical damage.[6] For example, according to a new study done by researchers at Florida State University, eating blueberries lowers diastolic pressure (number on bottom) by 7% and systolic pressure (number on top) by 6%.[7] The phytochemicals in blueberries increase nitric oxide production which lowers blood pressure. A diet high in plant-based foods increases nitric oxide levels. Nitric oxide penetrates the underlying smooth muscles and makes the arteries expand, lowering blood pressure and decreasing inflammation and oxidation. It also helps lower the production of excess white blood cells that would otherwise thicken the blood and cause further inflammation and oxidation. Phytonutrients help put a stop to heart disease, sexual dysfunction, and brain neurodegeneration by improving blood flow and preventing damage to the endothelium (inner lining of the arteries).[4]

Functional Alert: Vitamin and mineral deficiencies are not the biggest problems in America. The biggest problems are obesity, an unhealthy diet, a lack of Functional Training, and low hormones, which cause type-2 diabetes, heart disease, cancer, etc.!

CHAPTER 9

Functional Hormone Replacement

As you read through this chapter, we would like you to keep this thought in mind: Ignorance is when you refuse to accept something you don't know anything about! It is important to stand back, look at the real facts and use a little common sense. There is still a lot of controversy among physicians as to whether the benefits of Hormone Replacement outweigh the risks. Collective research and our experience dealing with ourselves and others proves that the benefits derived from Functional Hormone Replacement (FHR) most definitely outweigh any risk that may be involved. Functional Hormone Replacement is defined as treatment by a well-trained physician based on your symptoms, not by a scale that supposedly predicts what is considered to be normal hormone levels for your age. FHR is for males and females who want to grow old gracefully and try to extend their life spans. Let us be clear: We don't think that hormones alone can automatically add 20 years to one's life expectancy. On the other hand, we certainly don't believe that Functional Hormone Replacement such as testosterone for men and testosterone for women will shorten your life span when they are administered properly. In fact, low or an imbalance of hormones are linked to obesity, lack of libido, depression, osteoporosis, lack of muscle tone and strength, type-2 diabetes, heart disease, cancer, immune system dysfunction, autoimmune disease, and dying sooner![1]

Functional Alert: Taking testosterone for a testosterone deficiency is the same as taking insulin for type-1 diabetes. Just because you are healthy doesn't mean you'll remain that way if you have low testosterone levels. Hormones help ease the symptoms of many diseases and prolong life span, but they won't cure the damage that's already taken place from having low hormones (e.g., damage to the endothelium).[2] This means you need to start taking them before the damage occurs!

Men around the age of 30 and older (pre-andropausal, peri-andropausal, and post-andropausal) and women around the age of 35 and older (pre-menopausal, peri-menopausal, and post-menopausal) usually start showing signs of some kind of hormone deficiency.[3,4] The symptoms of low hormones, especially testosterone, are subtle, affecting the mood of both men and women. It often happens so gradually that most people are not aware of what is going on.

The symptoms of low testosterone are often mistaken as signs of depression, anxiety, or chronic fatigue syndrome. It's common for physicians to put their patients on antidepressants when hormone treatment would have been much safer, void of nasty side effects, and often fixed the root cause of the problem.[5] Prescribing antidepressants for everything is not the answer! Low testosterone is a subject that some in the medical profession are still avoiding, especially when it comes to the female population. Most middle-aged males are low on testosterone but don't know it! Likewise, most middle-aged females are low on testosterone and don't know it!

Functional Alert: Everyone will experience low testosterone in their own way. People can have very different symptoms yet have the exact same hormone levels. We think this is where a lot of people tend to get confused!

The stereotypical person who is low in hormones is a man in his 30s or a woman in her 40s who can no longer keep up with their younger friends or with their spouse in the bedroom. FHR helps change all that! It improves your quality of life and it also improves longevity because it gives you the energy and motivation to eat and exercise properly. Our clients want to be lifting weights, having sexual intercourse, going for walks, working in the yard, swinging their golf clubs, and riding horses into their 90s. The odds of being able to do these things without the aid of additional hormones are slim to none.

It's not fun when your body gets softer as you gain body fat. It's even more frustrating when you have been exercising hard for years without seeing improvements or begin experiencing a decline in muscle tone and strength due to a hormone deficiency. Your bones become deformed and brittle. You develop structural defects such as osteoporosis (bone loss) and kyphosis (forward curvature at the top of the spine).[6] You experience abnormal gait, a loss of balance, joint pain, fatigue, brain fog, depression, insomnia, anxiety, sexual dysfunction, weight gain in the form of body fat, increase in appetite, and insulin and leptin resistance.[7-9] You will also notice a decline in strength, endurance, and muscle tone, which significantly prevents the body from being able to perform its regular functions!

Functional Alert: Skeletal muscle mass declines approximately 1% per year after age thirty![10]

We sometimes meet people who don't want FHR because they are afraid of the long-term side effects. What they don't understand is that once hormones get low, it's impossible to feel great without taking them. Not taking the hormones creates the worst, long-term side effects of all: a poor quality of life! A word of caution: People who decided to stop FHR found that the negative side effects, such as depression, fatigue, and a low libido, returned with a vengeance! The vast majority of people in our society need FHR for the rest of their lives once they hit the dreaded andropause and menopause in order to maintain their previous lifestyle.

Hormones, combined with a Functional Diet and Functional Training, increases longevity by relieving mental stress, improving sex life, reducing body fat, lowering cortisol levels, improving sleep, improving insulin sensitivity, keeping the organs functioning properly, reducing LDL cholesterol, and preventing cancer. Low testosterone and a lack of Functional Training will cause the core and leg muscles to weaken, resulting in poor balance and posture, especially in the elderly. As you age, your balance and posture can be maintained with Functional Hormone Replacement, Functional Training, and a Functional Diet!

Men produce roughly 13 times more testosterone than women.[9] In a woman's early reproductive years, she has approximately 10 times more testosterone than estrogen running through her body.[11] It should come as no surprise that this is a time when a woman's muscle tone, health, functionality, and sex drive is usually at its peak!

It's no secret that both a male's and a female's testosterone and estrogen decline as they age; unfortunately, that can be where many of life's troubles begin! When testosterone and estrogen levels plummet, our voices change, but not in a good way! We develop sexual arousal disorder from a lack of genital blood flow during the sexual response. Our core temperature drops. As a result, we tend to be cold even when others around us are warm. We often eat more calories to try to recover some of the lost energy. We feel exhausted after what is considered a normal workout!

Functional Alert: It's very common for people lacking in testosterone to have forgotten what it was like to have great sex!

Our bodies require testosterone and estrogen for normal metabolic functions. Only estrogen can be found elsewhere. The fat cells in our bodies are able to produce a small amount of estrogen from testosterone.[12] The fatter we are, the more estrogen we produce and the less testosterone our bodies produce.[13] Hormonal changes prior to and leading up to andropause and menopause tend to create weight gain and various kinds of dysfunctional issues inside the body. There is substantial evidence that this weight gain, often manifested around the midsection, causes chronic inflammation/oxidation and dysfunction throughout the entire body.

Having healthy testosterone and estrogen levels will decrease your appetite and allow you to eat smaller meals because of their ability to help the brain block out stress.[14] Testosterone also helps you control your appetite by preventing leptin and insulin resistance through body-fat reduction.

Functional Alert: When it comes to a medical condition, just because doctors can't diagnose it, doesn't mean there's not a problem!

Just because you are in your 40s and beyond doesn't mean you have to look and feel like it! We agree with the antiaging specialists because we have read enough studies and seen enough anecdotal evidence to know that when your testosterone and estrogen decline, your functionality all across the board decreases. If you wait for researchers to agree on whether hormone therapy is 100% safe, it will probably be too late. This lack of common sense hurts a lot of people!

There are many well-known benefits for both males and female who use testosterone alone when incorporating FHR. FHR:

- Improves core strength and balance.

- Enhances brain function. Testosterone increases blood flow through the cerebral artery that feeds the brain. Cerebrovascular inflammation is reduced by a small portion of the testosterone that turns into estrogen.[15,16]

- Increases bone marrow activity and red blood cell count, which enhance nutrients and oxygen being delivered to cells, helping prevent a weakened immune system.[17]

- Increases metabolism without having to take harmful stimulants.[18,19,20]

- Improves sexual desire, function, and performance.[21]

- Increases the frequency and intensity of orgasms, making you smarter by promoting nerve growth in the brain.[22,23]

- Prevents hot flashes, cold chills, and hair loss. [24,25]

- Improves workout capacity and muscle/connective tissue recovery.[26]

- Increases nitric oxide production to suppress damage to the endothelium which helps prevent chronic inflammation and oxidation.[27]

FUNCTIONAL HORMONE REPLACEMENT

- Acts as an anti-inflammatory for treating arthritic conditions.[28]

- Lowers LDL (bad) cholesterol and heart attack risk by restoring estrogen levels.[29,30]

- Increases HDL (good) cholesterol.[31]

- Improves bone density by increasing mineral absorption. Bone mineral density decreases approximately 1% per year during and after andropause and menopause. This also increases your risk of tooth loss.[32,33]

- Lowers the risk of developing cancer.[34-39]

- Helps calm symptoms of autoimmune disease by making an overactive immune system less active.[40]

- Increases muscle tone and strength.[41]

- Decreases body fat, especially around the midsection by enhancing the metabolism.[42]

- Enhances mood and improves sense of well-being, leading to a better quality of life.[43]

- Prevents aging of skin (e.g., face, neck, and chest) where it's most noticeable by excreting extra oil from the glands.[44]

- Provides more energy and better sleep.[45]

- Enhances blood sugar regulation and lowers insulin production; decreases risk of diabetes, heart disease, sexual dysfunction, and Alzheimer's; and lowers the risk of developing cancer that is more aggressive.[46-50]

- Improves cardiac function by making the heart muscle stronger, decreasing the chances of your heart stopping if you have a heart attack.[51,52]

- Enlarges blood vessels, allowing blood to flow more easily through arteries and the heart to use less force while pumping which results in lower blood pressure.[53-55]

- Acts as a better antidepressant in many cases than mainstream antidepressants. This helps manage PTSD.[56,57]

- Improves kidney and liver function in order to purge Dysfunctional Toxins from the body.[58-60]

- Prevents degenerative disc disease by making the core stronger.

- Helps nerve regeneration, and builds bones, muscles, and connective tissue by conversion of IGF-1 (insulin-like growth factors).[61]

- Helps alleviate migraine headaches.[62-64]

- Enhances androgenic-induced brain function, which improves memory and the ability to train hard. Testosterone also helps preserve brain tissue.[65]

- Causes a significant decrease in chronic pain by increasing opioid activation in the brain.[66,67]

- Decreases sugar cravings by lowering depression and perceived stress.[68]

- Lowers anxiety once your body adjusts to the proper dosages.[69]

- Decreases appetite by helping stabilize blood sugar and insulin levels.[70]

- Regulates pro-inflammatory cytokine expression, which improves communication along the entire immune system.[71]

Hematocrit and Estrogen Levels for Males and Females

A knowledgeable hormone specialist will check hematocrit and estrogen levels. "Hematocrit" refers to the number of red blood cells in a specified amount of blood.[1] Hematocrit levels should be your primary concern when using testosterone! High hematocrit levels can increase your risk of deep vein thrombosis (a formation of a blood clot).[2] A small percentage of people experience a significant rise in hematocrit levels when using testosterone. If you have extremely high hematocrit levels, your blood can thicken from having excess amounts of red blood cells. Over the long haul, this can put you at an increased risk for heart attack, stroke, and blood clots. Elevated hematocrit levels are easy to fix and sometimes leave on their own once the body adjusts. The best options a knowledgeable physician will offer to lower hematocrit levels are as follows: lowering the dosage of testosterone you are using until the body adapts, donating blood every 2-3 months, drinking plenty of fluids, using a c-pap or a bi-pap if you have sleep apnea (because anything that lowers oxygen in the blood will stimulate Erythropoietin (Epo) production and the corresponding rise in hematocrit levels), losing body fat, implementing Functional Exercise, and using a daily form of testosterone gel, instead of weekly injections.[2]

Functional Alert: In order for hormone replacement to be considered functional, hematocrit levels must remain in a healthy range for your chemical makeup. High hematocrit levels (anything above 52%) can increase the production of pro-inflammatory cytokines and free radicals.[3] Taking a baby aspirin a day does not lower hematocrit levels, but it can thin out the blood and help prevent a clot.[4] Short-term, high-dose testosterone can increase hematocrit levels, but the body usually adapts to high doses long-term, causing hematocrit levels to stay within normal range![5]

The other potential side effect of hormone therapy is becoming estrogen dominant. We define estrogen dominance as having excessively high levels of estrogen. A certain percentage of testosterone gets converted into estrogen at the cellular level. Data supports that low testosterone and extremely high levels of estrogen are associated with cancer (e.g., prostate and breast) and heart disease. This is because estrogen dominance increases the body's production of pro-inflammatory cytokines and free radicals![6]

Your blood levels of estrogen aren't accurate in reflecting what is happening at the cellular level, which is where aromatization (testosterone converting to estrogen) takes place. This means estrogen dominance can't accurately be diagnosed through blood work. The best way to tell if you are estrogen dominant is by gauging your sex drive, mood, and energy levels. If your sex drive is high and you aren't experiencing extreme anger or fatigue, then you are not estrogen dominant for your body's chemistry![7,8] It doesn't matter if your estrogen levels appear high on the estrogen scale as long as your sex drive is high and you are not extremely angry or fatigued. If your sex drive is low and/or you are experiencing excessive anger and/or excessive fatigue, then you have reason for concern, regardless of your numbers. In the vast majority of cases, the only people who are at risk for estrogen dominance are people who are insulin resistant, avoid Functional Exercise, consume too many foods at the lower end of the Functional Food Spectrum (foods that lower testosterone and increase estrogen mimickers), allow body-fat levels to remain high for their body type, and use too much testosterone for their body chemistry.

Functional Alert: The use of HCG significantly increases estrogen levels!

In the vast majority of cases, non-breast cancer patients who follow a Functional Diet and keep their body-fat levels in check, yet become estrogen dominant while using testosterone, are better off lowering the dosage of testosterone than using an aromatase inhibitor (medication that stops the production of estrogen). The same rule applies to breast cancer patients who are estrogen receptor-negative and/or progesterone receptor-negative.

Functional Alert: In order for hormone replacement to be considered functional, estrogen dominance must be avoided. Estrogen dominance increases the production of pro-inflammatory cytokines and free radicals. Estrogen dominance is linked to strokes, heart attacks, and cancer.[9, 10] In addition, low estrogen must be avoided. It's ironic that the signs of having very low estrogen can be the same as being estrogen dominant—excessive fatigue, extreme anger, and having a low sex drive!

Synthetic vs. Bioidentical Hormones

The only natural hormones are the ones in your body! "Synthetic hormones" simply means they are synthesized or made in a laboratory. They mimic the effects of hormones produced in the human body. "Bioidentical hormones" are also synthesized in a laboratory by converting plant compounds into chemical molecules identical to those made in the human body.[1-6] All synthetic hormones are regulated and tested for purity and potency; however, some bioidentical hormones from compounding pharmacies are not.[7, 8]

Synthetic hormones and bioidentical hormones can act differently inside the body, but they all do basically the same thing in the end.[9] For example, the synthetic version of progesterone is actually progestin. Progestin binds in a much stronger way to the estrogen receptor than progesterone, which can promote cell proliferation.[10, 11] The body can make use of bioidentical progesterone and estrogen better than synthetic versions because it's more readily metabolized and excreted from the body.[12] However, any substance that stimulates the testosterone, estrogen, and progesterone receptors sets off a series of biochemical reactions with a similar end result.

Doctors have disagreements about whether bioidentical hormones are safer and more effective than synthetic hormones and vice versa. Any hormone administered in pill form causes a broader range of hormonal effects and increases pro-inflammatory cytokines and free radicals.[13, 14] We have known for a long time that oral derivatives of testosterone are much more difficult for the liver to metabolize than injectable or implanted testosterone. Common sense tells us that oral progestin and estrogen can thicken the blood and cause chronic inflammation and oxidation inside the body. This is caused from the release of excess pro-inflammatory cytokines/free radicals and subsequent white blood cells.

The only conclusive evidence in regard to hormones is that oral formulations can be dangerous and prolonged exposure to excessive amounts of any hormone for your chemical makeup or the lack thereof can cause serious illnesses. Each person has a different chemical makeup and you have to listen to your body. We believe oral progestin is bad and most women get enough estrogen from taking testosterone alone! We believe that all people should avoid using oral synthetic hormones in order for the hormone replacement to be considered functional. [15-18]

Testosterone is more potent and cost effective by injection, but those who don't like needles or do well with injectables should use implanted pellets or the transdermal method of delivery. We want to make sure you spend your money wisely and get positive results. Don't fall for advertising gimmicks that claim to be selling a safe and effective natural testosterone booster. The only safe and effective testosterone booster comes in the form of a prescription, not an over-the-counter supplement! [19] Likewise, you can't take other hormones, such as DHEA, and derive the same benefits as testosterone. They are two different hormones altogether. [20]

You should get a blood test to get the most accurate reading of your hormones. [21] Saliva testing from certain labs is also accurate. However, a saliva test is more expensive than blood work and some insurance companies won't cover the cost. Both serum and saliva levels vary significantly throughout the day, even within minutes.

Functional Alert: A hematocrit test must be done using a sample of your blood, not your saliva!

We feel that anyone who thinks hormone replacement might be bad for their overall health as they get older has been misled. How can having more sex, less depression and anxiety, a leaner body, a stronger heart, and less chances of developing type-2 diabetes and cancer be bad? We are convinced that you need to be concerned if FHR isn't implemented for life starting around menopause and andropause. The balance of hormones, diet, and exercise has a soothing effect on inflammation and oxidation, which helps keep the immune system strong. Symptoms of excess chronic inflammation/oxidation often become apparent during and after both andropause and menopause due to decreasing testosterone and estrogen levels in men and declining testosterone, progesterone, and estrogen levels in women. [22] Some people develop low testosterone before andropause and menopause due to genetics or from using recreational drugs, prescription drugs, and over-the-counter medications; from being overweight; giving birth; and from having various illnesses. Some drugs block the signal to the glands that tells your body to produce testosterone. [23] As many men and women will tell you, without any changes in their diet or exercise, they all of a sudden began gaining body fat, losing muscle tone and bone mass, and feeling tired and depressed. There are mornings they don't feel like getting out of bed. They no longer feel like themselves at all. Hormone imbalances are the reason!

Functional Alert: People with testosterone deficiencies shorten their life span and have a lower quality of life. In fact, taking testosterone in amounts greater than normally found in the body is healthier than having low to borderline low testosterone levels! [24]

The extra visceral fat around the liver from having low testosterone levels increases fat around and inside the liver, making it difficult for it to function properly. This reduces the liver's ability to filter harmful Dysfunctional Toxins and causes an increase in bad cholesterol (LDL) and triglycerides. The heart is a muscle and if it gets weak from low testosterone and/or a lack of exercise, your odds of dying from a heart attack are significantly higher.[25] Clinical data shows that the majority of men who have heart attacks also have low levels of testosterone.[26, 27] As testosterone levels decline, our bodies become less efficient at burning blood sugar for fuel due to a loss in type-2 muscle fibers and liver dysfunction.[28] This causes our cells to become less sensitive to insulin and OxLDL cholesterol increases.[29] Insulin sensitivity plays a major role in determining how healthy you will be and how long you are going to live! We believe insulin sensitivity may determine the rate of aging more than any other factor. Glucose or blood sugar dominance must be avoided at all costs if you want to live a long, healthy life. We also know that FHR, when coupled with the proper type of Functional Training will help prevent the decline of type-2 muscle fibers. These muscle fibers play a significant role in keeping our bodies hydrated in order to bring oxygen and other nutrients to the cells of the body's tissues and organs.

Functional Alert: Having a weak heart and/or high blood pressure can cause your heart to become enlarged! The most common causes of a weak heart and high blood pressure are a lack of Functional Exercise (Functional Training and Functional Cardio), eating a poor diet and/or obesity, and having low testosterone and/or estrogen levels!

Insulin-Like Growth Factors

Insulin-like growth factors (IGF-1) play a huge role in slowing down the aging process. They are important chemicals in your body because they help regulate the growth, repair, and replacement of cells that keep your body functioning properly.[30] Your liver converts growth hormone into IGF-1, which is directly responsible for the benefits derived from using growth hormone.[31] The downfall of using excessive amounts of growth hormone is that it increases IGF-1 levels too much. This could be unhealthy and actually stimulate cancer and diabetes. However, healthy amounts of IGF-1 from using testosterone actually lowers your risk of cancer, heart disease, diabetes, Alzheimer's, etc.[32-34]

IGF-1 deficiencies and a lack of Functional Training are associated with poor health outcomes, such as fibromyalgia.[35] IGF-1 is necessary for immune system function. We see a lot of people, who can barely get around as they get older. They have kyphosis (necks protruding forward) and walk very gently with a poor gait.

Ronnie: *At age 49, my IGF-1 levels are at the upper end of the scale of what is considered to be normal without having to use synthetic growth hormone. Functional Hormone Replacement is all I need to maintain healthy IGF-1 levels!*

Testosterone therapy increases IGF-1, but to a much lesser degree than pharmaceutical-grade human growth hormone therapy.[36] It's important to note that the use of testosterone alone, without the use of synthetic human growth hormone, usually produces enough IGF-1 to regulate the growth, repair, and replacement of cells that keep your body functioning properly. A major drawback of pharmaceutical-grade growth hormone is the cost! It generally costs around $15,000 per year, which makes it unaffordable for most people.[37] Luckily, testosterone is inexpensive and just about everyone can afford it. Furthermore, using too much synthetic growth hormone can cause some people to experience severe joint pain, swelling, and carpal tunnel syndrome, preventing them from exercising as needed.[38] The use of excess growth hormone has been linked to diabetes in some people because it can cause insulin resistance. Growth hormone is a counter-regulatory hormone to insulin.[39] It decreases the effect insulin has on the cells, meaning the ability of the cells to take in blood sugar can be compromised. Therefore, your blood sugar can increase! Excess growth hormone can also reduce blood sugar synthesis in the liver. It's important to remember that diabetes leads to heart disease and a host of other serious problems such as amputation of a limb!

How to Properly Balance Female Hormones

The basic foundation for all FHR should begin with the hormone testosterone! During a woman's normal menstrual cycle, testosterone levels skyrocket at ovulation, which is around day 14 of a 28-day cycle.[1] This is Mother Nature's way of increasing a woman's sex drive so she will be encouraged to reproduce. Sex is natural. It comes from God himself and it's the only reason we all exist. The testosterone surge that occurs during ovulation is when a female is at her sexual peak. This sexual peak is what females should be striving to duplicate with FHR.

Functional Alert: FHR for women is a big body-fat loss factor for those who are pre-, peri-, and post-menopausal!

On average, women produce 13 times less testosterone than men. If you are a female experiencing symptoms of low testosterone and your hormone specialist is happy with your replacement numbers because they fall within the normal range, we highly recommend you change to a different doctor, one who is willing to treat your symptoms. Unfortunately, the logical basic math approach doesn't work when it comes to human pharmacokinetics because everyone metabolizes hormones differently. Higher dosages are necessary for some to get their testosterone to a certain level because they metabolize hormones faster than others. The primary focus is to treat the symptoms, not some mythical number on a scale!

> **Kathy:** *I inject testosterone cypionate once a week and use progesterone cream every night. I take the progesterone to prevent having endometrium problems. I currently don't need to use estrogen to be functional because I use enough testosterone to take care of my estrogen needs through aromatization. At age 52, I feel great with my testosterone levels around 90 ng/dl, my progesterone levels around 10ng/ml, and my estrogen (estradiol) levels around 35.*

The vast majority of hormone experts now realize that it's the loss of testosterone/estrogen, more than the progesterone that causes females in midlife to gain weight; to feel fatigued; and to lose mental focus, libido, muscle tone, and bone density—all of which hurt their ability to function mentally, physically, and sexually!

Functional Alert: Higher blood levels of testosterone equate to an improved mood, enhanced functionality, and a higher level of sexual desire and satisfaction. "Free testosterone" is the amount of the hormone that is active in the body.[2] Blood levels of total testosterone and free testosterone vary among each individual, making it impossible for doctors to use a scale to establish precisely how much testosterone to prescribe. The focus should be on how you feel. Your free testosterone levels are what matters most. High total testosterone numbers on a scale mean nothing if your free testosterone levels are low. The more testosterone you take, the higher your free testosterone will become!

The best FHR we know of for most females is testosterone cypionate injected once a week, topical testosterone cream used daily, or testosterone pellets injected every 3 months. There is no set limit to how much testosterone you can use as long as your hematocrit levels stay in normal range, you don't become estrogen dominant, and you don't experience a deeper voice or any unwanted facial hair.

FUNCTIONAL HORMONE REPLACEMENT

Functional Alert: There are a lot of females who are willing to deal with a little extra facial hair growth in order to reduce body fat, improve muscle tone, and have an amazing sex drive. They use facial creams, waxing, plucking with tweezers, etc., to get rid of any unwanted hair!

Testosterone is basically nontoxic since it's a naturally occurring substance in your body. Dosages must be determined by your response! Those who take the testosterone cream route, instead of the weekly injections, will need to use it every day, and higher dosages are often needed due to a lack of absorption. The injections are less expensive and more potent, but the cream or implanted pellets are the preferred choice for some women. If you decide to go the injection route, ask your doctor to prescribe a 10 ml bottle of testosterone cypionate containing only 100 mgs per ml if your insurance will cover it. The lower-dosed vials are less difficult to measure out for injection. You don't want to buy the 1 ml bottles because you get less for your money. Women who do a bi-weekly testosterone injection (a shot every 2 weeks) find that by the time the second week rolls around, their testosterone/estrogen has become too low or unstable at around day 10. This leads to poor testosterone/estrogen levels, mood swings, hair loss, and loss of libido. We strongly recommend that you ask your doctor about switching to once-a-week injections in order to obtain stable testosterone and estrogen levels!

A physician or nurse will teach you or someone else how to inject the testosterone so it can be done at home. The smallest needle that can be properly used to inject testosterone is a tiny 1 inch 25 gauge needle. Use an 18 gauge needle to draw it into the syringe. The testosterone is easier to inject after it has been heated. It's best to heat the testosterone with a hair dryer for about 30 seconds once it's in the syringe.

Functional Alert: Testosterone helps reduce vaginal dryness, which can cause pain during sex. We believe that if additional estrogen is needed in addition to your test base, it should come in the form that is inserted vaginally to help prevent vaginal dryness and estrogen dominance![3]

Progesterone and/or estrogen can be added to your testosterone base if needed to prevent hot flashes and help functionality all across the board. The three hormones (testosterone, progesterone, and estrogen) in women are comparable to the three macronutrients (protein, carbs, and fats) in our diet. With hormones, testosterone is the base hormone and estrogen and progesterone are considered accessories. With diet, protein is the base macronutrient while carbs and fats are considered accessories. A very small percentage of women don't need to take testosterone because their levels are naturally high due to having polycystic ovary syndrome (PCOS). PCOS is usually caused by excessively high insulin levels.[4, 5]

FHR makes females feel 100% better. Dysfunctional Hormone Replacement makes them feel the same or worse. If you can get by with just taking testosterone alone, then that is the preferred choice! Aromatase (an enzyme located in the many tissues) converts testosterone to estrogen. Therefore, when you take testosterone alone you also get some estrogen. This makes a huge difference in your sex drive, energy levels, and bone density!

We recommend that females who need estrogen and/or progesterone in addition to their testosterone base, take the lowest effective doses of progesterone and/or estrogen as possible. Some women feel lousy using progesterone because they weren't low to begin with or they are taking too much for their body chemistry. Likewise, some women feel lousy using estrogen because they weren't low to begin with or they are taking too much for their body chemistry. Too much estrogen can cause causes sugar cravings, a lack of sexual desire, a lack of sensitivity in the genitalia, and can delay or prevent the ability to reach orgasm. Too little estrogen can cause sugar cravings, joint pain, lethargy, increased LDL cholesterol, damage to the endothelium (inner lining of the arteries), a loss in libido, a lack of sensitivity in the genitalia, and vaginal dryness, and can delay or prevent the ability to reach orgasm.[6, 7] Too much progesterone (progesterone dominance) causes mood swings, vaginal dryness, low sex drive, and breast tenderness.[8] But too little progesterone can cause anxiety and endometrium problems that lead to painful sex.[9] Low testosterone can make females indecisive. The vast majority of women function best using testosterone alone with no added estrogen and sometimes a very small amount of progesterone to prevent endometrium problems. This helps them become more functional while avoiding estrogen dominance!

Functional Alert: Excessive fatigue, extreme anger, and low sex drive are symptoms of both low estrogen and estrogen dominance in males and females!

Endocrinologist professor Jerilyn C. Pryor, MD, at the University of British Columbia, found that 50% of women in North America have a serious deficiency in progesterone by age 35, and during menopause, levels decreased to almost nothing. She also found through studies that estrogen levels in these same females during menopause decreased by 40-60%.[10-12] Other studies have shown that some female's testosterone levels get low by age 35.[13] These studies show us how each woman's body reacts differently and must be treated on an individual basis.

FUNCTIONAL HORMONE REPLACEMENT

Dr. Allen Kirchner of Aiken, SC, is a retired gynecologist with 40 years of experience. He is certified by the American Board of Obstetrics and Gynecology, and is a Life Fellow of the American College of Obstetricians and Gynecologists. Dr. Kirchner received his M.D. and post-graduate training at the University of Maryland, and formerly served as Clinical Assistant Professor of Obstetrics and Gynecology at the Medical College of Georgia.

There is no doubt that proper hormone balance is key to healthy living and graceful aging. There is, however, much disagreement and much misinformation about how to achieve that goal of proper hormone balance. In prior times, it was perhaps less of an issue. Life expectancy of a female in the 19th century was 50 years, not coincidentally approximately the age of menopause. Evolutionarily speaking, as the authors have suggested, it makes sense that when an organism can no longer reproduce, its purpose and role in the world is over. We have come a long way in the last hundred years. Life expectancy of a woman in America now exceeds 80 years. How can we expect to survive nearly twice as long as evolution would dictate, and do so with an acceptable quality of life? The answer lies in fitness, diet, healthy living and adequate levels of vital hormones. But the truth is that hormone function begins to deteriorate long before the average age of menopause in women and before the point of evolutionary uselessness in men.

I owe much of my understanding of this subject to a true visionary in antiaging hormone therapy, Dr. Edwin Greer who, 30 years ago, was preaching to predominately deaf ears much of what is now commonly accepted.

My outlook and goal of hormone replacement has always been to titrate [continuously measure and adjust the balance] to physiologic effect rather than to a specific laboratory test result. The laboratory ranges of normal for most hormones is extremely wide. For example, "normal" female estrogen levels may vary 200-300%. The point is that what is "normal" for one person may be too high or too low for another. A baseline laboratory test is very useful to determine where on the scale a particular person may be, but it has very little usefulness in determining the end point of treatment.

Rather, physiologic effect, or resolution of adverse symptoms, or improvement of perceived well-being should be the goal of treatment. There are many hormones that decline with age, including, but not limited to, testosterone, estrogen, progesterone, and thyroid hormone. Estrogen in post-menopausal women is key to preventing osteoporosis, a debilitating and life-threatening disease. Less well recognized, but increasingly more accepted, is the need for testosterone in both men and women in order to maintain health and quality of life.

Replacement of any of these hormones requires medical supervision and prescription medications. You may have to actively search for a physician who will share your goals regarding hormone replacement; not all have seen the light, but enough have. Do not be misled by the many TV and magazine advertisements for "natural" hormones that you can buy online or over the counter. They are useless at best, and dangerous at worst.

Quality of life is a balance that is achievable, but one that requires effort on your part. Proper diet, exercise, fitness, appropriate preventive medical care, and in many cases, hormone supplements should allow all of us to survive and enjoy many decades of life beyond the age at which we have ceased our evolutionary purpose.

The Women's Health Initiative Study

The Women's Health Initiative (WHI) study claimed that women between the ages of 50-79 who took the oral version of estrogen and progestin (synthetic progesterone) were more likely to have breast cancer, strokes, and heart attacks.[1]

We believe the study showed us seven things:

1. Giving females large amounts of estrogen and progestin in pill form without any testosterone to balance out the other two hormones is counterproductive. It results in their bodies producing excess amounts of pro-inflammatory cytokines and free radicals.[2] Testosterone regulates cytokine expression and increases oxygen levels in cells, helping prevent cancer, stroke, heart disease, etc.

2. Synthetic hormone pills increase the production of pro-inflammatory cytokines and free radicals, increasing the risks of breast cancer, stroke, heart disease, etc.[3]

3. Synthetic progestin (not to be confused with progesterone) is linked to sugar imbalances and insulin imbalances that increase the production of pro-inflammatory cytokines and free radicals.[4]

4. The high dosage of oral estrogen had a number of physiological effects that

were amplified by adding a high dosage of oral progestin and vice versa. Some of the participants were unknowingly over-dosing on estrogen and/or progestin, increasing the production of pro-inflammatory cytokines and free radicals.[5]

5. Some of the women in the study became estrogen dominant. Estrogen dominance restricts oxygen exchange in cells which results in oxygen levels getting too low, leading to the development of cancer, stroke, heart disease, etc. The lack of oxygen from estrogen dominance increased the release of pro-inflammatory cytokines and free radicals.[6,7]

6. Oral hormones can accelerate damage caused by bad lifestyle habits.[8,9]

7. Some of the females in the study drank alcohol on a frequent basis. Females who have more than one alcoholic beverage per day are at a much greater risk of high blood pressure, stroke, heart disease, and breast cancer. One drink consists of one 4 oz of wine, 12 oz beer, or 1 oz of liquor.[10-12]

When a female's sex drive, energy, and mood are at their peak while using a particular dosage of hormones, then she is considered functional, not estrogen dominant! On the other hand, if sex drive drops or remains the same if already low, the dosages given or the combinations thereof, would be considered dysfunctional because of estrogen dominance and/or a lack of testosterone.

As stated previously, some of the females in the WHI study became estrogen dominant. We believe that was probably true for some of the women who developed medical problems, but certainly not for all of them! Some of them would have gotten breast cancer or had a stroke or heart attack anyway due to genetics, bad lifestyle habits, and obesity.

There have been numerous studies showing the health benefits of taking non-oral hormones in proper dosages.[11,12] It's very important to take the sum of all studies and interpret them using common sense. You must be very wary of contradictory information on complicated issues. We believe that the millions of women who are now suffering from hormonal imbalances and a poor quality of life should be outraged because the WHI study has made some doctors afraid to prescribe non-oral hormones!

The average age of the women in the WHI study was around 60 years and older. Many of the women who participated in the study were former smokers and overweight, and some had to take medications to help control their already damaged arteries (e.g., high blood pressure and cholesterol medications).[13] The most important thing we have learned from the WHI hormone therapy study is that oral progestin and oral estrogen can add to the damage that's already been done. In addition, these hormones won't reverse the damage that has already been done to the endothelium (inner lining of the arteries) due to poor lifestyles (e.g. unmanaged stress due to a lack of Functional Exercise, obesity, poor diet, high blood pressure, imbalanced hormones, smoking, excess alcohol, and/or use of birth control pills) prior to taking hormones.

Functional Alert: Researchers have known for a long time that prolonged exposure to excessive amounts of estrogen (whether from hormone replacement or a woman's own ovaries) elevates pro-inflammatory cytokines and free radicals. This exposure increases the risk of breast cancer, heart disease, and other serious medical conditions. Many are surprised to learn that a lack of fiber in the diet increases estrogen levels in the body! [14, 15]

Ronnie: *I have been studying exercise, nutrition, and hormones for many years. My view of the WHI hormone study done on women with low hormones is that it was set up like a faulty diet plan for pre-diabetics. I believe that giving these women high dosages of oral estrogen and progestin combined was comparable to giving a pre-diabetic a diet high in refined carbs and saturated fats. When you leave out the most important ingredient of the study (testosterone) and combine the two known villains (oral estrogen and progestin in high dosages), the end results are practically meaningless. It's similar to putting a pre-diabetic on a diet void of protein and high in the two known villains; refined carbs and saturated fats. However, in this particular study, it wasn't meaningless because it backs up what we are saying, so women can move forward using the functional approach for hormone replacement. Some of the most important discoveries in the medical community have come from mistakes made by others. We now know that being glucose dominant poisons our bodies; estrogen dominance does the same! Estrogen is like glucose (blood sugar). Your body needs both for overall mental health (e.g., to maintain healthy serotonin levels) and physical health (e.g., to prevent chronic fatigue), but excessive amounts can cause a host of health problems. It really is that simple, but some people are trying to complicate the entire issue, making some women anxious about taking hormones. As long as it's Functional Hormone Replacement, there is no need to give it a second thought!*

The side effects from being estrogen dominant may show up before females hit peri-menopause, menopause, or post-menopause. Progesterone, like progestin, magnifies the effect by making the estrogen receptors more sensitive. In today's toxic world, more Dysfunctional Toxins are being stored in female's fat tissues. These Dysfunctional Toxins act as estrogen mimickers called xeno-estrogens that can further add to the estrogen already in the body and lower testosterone levels.[16] Estrogen dominance is associated with heart disease, strokes, cancer, extreme mood swings, excessive fatigue, sexual problems, endometriosis, aggression, and fat buildup around the stomach, legs, and hips. Estrogen dominance can interfere with the thyroid gland and cause severe PMS-like symptoms comparable to bipolar disorder.[17] Functional Hormone Replacement puts people in a better mood. According to a study published by Rebecca L. Glaser MD, Functional Hormone Replacement with implanted testosterone pellets decreases anxiety, irritability, and aggression in over 90% of all female patients![18] Losing body fat and gaining muscle tone are always needed in addition to the hormone treatments in order to receive maximum antiaging benefits. Losing body fat with the aid of hormone therapy and a high-fiber diet helps fix the liver metabolism so that when the body breaks down estrogen mimickers (xeno-estrogens), it doesn't leave harmful Dysfunctional Toxins (e.g., atrazine, a commonly used high-risk pesticide/herbicide) that retain excess estrogenic properties linked to cancer.[19-21]

Functional Alert: FHR prevents estrogen dominance and potential health problems!

Birth Control Pills

Birth control pills can greatly affect how your body functions. Some women have a surge in sex drive using estrogen-only birth control pills, whereas others lose their sex drive altogether. Other women have a surge in sex drive using progestin-only birth control pills and others lose their sex drive altogether. Then there are those who use a combination of estrogen and progestin birth control pills and the same scenario happens.[1] If you are taking a birth control pill that is causing you to lose your sex drive, it's a sign your body has become estrogen dominant and/or progesterone dominant and you need to change over to something else. We believe some women get breast cancer during peri-menopause, but it doesn't show up until they reach menopause or even later in life. We believe it's the estrogen- and/or progestin-based birth control pills that have caused some breast cancer cases.[2] Females who have an increase in sex drive are not becoming estrogen or progesterone dominant and, for them, the birth control pills are safer. Some females have more estrogen and progesterone receptors or better sensitivity that allow them to make better use of the hormones. Sometimes these same females have higher natural testosterone levels that help keep things in balance. However, all this is subject to change at any time due to age, weight gain, child birth, medications, illnesses, etc. Clearly there are numerous factors that determine your sensitivity to the hormones testosterone, estrogen, and progesterone.

Functional Alert: Oral birth control pills, Norplant implants, and vaginal rings suppress the ovaries, reducing testosterone production and preventing many females from being able to functional optimally.[3-6] For example, they have less ability to manage their pain perception and response. A better option is the IUD.[7] Females using any form of hormones for birth control may be helped with testosterone therapy or testosterone therapy used in conjunction with an aromatase inhibitor. We believe birth control pills are causing many females to become estrogen dominant!

Preventing Hair Loss in Females

FHR helps prevent hair loss, facial hair growth, and voice changes in females. According to the America Academy of Dermatology, hair loss is a condition that affects about 30 million females in America.[1] The psychosocial impact of hair loss can be traumatic. Hair loss may occur through several pathways, but its primary cause is low hormones! Most women experience some hair loss with aging and their rate of hair growth slows down as well. In a few females, hair loss can occur as early as their 20s. These women notice thinning on the top half of the scalp and some on the frontal line. Hair loss occurs in about 50% of females as hormones decline.[2] Once women reach their mid-50s, hair growth usually begins to slow down.

    A female can have high, normal, or even low testosterone, yet still experience thinning of the hair on the scalp. This is because testosterone does not cause hair loss, but rather Dihydrotestosterone (DHT)![3] DHT binds to receptors in the scalp follicles, making it nearly impossible for hair to survive. DHT levels can be within what doctors consider "normal range" on a scale, but still cause a problem. Hair loss in the young female population usually occurs for the same reasons as in the older female population: hormonal imbalances! Hair loss in the young is usually caused by excessive activity of an enzyme called 5-alpha reductase, which converts testosterone into DHT, or it can be caused by having low sex hormone-binding globulin (SHBG) levels from a lack of estrogen, which also increase free testosterone levels and DHT.[4,5] The vast majority of females won't start showing hair loss until they approach menopause and begin experiencing hormonal imbalances. During menopause, most females will become low in either testosterone, progesterone, estrogen, or a combination thereof. These sudden hormonal changes can result in facial hair growth, voice changes, and hair loss on the scalp.

Functional Alert: It's important to note that Functional Hormone Replacement doesn't cause hair loss in women. In fact, according to Dr. Rebecca L. Glaser of Dayton, OH, who specializes in implanting testosterone pellets, two of three patients regrow hair on Functional Hormone Replacement![6]

It's very important to tackle hormonal imbalances before irreversible damage occurs! Sudden hormonal changes or imbalances often cause excessive activity of the enzyme 5alpha-reductase that leads to more DHT conversion. Sudden hormonal changes can also lead to the testosterone-to-estrogen ratio being out of balance. When estrogen levels are too low in relation to testosterone levels, it lowers SHBG, which binds up to 98% of testosterone in the blood.[7, 8] It also binds up DHT.[9] DHT can be free or bound, just like testosterone. DHT has more attraction for SHBG than testosterone.[10, 11] DHT levels will increase if your testosterone levels are too high in relation to estrogen.

Progesterone also inhibits 5-alpha-reductase, the enzyme that converts testosterone to DHT.[12] The bottom line: Estrogen and progesterone work in opposition to the testosterone in the female body. They help prevent hair loss on the scalp, facial hair growth, and voice changes that's caused by excessive amounts of DHT being converted from testosterone.

Functional Alert: Estrogen protects against hair loss and stimulates new hair growth! The relationship between estrogen and hair is seen during pregnancy, when a female's hair becomes thicker and shinier due to estrogen levels increasing.[13] However, the extra hair grown during pregnancy is quickly lost when estrogen levels drop back to normal after childbirth. A hormonal change during pregnancy is comparable to a hormonal change during menopause!

We recommend that females who are experiencing thinning hair or want to help prevent it, use shampoos that help prevent DHT buildup on the surface of the scalp. However these shampoos don't work for everyone. We do not recommend using drugs such as finasteride to lower DHT due to the potential sexual side effects that can occur during use and even after discontinuing the drug.[14-19] The newest treatment for hair loss is platelet rich plasma, which supposedly stimulates dormant hair follicles.[20]

Functional Alert: Thyroid dysfunction can cause hair loss. Be sure to have your thyroid levels tested by your physician.[21] Hypothyroidism is a silent killer because it lowers testosterone and elevates estrogen levels!

Testosterone and Breast Cancer

Chronic inflammation and oxidation have become a living nightmare for many. When the body releases excess amounts of pro-inflammatory cytokines and free radicals, its cells become low in oxygen, leading to the dreaded diagnosis: breast cancer.[1-3] Hearing that diagnosis is one of females' biggest fears. Testosterone helps prevent breast cancer because it improves team communication among the entire immune system, which lowers inflammation and oxidation. Effective communication allows team members of the immune system to understand their roles and the roles of everyone else. The increase in oxygen levels deters the formation of benign cells in local tissues and malignant cells in other locations.[4]

How does testosterone lower inflammation and oxidation? First, it regulates pro-inflammatory cytokine expression, specifically TNF-a, and IL-1B.[5] Inappropriate cytokine expression creates an immune response that is associated with cell proliferation.[6] In addition, it stimulates the anti-inflammatory effects of sIL-6r that deter cell proliferation.[7] Second, it improves insulin sensitivity that dramatically lowers inflammation and oxidation.[8] Third, testosterone improves blood sugar metabolism and decreases the risk of developing insulin resistance and hyperinsulinemia.[9] Sugar imbalances always cause some degree of insulin resistance and/or hyperinsulinemia, provoking the body to produce excess amounts of pro-inflammatory cytokines and free radicals.[10] This causes cells to become low in oxygen. Fourth, the testosterone that gets converted into estrogen increases nitric oxide. Nitric oxide helps counterbalance chronic inflammation and oxidation at the cellular level.[11] Fifth, testosterone reduces depression and overreacting to stress in our lives, which lowers the body's production of pro-inflammatory cytokines and free radicals. [12-16] The bottom line is that testosterone helps decrease the risk of breast cancer by improving communication among the various links of the immune system and increasing oxygen in the cells!

Dr. Rebecca L. Glaser, MD, a researcher on testosterone therapy, who treats pre- and postmenopausal women (with or without a history of breast cancer) states, "Pre-clinical and clinical evidence supports that testosterone is breast protective and can reduce the risk of breast cancer." It's important to note that her conclusions were based on patients who were not, or were prevented from becoming, estrogen dominant while using testosterone pellets. Approximately 40% of Dr. Glaser's non-breast cancer patients had to use aromatase inhibitors to alleviate symptoms of estrogen dominance. Most (95%) of Dr. Glaser's breast cancer patients are treated with aromatase inhibitors.[17] The use of aromatase inhibitors is based on disease stage and symptoms.

Functional Alert: Improving functionality and getting an anticancer effect requires taking a large enough dose of testosterone to sufficiently stimulate the androgen receptor![18]

About 2 out of 3 of breast cancers are estrogen receptor-positive and/or progesterone receptor-positive: Their cancer feeds off of estrogen.[19] Recognizing women who are at an increased risk for estrogen dominance (including breast cancer survivors) and treating them accordingly is very important for cancer prevention. It is an essential part of administering Functional Hormone Replacement. We believe, however, that the vast majority of non-cancer patients and about one-third of breast cancer patients wouldn't need to use harsh drugs called aromatase inhibitors along with their testosterone if they would simply lower their body-fat levels using a Functional Diet and Exercise program. This usually makes their estrogen dominance symptoms go away!

Functional Alert: Testosterone alone, without the use of aromatase inhibitors, can help breast cancer patients whose tumors are estrogen receptor-negative and/or progesterone receptor-negative (about one-third of all breast cancer patients), given they are not estrogen dominant![20]

If your physician tells you that Functional Hormone Replacement might promote breast cancer instead of helping prevent it, we highly recommend you find another doctor who has a better understanding of testosterone. It's disappointing to see a physician reject something they know little or nothing about. Take a long, hard look at how many females died with low testosterone levels versus those with healthy ones. Do the research and you will find that when the vast majority died from diseased conditions, their testosterone levels were low when compared to the levels of their youth. You will find a pattern that can't be denied!

Functional Alert: Anabolic receptors are located in most tissues of the human body (e.g., the breast and bones) and need adequate amounts of testosterone to remain functional![21]

Some doctors don't believe females need progesterone if they don't have a uterus; others do. We know females who have benefited from using it. A combination of progesterone and testosterone can be very beneficial for females with endometriosis because without the hormones, sexual intercourse can be very painful. Progesterone does a lot more things than just protect the endometrium, which is the uterine lining. It helps to improve sleep, lubricate the vagina, control anxiety by producing a calming effect, and balance out estrogen and DHT levels.

Functional Alert: Some women with anxiety due to low testosterone, estrogen, and progesterone may think they have a mental illness, but this is not the case. It's simply their bodies telling them they need hormones!

The imbalance of testosterone, progesterone, and estrogen in females can cause damaging inflammation and oxidation throughout their entire bodies. For younger women who are not approaching menopause, yet feel sluggish, depressed, and sexually dysfunctional, the answer isn't always to mess with their hormones, but rather to lose body fat and build muscle tone through a Functional Diet and Exercise program! This will increase testosterone to a small degree and significantly reduce the amount of estrogen circulating in the system. If that doesn't work, then it's time to add hormones!

Functional Alert: We recommend that you see a qualified expert in this field and get your levels measured. Have your doctor make any necessary adjustments from there in accordance with how you feel, not some number on a scale. Hormones are best taken at night because of their potential calming effect!

Women's Intimate Relationships and Hormones

A high-frequency sex life is common when people begin to fall in love. At the beginning of their intimate relationship, their sex drives are often compatible and they have what we refer to as a Functional Sex life. As time progresses, a decline in their hormones can change the way partners feel about their significant others. All too often, women tend to wrongly associate their lack of sex drive with headaches, lack of time or energy, or feelings of depression and irritability. In reality, their hormones, especially testosterone, are out of balance, causing them to become disinterested. Extremely low testosterone and estrogen levels can also cause a lack of libido, anxiety, depression, chronic fatigue, etc., in females. When your hormones are low or out of balance, you can go without sex and not miss it. If you are content with having sex only 1-2 times per week, you definitely need FHR! It changes all this because it brings back the desire to have Functional Sex daily.

Functional Alert: Some women are left with hormonal imbalances after childbirth. They are unable to recapture their pre-childbirth sex drive until they get their FHR!

It's not uncommon for some women to avoid sex because they have trouble orgasming. They like sex, but they fear they'll disappoint their man with endless attempts to bring forth an orgasm that will never happen. Several men have told us in private that they have to beg or bribe their women for sex and then when they agree, it seems like a chore. Most of these men are secretively on the prowl, looking for other females to have sex with, and their women haven't a clue! A lack of sexual desire is more than just staying tired all the time because of work, household chores, taking care of kids, etc. Life doesn't have to be this way. Men, when you see the key signs of your woman struggling with imbalanced hormones, you can help her through this tough time by persuading her to go to the doctor. Ladies, it's your responsibility to get your hormones straightened out. You can't hold an uncooperative doctor accountable if they decline to treat symptoms. It's up to you to find a doctor who will!

Functional Alert: Having a functional relationship requires saving each other during times of need. Gentlemen, if your woman's sex drive isn't completely resolved by FHR and you getting fit, it's a sign that she feels overwhelmed and upset about the excessive responsibilities she has taken upon herself. In these particular cases, you'll need to help out more around the house, etc., so she can slow down in this fast-paced society. In addition, you need to focus on her needs first in the bedroom!

Ladies, your men will still want to be intimate when you grow old together, so you'll want to keep up sexually to maintain the relationship! Although testosterone therapy was introduced into clinical practice to improve sexual function in males, there is an increasing use of testosterone to fix the array of sexual dysfunctions associated with low testosterone in females. Many men want to be intimate every day and they usually want to have passionate-adventurous sex. It's difficult for women with imbalanced or low hormones to want to have sex. If men have to bother and pester for sex, you can be assured they will search elsewhere! They may really try hard to avoid having an affair at first, but it's inevitable in the vast majority of cases. They will often have a fling with a woman at work, with someone they met on the Internet, etc. Since your man has been feeling denied, the sex during the affair will seem astounding to him! There is a great chance he will walk away from the marriage or relationship and not have a single regret. Why? Men often equate passionate-adventurous sex with love and being desired!

Functional Alert: Men get angry if they are denied Functional Sex!

A deficiency in testosterone will usually cause many problems for females. Along with losing their sense of security, they experience a lack of sexual desire, sexual fantasies, sensitivity to sexual stimulation, and orgasms. Yet we have known of doctors who have told women their testosterone levels were normal for their age, when, in fact, they had hardly any testosterone at all. Ironically, these doctors wouldn't tell these same women not to use injectable insulin if their pancreases weren't producing enough of the hormone insulin! Even though we believe many people are being overmedicated, we also believe that taking hormones is much better than having your life taken away by the side effects of low hormones.

On the other hand, if a woman is highly sexed, it's usually a sign she has more testosterone and/or dopamine than the average female. Some females get lucky and produce a lot of testosterone, while others get short-changed and struggle emotionally and sexually from the time they reach puberty until they reverse the problem.

We have heard women say they are afraid of taking testosterone because they fear getting manly muscles. The fact, is, having high testosterone levels doesn't automatically equate to having big muscles. The size of your muscles actually has more to do with how many type-2 fibers you were born with than your testosterone levels. There are plenty of females and males with high testosterone levels who work out with heavy weights, yet still have small muscles. We put some of them on Slingshot Functional Training (bodybuilding programs) and they still couldn't bulk up with muscle!

We'd like to end this section by saying that many men have told us they are afraid to commit to marriage. Why? Because they have bought into the idea that females lose interest in having frequent Functional Sex after marriage and/or allow themselves to become overweight and out of shape. They also fear that one day their wife will prefer other activities, such as gardening and shopping, over having frequent Functional Sex. This should not be the case unless a female's hormone levels are out of balance, they allow themselves to become overweight and insecure, or they were faking their high sex drives from the beginning. Unfortunately, plenty of females have low testosterone before getting married and are clueless about what it's like to have a strong libido. We believe that hormones are usually the reason for sudden changes in sex drive directly after marriage. Wanting to have a happy marriage, along with the best sex of your life, is certainly nothing to be embarrassed about.

Functional Alert: Functional Sex is probably the most important aspect of a marriage. Sexual incompatibility will destroy a marriage!

How to Properly Balance Out a Man's Hormones

When it comes to a man, all that's needed for hormone replacement is testosterone. The best hormone replacement we know of for men is to inject testosterone cypionate once a week! There's no set limit to how much testosterone you can use as long as your hematocrit levels remain in a normal range and you avoid becoming estrogen dominant. Testosterone is basically nontoxic since it's a naturally occurring substance in your body. Dosages must be determined by your response! If men desire to go the cream or gel route, they'll need to take a considerable amount daily in order to get their testosterone levels high enough to experience a noticeable effect. Some men can't use the transdermal version because it irritates their skin or won't absorb well enough to give them a positive response. Gels/creams or implanted testosterone pellets can be good options for men who experience high hematocrit levels and/or estrogen dominance with the injectable version of testosterone. The injections are a lot less expensive and less hassle for those who aren't afraid of needles. You don't want to buy the 1 ml bottles because you get less for your money. Ask your doctor for the 10 ml bottles that contain 200 mgs per ml.

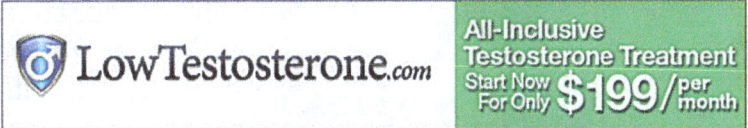

Functional Alert: Higher blood levels of testosterone equate to an improved mood, enhanced functionality, and a higher level of sexual desire and satisfaction. "Free testosterone" is the amount of the hormone that is active in the body. Blood levels of total testosterone and free testosterone vary among each individual. This makes it impossible for doctors to use a scale to establish precisely how much testosterone to prescribe. The focus should be on how you feel. Your free testosterone levels are what matters most. High total testosterone numbers on a scale mean nothing if your free testosterone levels are low. The more testosterone you take, the higher your free testosterone will become!

Dysfunctional Hormone Replacement is running rampant among males! It can stem from doctors not giving them enough testosterone or giving them one huge injection of testosterone cypionate every 2 weeks. Men who do a shot every 2 weeks find that by the time the second week rolls around, their testosterone has become too low or unstable at around day 10. This leads to poor testosterone levels, mood swings, hair loss, and loss of libido. We strongly recommend that you ask your doctor about switching to once-a-week injections in order to obtain stable testosterone and estrogen levels!

A physician or nurse will teach you or someone else how to inject the testosterone so it can be done at home. The smallest needle that can be properly used to inject testosterone is a small 1 inch 23 gauge needle. Use an 18 gauge needle to draw it into the syringe. The testosterone is easier to inject after it has been heated. It's best to heat the testosterone with a hair dryer for about 30 seconds once it's in the syringe.

Ronnie: *At age 49, I feel great with my testosterone levels around 1300 ng/dl. I've been taking testosterone for over 20 years and haven't experienced any negative side effects. I inject testosterone cypionate once a week.*

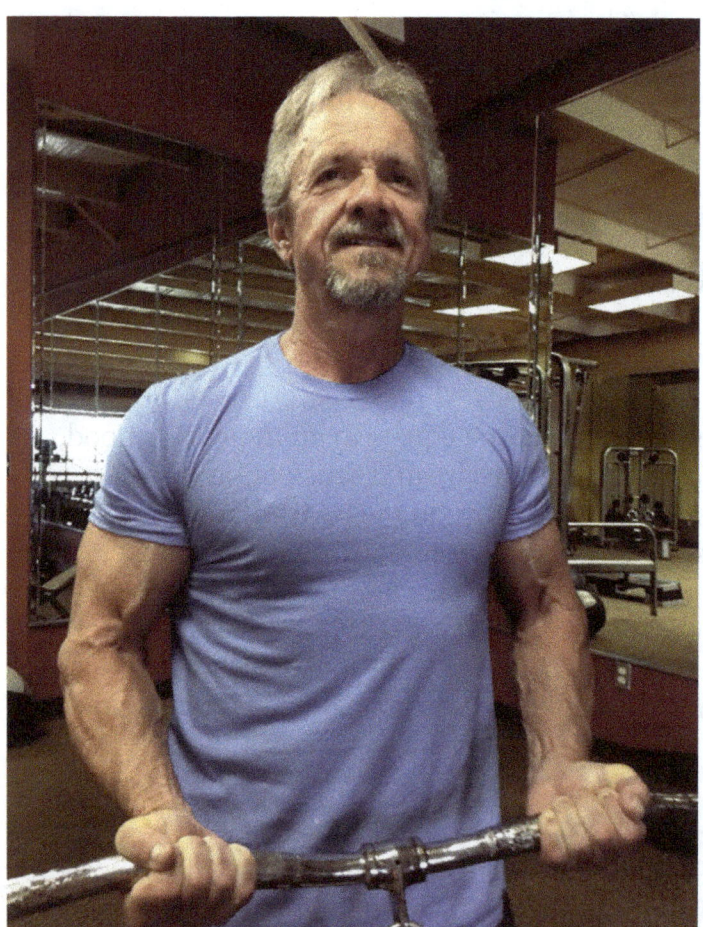

Earl Lenderman, age 66

Once in a lifetime, a special personal trainer comes along in your life that connects with you, guides you, and has tremendous character. I am lucky to have this personal trainer named Ronnie Rowland. He's very down to earth and easy to talk to. You can't miss Ronnie and his wife Kathy Rowland in the gym. His arms are inspiring and her leg development is remarkable. They represent what a happy marriage really looks like.

I met Ronnie Rowland approximately seven years ago while attending a nutritional seminar he was giving at the gym. After the seminar, I explained to him about my chronic lower back pain from two degenerative discs and my desire to lose body fat and gain more muscle. Ronnie said he could help me if I would follow his instructions. My only regret was not hiring him sooner! The muscle magazines I was reading had me extremely frustrated. I thought I could get as big and lean as the guys in those magazines if I followed their workout and nutritional/

supplement programs. Ronnie explained to me that it was impossible to become like them unless you are born with an abundance of type-2 muscle fibers. But he said he could teach me how to max out my genetic potential. I learned I had been overtraining, lifting too much weight, performing too much cardio, eating the wrong kinds of foods, and using the wrong exercises for my chronic lower-back condition, and needed Functional Testosterone Replacement.

I always thought it took free weights to gain muscle and strength, but Ronnie taught me that machines were actually more productive in my case. At age 66, I am stronger, more energetic, and more muscular/vascular than ever. The only prescription medication I take is testosterone cypionate once a week. Every time I tried to lose body fat in the past, I lost more muscle than fat. We solved that problem with Slingshot Functional Training, a Functional Diet, and Functional Testosterone Replacement. My lower back pain has improved significantly and my leg pain has completely disappeared. The boost in testosterone, combined with the proper training and diet, has made my entire core stronger and lowered inflammation in my body. I am no longer a candidate for back surgery! I can play more rounds of golf before my lower back begins to hurt and I can hit the ball farther. **Functional Training with a Fork** *has put me on the right path. My stress levels would be unmanageable if I were not following the principles found in this book. I hope people who are dealing with various health issues will give* **Functional Training with a Fork** *a try. I see a lot of my friends suffering needlelessly because they are not following the principles found in this book!*

Low Estrogen in Males

Low estrogen causes sexual, physical, and mental side effects for males. It's not just low testosterone that men have to worry about as they age; they also have to worry about low estrogen! A lack of testosterone translates into a lack of estrogen because some of the testosterone converts into estrogen. Low estrogen levels, even in the presence of high testosterone levels, can destroy a male's sex drive; cause depression, joint pain, and lethargy; increase LDL cholesterol; make arteries less flexible; and cause hair loss on the scalp. This has been proven by guys using testosterone who took aromatase inhibitors to reduce estrogen levels and free up more bound testosterone.

Increased estrogen levels should be welcomed during Functional Hormone Replacement, not feared. As stated previously, some of the symptoms of low testosterone in males (e.g., low sex drive) are partially caused by low estrogen levels! [22] Estrogen improves blood sugar metabolism and decreases the risk of developing insulin resistance, hyperinsulinemia, and heart disease. It also protects against undesirable changes in the electrical pulse controlling the heartbeat, as well as protecting against an enlarged heart. [23, 24] Moreover, a lack of estrogen increase the production of pro-inflammatory cytokines and free radicals. [25]

The only time estrogen levels should be a major concern is if your body has excessive amounts of estrogen (estrogen dominance). It's rarer for males to experience estrogen dominance than females because they usually have more muscle and less body fat. Gynocomestia (a lump located near the nipples) is often a sign of estrogen dominance in males. In these rare cases, we feel it's better to try and get by with using less testosterone and/or losing body fat instead of using aromatase inhibitors that can have undesirable side effects (e.g. joint pain, a loss of libido, and bone loss). [26-30] The body will often adjust to the increased hormones on its own over time and the gynocomestia can disappear on its own. Gynocomestia can also be caused from high body-fat levels stemming from a lack of testosterone.

Functional Alert: Functional Hormone Replacement prevents low estrogen levels in males and potential health problems (e.g., heart disease). Males who use aromatase inhibitors along with their testosterone therapy are at increased risk of heart disease.[31-35] The bottom line is, using aromatase inhibitors is probably just as bad for your heart, if not worse, than being estrogen dominant. Therefore, body fat should be kept relatively low while using testosterone so you can avoid having to use these harsh drugs.[36] Obese people who need them should only use them short-term until they get their body-fat levels down!

Testosterone and Prostate Cancer

Chronic inflammation and oxidation have become a living nightmare for many. When the body releases excess amounts of pro-inflammatory cytokines and free radicals, its cells become low in oxygen, leading to the dreaded diagnosis: prostate cancer.[1-4] Hearing that diagnosis is one of males' biggest fears. Testosterone helps prevent prostate cancer because it improves team communication among the entire immune system which lowers inflammation and oxidation. Effective communication allows team members of the immune system to understand their roles and the roles of everyone else on the team. The increase in oxygen levels deters the formation of benign cells in local tissues and malignant cells in other locations.[5]

How does testosterone lower inflammation/oxidation? First, it regulates pro-inflammatory cytokine expression, specifically TNF-a, and IL-1B.[6] Inappropriate cytokine expression creates an immune response that is associated with cell proliferation.[7] In addition, it stimulates the anti-inflammatory effects of sIL-6r that deter cell proliferation.[8] Second, it improves insulin sensitivity that dramatically lowers inflammation and oxidation.[9] Third, testosterone improves blood sugar metabolism and decreases the risk of developing insulin resistance and hyperinsulinemia. Sugar imbalances always cause some degree of insulin resistance and/or hyperinsulinemia, provoking the body to produce excess amounts of pro-inflammatory cytokines and free radicals.[10] This causes cells to become low in oxygen. Fourth, the testosterone that gets converted into estrogen increases nitric oxide. Nitric oxide helps counterbalance chronic inflammation and oxidation at the cellular level.[11] Fifth, testosterone reduces depression and overreacting to stress in our lives, which lowers the body's production of pro-inflammatory cytokines and free radicals.[12-16] The bottom line is that testosterone helps decrease the risk of prostate cancer by improving communication among the various links of the immune system and increasing oxygen in the cells!

Dr. Abraham Morgentaler, a practicing urologist and an Associate Clinical Professor of Urology, at the Harvard Medical School, has done a lot of research on testosterone and prostate cancer. He states, "I no longer fear that giving a man testosterone therapy will make a hidden prostate cancer grow or put him at increased risk of developing prostate cancer down the road. My real concern now is that men with low testosterone are at an increased risk of already having prostate cancer."[17-20] Furthermore, Dr. Joel Kaufman and Dr. James Graydon, in an article in The Journal of Urology in 2004, reported that they treated men with testosterone therapy after they had undergone surgery to remove all of the prostate gland and some of the tissue around it. None of the men had developed a recurrence of their prostate cancer. Another group from Baylor College of Medicine reported the same results! [21, 22]

Functional Alert: Research carried out in the past 10 years has shown that testosterone therapy doesn't cause a recurrence of prostate cancer! [23-25]

If your physician tells you that Functional Hormone Replacement might promote prostate cancer instead of helping prevent it, we highly recommend you find another doctor who has a better understanding of testosterone. It's disappointing to see a physician reject something they know little or nothing about. Take a long, hard look at how many males died with low testosterone levels versus those who had healthy levels. Do the research and you will find that when the vast majority of men died from diseased conditions, their testosterone levels were low when compared to the levels of their youth. There is a pattern that can't be denied!

Functional Alert: Anabolic receptors are located in most tissues of the human body (e.g., the brain and heart) and need adequate amounts of testosterone to remain functional! [26]

Men's Intimate Relationships and Hormones

We've noticed that men who are low in testosterone begin to have a change in priorities. They decide they need to get into shape, but they don't have the energy and drive to stick with it. Others who are already working out, find themselves facing the same problem. They also struggle because of a lack of energy and drive.

Low testosterone can be the reason a man leaves a relationship after many years of dating or marriage because he has lost his sex drive and believes that finding another woman will restore it. Unfortunately, a lot of women never see it coming! Ladies, when you see the key signs of your man struggling with imbalanced hormones, you can help him through this tough time by persuading him to go to the doctor. Men, it's your responsibility to get your hormones straightened out. You can't hold an uncooperative doctor accountable if they decline to treat the symptoms. It's up to you to find a doctor who will!

Functional Alert: Having a functional relationship requires saving each other during times of need. Ladies, if your man's sex drive isn't completely resolved by FHR and you getting fit, it's a sign you need a better understanding of his sexual desires. Men will lose their romantic connection if you are uptight and/or boring in bed. Make each sexual encounter a memorable experience so he's eager to have sex again!

For most females, an affair is more about being emotionally connected with someone than sex, whereas for most males, it's more about sex than an emotional connection. However, both sexes need strong emotional and sexual connections to be happy in a relationship. When a male doesn't get enough sex because he's low on testosterone and/or his woman is low on testosterone, he becomes emotionally disconnected. This not only leads to him cheating on his woman, but also his woman cheating on him! As you are seeing while reading this book, a lot of the things that appear to be complicated on the surface are actually very easy to fix!

Functional Alert: Contrary to popular opinion, males who have a high sex drive are less likely to cheat as long as they are being emotionally and sexually satisfied. This is because they are not going to risk losing their most valued treasure!

One of the most common problems a male faces when experiencing low testosterone and estrogen is a low libido coupled with irritability, anxiety, and depression, leading to weight gain. Television and movies portray a middle-aged male with his libido at an all-time high. Instead, the opposite is actually true in most cases. Negativity overcomes them and they begin to think they can't satisfy their women or their employers. In other words, they tend to run away from their responsibilities. Several females have told us that their men no longer show interest in them sexually and emotionally. When they are confronted, men often change the subject by saying they are just tired from working so many hours.

> **Kathy:** *Men with higher testosterone levels are more assertive and more attractive to women. Men with low testosterone have a lesser chance in winning the attention of a woman.*

We'd like to end this section by saying that many women have told us they are afraid to commit to intimate relationships and marriage. Why? Because it's hard for them to let go of insecurities and trust a guy they are interested in. They have been hurt in the past and they believe most guys only want one thing (sex) and the women are afraid of being hurt again. They fear that guys are going to use them for sex until something better comes along. This really is the hardest part for a woman in any intimate relationship! When they let go and trust, they risk some very bad heartaches because their brain works on a higher emotional level than males. Guys, you need to make sure you are trustworthy and provide your woman with the constant attention she needs to feel good about herself, and you need to maintain your testosterone levels if you want to get into a long-term, intimate relationship with a female and make it last.

Functional Alert: Women take it personally if you lose interest in having Functional Sex with them!

Defensive Hormone Therapy

Many doctors are practicing defensive hormone treatment (avoiding high-risk patients and Functional Hormone Therapy) to try to reduce their exposure to malpractice liability. Concerns regarding malpractice liability cause doctors to become very uncertain about medical outcomes. Therefore, some tell their patients hormone replacement can be dangerous and is not recommended. Defensive hormone treatment is causing the cost of health care to rise for everyone because some doctors are not treating the problems and the patients will remain or become sick.

It's not uncommon for reputable doctors who often go above and beyond their duties, to tell their patients their hormones are fine for their age and they don't need any. The truth of the matter is, some doctors are now reluctant to administer Functional Hormone Replacement. Why? We believe America has too many lawyers![27] Some of the lawyers are struggling to make a living in their profession, especially the younger ones who are in debt up to their ears from student loan payments every month. We believe this has led to an overabundance of frivolous lawsuits against the medical community. It has also caused a lot of reputable doctors to begin practicing defensive medicine or stop practicing medicine altogether.

In addition, doctors have to use their DEA numbers when prescribing medications, and medications such as testosterone are tracked more than others due to all the steroid scandals in sports.[28,29] Testosterone is now a scheduled 3 drug on the DEA's list of controlled substances.[30] Doctors don't want that kind of attention. Many people (doctors included) think it's unfair that the DEA and FDA are harming others by overly enforcing misguided drug laws.[31-36] They've made it especially hard for a female to get a prescription for enough testosterone to have a positive effect. It appears this is due to gender bias! [37]

There's no disputing the effectiveness of Functional Hormone Replacement in both males and females! Therefore, we strongly believe the FDA has wrongly stated that there's no clear scientific evidence showing testosterone therapy can reverse some of the effects of aging. [38-40] We believe it's all based on erroneous assumption and that facts and data are being ignored. We also believe this is a clear case of government regulation without a reason. Now insurance companies are beginning to limit coverage for the use of testosterone to help people who are suffering from low libido, low energy, depression, etc. Insurance companies are telling doctors what they can and cannot do, and it's affecting you!

Don't allow the opinion of others make you feel ashamed about using testosterone. When you keep it a secret, you are letting other people control you! It's good to let others know what testosterone has done for you. We would also like to encourage doctors who understand the benefits of Functional Hormone Replacement to not let other doctors make you feel as if you are wrong for helping millions of people by prescribing testosterone. Doctors need to voice their opinions on how testosterone has helped their patients!

Functional Alert: We see a lot of people on the Internet (doctors included) who are in favor of testosterone therapy, but they are hiding behind Internet screennames. What are you afraid of? Take a stand for what you believe in! It's time for everyone (doctors included) in favor of testosterone to voice their opinions to others and contact their local congressman. It's very important that you tell them you want access to Functional Hormone Replacement. If you don't, there's a good chance the government and insurance companies will make it almost impossible to get or prescribe in the future!

We encourage you not to allow some people in the media to persuade you to make poor decisions. Also, a lot of primary care physicians are inexperienced when it comes to hormones and don't want to get involved in working with patients to try to figure it all out. There are some doctors who tell their patients that Functional Hormone Replacement is dangerous. It's disappointing for us when we hear about doctors who are overconfident and in direct conflict with reality. We think the problem is that some of their patients haven't done their homework and will accept whatever doctors say. Quite often, the patients end up not getting the proper treatment they need! Even doctors who have a pretty good knowledge of hormone replacement often figure it's high risk for their careers if they raise their patients' hormone levels to the higher end of the scale or beyond, even though it often cures their symptoms. In addition, there is not a lot of money in it for the majority of doctors because they can't charge high consultation fees.

These days, it seems our money is often more sought after than our well-being. For example, in 2009, some of the FDA's own scientists admitted that they are often threatened by those in authority to cover up study data.[41] We believe this results in everyone getting corrupted information and the FDA getting a huge kickback by charging money for new drug application fees being submitted by pharmaceutical companies.[42] We feel it's time for everyone to take a stand for Functional Hormone Replacement so the FDA stops targeting doctors, etc. The bottom line is, Functional Hormone Replacement, combined with Functional Exercise and Diet can help prevent medical conditions that cause healthcare cost to rise and lower the amount of medications needed. We believe that the proper use of testosterone, combined with Functional Exercise and Diet would drastically lower overall profits for both the FDA and pharmaceutical companies. We believe this is the #1 reason the FDA is trying to control what doctors can and can't do in regard to hormone treatment! If that were not the case, then why are they not regulating harmful drugs such as tobacco and alcohol?

We remember around five years ago when we first started seeing and hearing TV and radio advertisements for what was essentially testosterone therapy. They talked about low testosterone and how restoring testosterone levels would improve our functionality. Later on down the road, some of the people taking testosterone had heart attacks and strokes. This generated a class-action lawsuit against the companies making testosterone. Unfortunately, some people jumped on the bandwagon and sued for things such as stroke and heart attacks. It was highly unlikely that hormone replacement caused any of their problems in the first place if their hematocrit levels were in normal range and if they weren't estrogen dominant. We believe that most of these people would have had a heart attack or stroke without the use of hormones. In fact, health problems almost always occur much sooner for those low in hormones because they are sitting around not exercising, losing muscle tone, and eating fattening foods.

Functional Alert: The new concerns over testosterone therapy are mostly due to methodological limitations and data errors. The most current research shows that testosterone lowers the risk of strokes and heart disease. In fact, mortality is reduced by approximately half in people who take testosterone by prescription compared to those who don't! [43]

There is a dirty little secret that was kept by some patients who have sued testosterone manufacturers for stroke or heart attack. In some cases, it appears drugs did cause heart attacks and strokes even when hematocrit levels and symptoms of estrogen dominance were being checked periodically by doctors. However, it wasn't the testosterone being prescribed by their physician that caused the stroke or heart attack. It was over-the-counter drugs, prescription drugs, and the use of recreational drugs.[44, 45] The doctors and lawyers probably had no clue about their use of these drugs or the damage being caused, so the testosterone manufacturers got the blame! These patients joined the class action lawsuit to cover their medical expenses. In the long run, they not only hurt themselves, but others who need testosterone therapy to remain healthy. This is because medical problems stemming from hormonal imbalances or low hormones leads to a lack of exercise and muscle tone, a poor diet, obesity, and an increase in inflammation and oxidation. Without the hormones their life-cycle becomes: overeat, take medicines, work, and die! Approximately 70 million Americans use mind-altering drugs.[46] About 70% of all Americans are taking some form of prescription medication and at least 50% are on two or more! [47]

Functional Alert: Recreational drug use is the driving force behind poverty, crime, and violence in America! Having a drug addiction can make you feel as though there's no hope for getting better. When all else fails, increasing dopamine levels by combining Functional Hormone Replacement, Functional Diet, and Functional Exercise (Functional Training and Functional Cardio) helps people stop using drugs!

Regardless of what anyone may claim, doctors included, there is no clear evidence that FHR alone causes heart attacks or strokes when hematocrit levels are kept in normal range and estrogen dominance is avoided. We suspect that most of the people who thought testosterone replacement caused their heart attack or stroke were never absorbing enough on a frequent basis to actually do anything positive. In other words, they were taking so small of a dose or taking it so infrequently that their bodies were still low in the hormones needed to help counteract inflammation, oxidation, and heart disease.

If you are not experiencing a noticeable increase in energy, mood, and libido with hormone therapy, then your therapy is dysfunctional and needs to be adjusted by a willing physician until you feel something very positive happening. Your body's response is the only gauge for whether or not the amount of hormones you are taking is right for your chemistry. You will know if your overall health and performance are improving or worsening by the way they make you feel. Hormone therapy is one of the few areas of medicine where a patient will go back to their doctor and say, "You really helped me feel great!" Men and women around the world are in desperate need of FHR help from the medical community. Low hormones can be a life or death issue and they are most certainly a quality of life issue!

Functional Alert: Doctors need support from the FDA, DEA, and insurance companies!

The extent of dysfunctional medical practice by some doctors astounds us. Their dysfunctional thinking goes something like this: They tell their male and female patients that they don't prescribe hormones because they don't know the long-term effects of this substance that is already naturally occurring in their bodies. They only know the short-term effects, which are reduced pain from inflammatory conditions, stronger bones, enhanced muscle tone and strength, improved motor skills, body-fat loss, increased energy and mood, decreased risk of cancer and heart disease, increased mental clarity, a better sex drive, etc. So what do they do? They prescribe a drug that doesn't naturally occur in your body, knowing that the long-term side effects can be dangerous! They also know the short-term side effects of these drugs, which are almost always decreased energy, lowered testosterone levels, brain fog, decreased sexual performance, increased weight gain, decreased motor skills, and loss in muscle tone and strength.

Functional Alert: There's a lot to be said for finding a doctor who has common sense. Unfortunately, some of the doctors who score the highest on IQ tests have foolish ideas and behave inappropriately. Your best option is to find one with both common sense and a high IQ!

Insurance companies could save a ton of money if they persuaded the doctors to start prescribing hormones for their male and female patients instead of medications that deter people from a Functional Diet and Functional Exercise by taking away their drive and energy. In addition, low or imbalanced hormones can cause mental problems leading to violent actions and suicidal tendencies. People begin to feel worthless, unhappy, and lack confidence. These negative factors lead to obesity!

Antidepressants help increase serotonin levels that become depleted when hormones get low or out of balance. A lot of doctors are quick to hand out antidepressants for males and females because these drugs are not scrutinized by the DEA in the same way as testosterone. The lack of sexual function often caused by the antidepressants causes even more depression![48] On the other hand, testosterone helps eliminate depression while enhancing the libido, further eliminating depression!

Functional Alert: An actual antidepressant should not lower sexual functioning!

Testosterone also brings forth a "true" sense of well-being and allows you to adapt your lifestyle. Antidepressants such as selective serotonin reuptake inhibitors often bring forth a "false" sense of well-being that causes you to become disconnected from the real world. Healthy levels of testosterone are required in both males and females for healing and central nervous system support of opioid receptors.[49, 50] The opioid system controls both acute and chronic pain.[51] It also helps control addictive behaviors such as overeating. Testosterone levels also make you smarter and happier by maintaining the blood-brain barrier (a network of blood vessels that allows the entry of essential nutrients while blocking other substances) and activating dopamine activity, which helps make you happier by alleviating depression.[52, 53]

Functional Alert: Testosterone and estrogen work in harmony to enhance cognitive function by improving electrical activity in the brain. This lowers inflammation and oxidation in the brain and throughout the entire body![54]

A lot of older people look at younger people and say, "I would like to have some of their energy!" We are here to tell you that you can have some of that youthful energy back with FHR! However, Dysfunctional Hormone Replacement, which is being implemented by some doctors, isn't going to give you any extra energy. In fact, it might make you feel worse! The number of men and women who suffer from low hormones, especially testosterone, is very high because laboratory reference ranges accept low levels as normal. This only ends in disappointment and frustration for the patient. We have seen a lot of people who could not lose body fat and purge their bodies of Dysfunctional Toxins because they simply did not have the energy to exercise as needed. Willpower had nothing to do with it. Their hormones were the problem! We have learned that Functional Hormone Replacement, when combined with a Functional Diet, Functional Training, and Functional Cardio, is more effective for depression, anxiety, high blood pressure, type-2 diabetes, and obesity than any medications on the market.

Functional Alert: Aerobic and anaerobic function declines as people grow older. Newly conducted research by Thomas W. Storer, PhD, Director of the Exercise Physiology Laboratory at Brigham and Women's Hospital of Harvard Medical School in Boston, MA, and his colleagues shows that testosterone therapy significantly improves functional capacity in aging people. They discovered that there's a significant decrease in blood lactic acid during incremental load work levels in aging people who take testosterone.[55] This means better performance and less muscle pain during exercise and daily activities!

Emotional Connections

Emotional connections can end with weight gain and hormones! The inability to have an emotional connection like you once had with your significant other is often due to being overweight and/or having imbalanced hormone levels. Being in an unhappy relationship leads to poor health and stress-induced behavior such as overeating and alcohol addiction! The following is an illustration of what we have observed throughout the years as personal trainers. It is based on real people and real life experiences. Jack and Emily are a married couple. Jack was an engineer in his early 40s and needed to lose 100 pounds. Emily, a school teacher, was also in her early 40s and she needed to lose 75 pounds. Both had tried various diets, ab machines, cardio equipment, and boot camp DVDs they purchased off television. Jack could lose around 50 pounds in six months, but much of it was in the form of muscle and he always gained his weight back. Emily, on the other hand, could never lose any appreciable weight. She would get about 15 pounds off and her body would stagnate and she would just quit. She also began to think her husband no longer found her attractive because he no longer initiated sexual intercourse.

At our suggestion, both began following the Functional Diet, Basic Functional Training 3 times a week, and Functional Cardio 3 times a week. We also told them that testosterone therapy would help them reach their goals. It took a little persistence on their behalf because their primary care physician was reluctant to give either one of them testosterone. He told Jack it might cause prostate enlargement and that Emily could grow facial hair. Jack found another doctor who referred him to a reputable endocrinologist. The hormone specialist took care of Jack's needs. He was prescribed a topical version of testosterone for daily use. After 6 weeks, he noticed a little difference, but not nearly as much as he had hoped. We told him to ask his doctor about weekly testosterone injections. His doctor put him on a trial run of a once-a-week injection of testosterone cypionate. The injection was a 1 ml shot, which equals 200 mgs of test cypionate. At around 8 weeks, his testosterone levels were at around 1000 ng/dl and his energy levels picked up dramatically. His productivity at work increased. His libido dramatically improved to the point where he felt young again and was no longer having anxiety issues in the bedroom from not being able to perform up to par. He had increased sensitivity, better orgasms, and woke up with morning erections for the first time in years. He told the doctor, "I am staying with the injections!"

Emily finally found a knowledgeable gynecologist after her third attempt. He discovered that she was low in testosterone, progesterone, and estrogen. The female body is more complicated in terms of obtaining a nice hormonal balance and everyone is different in how they metabolize these hormones. This is why the scale doctors use is nothing more than a baseline to try and gauge what is going on. Emily was prescribed 2% testosterone cream daily, which took her levels up to 60 ng/dl. It took 4 months for her to get her hormones where they needed to be and to see positive effects on her libido, energy, and mood. She also made note of a few hot flashes for the first 2 months. It took around 3 months before her chronic migraines left and she could stop taking the migraine medicine. Her mood stabilized and she had a more positive outlook on life in general. She learned that making small adjustments in hormones and really listening to her body was the best guide she had.

Functional Alert: Both of these individuals' testosterone blood levels came back in the so-called normal range for their age group prior to beginning FHR!

Emily said that for some reason she had never had a sex drive like this her entire life. They went from having sexual intercourse once a week to once a day! Once the testosterone built up in their systems and they began to exercise and eat properly, they noticed it helped them control their appetites. Their ravenous sugar cravings eventually left, enabling them to stop eating before reaching the point of getting bloated and feeling sick. They also began looking forward to working out for the first time in their lives. Before they did not understand what people meant when they talked about being ready to go pump some iron or getting an endorphin high during training, but now they did! Their ability to exercise with great intensity caused a release of endorphins in their brains. Frequent endorphin releases are linked to remarkable changes in people who suffer from stress, anxiety, anger, severe panic attacks, depression, chronic pain, and emotional eating. The release of endorphins has been called life changing by many of our clients!

Ironically, Jack was very thin as a young child. So thin, in fact, that his parents forced him to eat when he wasn't hungry. He told us, "I suppose the extra food worked really well. I began to have a weight problem around age 16. I went from a skinny kid, to a heavy teen, to an obese young adult, and was embarrassed at what I had allowed myself to become." For many years, he had avoided his yearly medical checkup because he did not want to be told that he needed to lose some weight and get on medication to control his high blood pressure. Jack knew that he should lose weight and, thanks to the blood pressure machine at the local pharmacy, he also knew he had high blood pressure. He was well aware of the fact that his eating was out of control. Trying to lose weight was his subject of discussion until he was in his mid-30s. Then he just decided he was going to be fat all his life and gave up. He decided that he should accept himself for who he was, even though, deep down, he didn't love himself. So he bought larger clothes and tried to enjoy life even though he felt as if he were walking around with a 100-pound barbell on his back. He got winded just climbing a small set of stairs and his back constantly ached when he had to stand for longer than 5 minutes in one position. Jack's back felt as if it were going to give out when he got up from his chair. He lost his sex drive and began to rationalize it had to do with no longer being physically attracted to his wife who had also allowed herself to become obese.

By the time he turned 40, he was well past 300 pounds. He was miserable! There was a small voice in his head that kept telling him that he was killing himself with food. He stayed tired and in a bad mood. Due to his lack of libido from having high blood pressure and low testosterone levels, his appetite for sex had been replaced with an appetite for food. He began showing signs of an enlarged prostate from the lack of sexual intercourse. Little did he know the prostate gland is made up of fibromuscular bands that weaken when not worked out frequently, causing chronic erectile dysfunction. Nor did he know that low testosterone can cause problems with urination. Jack told us, "I remember sitting at a restaurant and my belly was touching the table. I was shocked at the size of my belly!" One day Jack took a long, hard look at himself in the mirror and decided that if he wanted to see his child grow up, he needed to do something now! He'd spent years of his life proving that he could not control his eating. Treating himself with just a bit of ice cream and cookies every night always led to overindulgence. His bad eating habits and the weight gained are what brought him to the gym to hire a Functional Personal Trainer.

Approximately 1 year went by and Jack lost around 100 pounds of body fat and gained 16 pounds of lean muscle! The majority of his weight loss appeared to come from his bloated stomach and face. He could buy clothes off the rack again instead of having to go to specialty stores. He began to have more confidence in himself and said he felt stronger and younger. His entire physique changed and he looked 10-15 years younger. When his feet hit the floor in the morning, he was ready to face the day, and his chronic lower-back pain had completely disappeared. He was more rational in his thinking and less argumentative with his wife. Jack was able to discontinue the high blood pressure medication he had been taking for the past year. Heart trouble ran in his family and he said he would never have been able to keep the weight off if he had not hired a Functional Personal Trainer. He continued taking 5 mgs of Cialis® at night along with the testosterone because his doctor told him it would help prevent further enlargement of his prostate from all the years of disuse and because it had a mild blood pressure-lowering effect. The sexual side effect was a bonus. Jack's appetite had decreased, while his metabolism and libido had increased. Lab work showed that his health had improved dramatically all across the board and he became functional again!

In college, Emily was a size 10. That is when she began taking diet pills and lost about 15 pounds, but she was concerned about the health risks. So, she went off them and gained all the weight back and then some! By the time she met Jack she was a size 12. The majority of their relationship centered on food. They went out to dinner a lot and ate junk food and drank alcohol. Emily stated, "The weight piled on for both of us. In just 1 year Jack and I both gained roughly 30 pounds each! Every time I got mad at him, I used it as an excuse to go eat and he did the same. I remember sitting on my couch watching television wearing shorts and being shocked at the size of my thighs. I thought to myself, Can my legs get any bigger? Emily took a long, hard look at herself in the mirror alongside Jack and got angry with what she saw and where life had taken them. Together they made the final decision that if they wanted to remain married and see their child grow up, they needed to do something quickly. They learned the hard way that good marriages don't just happen and, contrary to popular belief, love doesn't conquer all. Couples must continue to stay in shape to keep the attention of their partner and prevent early death.

Approximately 1 year later, Emily had lost around 80 pounds and gained 5 pounds of muscle! The majority of her fat loss came from her legs, hips, arms, and lower abs. Her glutes had a better shape. Emily went from a plus size to a size 8. She was ecstatic about buying new work-out clothes! In the past, she had been on an antidepressant for depression and an antianxiety drug for panic attacks. The panic attacks were so severe that she could not go out in public without having to take an antianxiety pill. Due to her lack of libido from the antidepressants and extra weight, food had replaced sex for gratification. Luckily for Emily, the Functional Hormone Replacement, Functional Diet and Functional Exercise allowed her to regain control. She has not been on any antidepressants, antianxiety pills, or medicines to control migraine headaches for more than 5 years. Her appetite decreased while her metabolism and libido increased. She told us, "I know now there's no faking a low libido!" Lab work showed that Emily's health improved dramatically all across the board and her overall functionality was better than ever!

CHAPTER 10

Chronic Pain

Ronnie: Attempting to alleviate chronic pain is frustrating for patients because they want relief and it's frustrating for physicians because they want to help people, but there's often no cure! Back surgery is notorious for its different outcomes because of each individual's different biomechanics and the degree their body grows scar tissue, surgical procedures, and the surgeon. I know what it's like to be a prisoner of chronic pain. I have been dealing with it to various degrees for over 30 years. There's not a day that goes by when I don't hurt! Until you have been there you can't possibly understand. It's like being trapped inside a body you don't want to be in. I was a professional motocross racer as a teenager. It seemed like a great idea at the time because it was a lot of fun and I was very good at it. Now I realize it was the worst decision I ever made in my life! I have had 11 surgeries on my lower back (a total of four discs removed and fused) stemming from a motocross accident I had when I was 18 years old. I endured multiple failed back surgeries; painful, invasive diagnostic tests; and hardships because none of the top spine specialist I visited could figure out how to make my back fuse together (a condition known as pseudoarthrosis) and others were afraid to accept me as a patient. Over the years, the financial loss has been overwhelming.

I know what it's like to pretend being limited doesn't bother you, but you just want to explode! I know what it's like to be pushed around the hospital in a wheelchair thinking you may never walk again. I have never been so scared in my life! I know what it's like to have electric-like shocks and burning pain that's so severe in both legs that it cannot be properly managed with medications. I know what it's like to have doctors give up on you and say there is nothing they can do to help ease the pain. I also know what it's like to be mad at a doctor when they tell you, "I don't know what's causing your pain; maybe it's all in your head." The last thing I needed to hear from a person who was supposed to try to help was that he didn't even believe my pain was real! I know what it's like to hurt so bad you push people away and just want to be left alone. I know what it's like to get to the point where you no longer care whether you live or die from not being able to control the pain, even though I drastically limited my daily activities. I know what it's like to have reoccurring nightmares that wake you up in a state of panic, soaked in sweat and with your heart pounding in your throat. The trauma I endured was so bad, I developed PTSD.

Fortunately for me, God heard my prayers and sent a doctor that was a pioneer in the spine industry. His name is Dr. David H. McCord, located at 1718 Charlotte Avenue,

Nashville, Tennessee, 37203. His office number is 615-329-0333. I am certainly not alone when I say he is the best orthopedic spine surgeon in the United States! God gave this man the gift of knowing how to treat complex back problems that most doctors are afraid to touch or often make worse. Dr. David H. McCord helped design the FDA-regulated cages that spine surgeons all across the world are now putting in patients' backs and necks. He also has an upright MRI in his office building. It allows all parts of the spine to be imaged in the weight-bearing state. This provides much better detail than a conventional supine MRI and problems with claustrophobia are eliminated. If I had not found Dr. McCord, I wouldn't be working today as a personal trainer. He figured out that my body had been rejecting the cadaver bone (bone in a tissue bank taken from a deceased person) that the other doctor had been using. Dr. McCord used bone from my hip and I had a successful fusion. With his help, I can walk again and my quality of life has improved dramatically!

The sad fact, is that all the prior surgeries before I found Dr. McCord caused arthritis and adhesive arachnoiditis that remain today. Adhesive arachnoiditis is from the buildup of excess scar tissue and it causes a chronic inflammatory condition. This inflammation causes constant scarring, swelling, and binding of nerve roots and blood vessels. The main symptoms of arachnoiditis is chronic pain in the lower back and lower limbs. Arachnoiditis is one of the most painful conditions imaginable. Arachnoiditis is a chronic disorder, with no known cure! Surgery is not recommended for arachnoiditis because it only causes more scar tissue to develop and exposes the already irritated spinal cord to further damage. I still experience subluxations from the vertebra that sits directly on top of my 4-level fusion (L2-L1). A reputable chiropractor combined with the proper Functional Training can often eliminate subluxations, but not in my case. On a positive note, as far as I know, I am able to function better than anyone else in the United States who has had eleven major lower back surgeries. This is because the last surgery I had by Dr. McCord was a success and I have persistently implemented the proper type of Functional Training, Functional Diet, and Functional Hormone Replacement.

It wasn't easy, but I have learned to accept my limitations and work around them to the best of my ability. I will always have substantial limitations and chronic pain from hurting my back racing motocross. The sensation-seeking, adrenaline rush from racing, and managing my emotions in an extreme environment was so great that there was no talking me out of it as a teenager. There was something about the element of danger that attracted me to the "high-risk sport" as a youth. The thrill of pushing boundaries in a group setting seemed exciting and adventurous. Adrenaline built inside to a level that made me feel alive. The feelings of my body were often in conflict with the known reality in my head. When my injury occurred it was a cold, lonely world. I was another young guy who thought he was invincible. If I could go back and change things, I would never have raced motocross bikes, even though I loved it and was very good at it. Many of us have to learn some things the hard way as we mature and I was one of those people when it came to contact sports. I found out later in life the human body wasn't nearly as tough as I once thought.

I admit, you can get hurt doing anything, but looking back on it now, I realize how stupid I was to think I would somehow get by with participating in a "high-risk sport" without paying a price. I was one of those that thought it would happen to the other guy and not me if I used caution. A lot of people have suffered injuries racing motocross and will live in chronic pain the rest of their lives. When people ask me what I think about racing motocross racing, I tell them that it's fun, but it's not worth it! Some have also asked me about my opinion of CrossFit®. I tell them I have never tried it as a way of fitness and never will. I have learned from my past mistakes, and I know that CrossFit® would put me in a wheelchair. CrossFit® is a dangerous sport like motocross and was never designed to be a lifestyle of fitness.

Functional Alert: When we are young we tend to do ignorant things that are very dangerous without looking at the long-term consequences. If you are young, I hope you will benefit from my bad experiences, so you don't end up like me or worse. If you listen now, you'll be so glad you did later!

I compare CrossFit® to motocross racing because it improves endurance, but destroys your body in the process. A lot of the younger generation don't understand just how dangerous it is, and I feel an urgent need to give them fair warning. Once you get severely injured, there is no going back to a normal lifestyle. There is no such thing as pain remission, only pain management. This is why people living in chronic pain have to visit pain management centers. They could not function otherwise! My wife and I know of a wonderful pain management specialist who helped keep our pain under control after surgery. His name is Dr. Hemant Yagnick, MD. He is the most knowledgeable and compassionate pain doctor we have ever met.

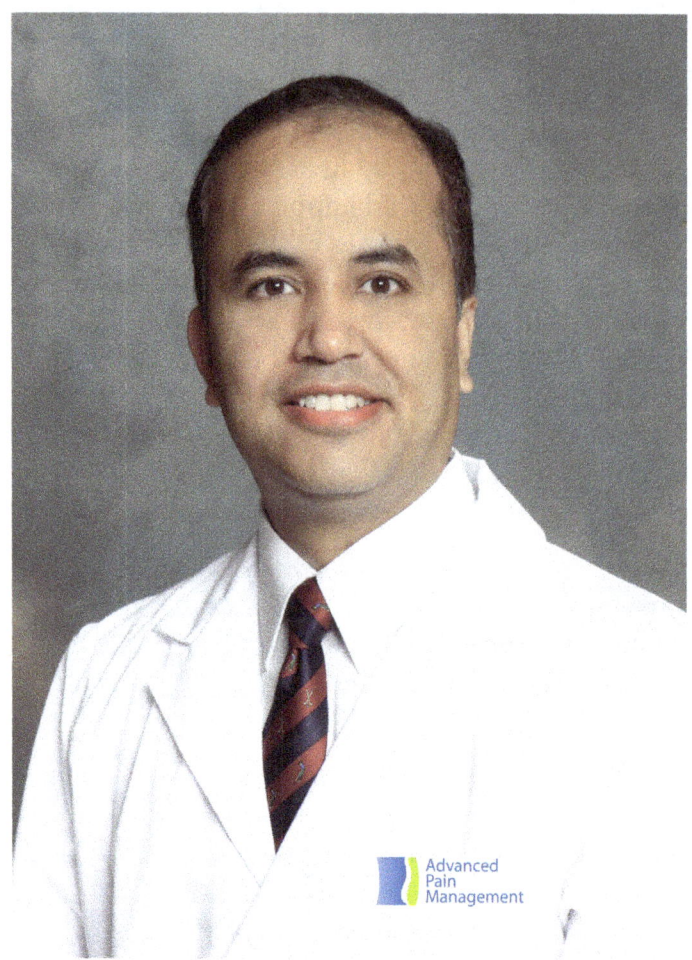

Hemant Yagnick, M.D.
Located at
404 Town Park Boulevard #101, Evans, Georgia 30809.
His office number is 706-922-7246.

*I am honored to write an endorsement for Mr. and Mrs. Rowland's book, **Functional Training with a Fork**. I have known them for several years personally and have had extensive discussions about fitness and chronic pain. I'm an Interventional pain physician by training and see personal fitness and activity improvement playing a key role in treating chronic pain every day. Better nutrition, exercises that improve and strengthen the core muscles, and increasing daily activity is what I advise my patients as well.*

*Mr. and Mrs. Rowland have done a marvelous job of collecting a lot of diverse information in one book about all of the above. It gives the reader a well-thought-out collection of information about the physiology and the reasons for proper nutrition, diet and exercise, and activity in our daily lives. Over the last several years in my private practice I have seen the best results in patients who used the multimodal approach of proper activity, exercise, injections, or medications if needed for their chronic pain issues. This book is sure to guide and inform a lot of patients about the important aspects of maintaining a healthy lifestyle and strengthening their core. Once again I'm very happy to endorse **Functional Training with a Fork** as it is surely going to help a lot of people!*

Ronnie: Weight training is the best form of Functional Training when performed sensibly and in moderation! Functional Training should be gentle at first, gradually increasing, and not taking huge risk in injury. I believe violent exercise such as CrossFit® should never be used as a way of fitness, only during CrossFit® games because the risk of becoming injured is too great. Group workouts can be motivating and put you in shape, but when fitness becomes competitive, an array of injuries start to happen. I learned this the hard way at age 18 from a motocross accident. Here's a question for all readers: How long do you want to be able to continue working out without having to work around chronic pain and limitations?

For those of you who make the decision to continue CrossFit® as a sport after reading this book, I encourage you to trust your own instincts instead of letting coaches and teammates push you beyond your limits. There is no sport on this earth that is worth it, especially when you are not getting paid millions of dollars to do it. Trust me when I tell you: Those once-sought-after trophies turn to dust collectors. Anyone who says, "I do not regret getting injured while doing CrossFit® and would do it all over again" is not being honest!

I am well-versed in helping teach others how to rehab and manage their chronic back and neck pain. I can also empathize with everyone on a different level, which would have been impossible if I had not endured so much pain myself. It has also greatly helped me in my abilities to rehab other parts of the human body. I have become more aware of how to prevent injuring myself and my clients while working out. I get great satisfaction knowing I have helped improve someone's overall functionality.

The eleven back surgeries have put me through physical and emotional pain that words cannot describe. It's a whole other book in its entirety! Sometimes I wake up in severe pain, and it always gets worse as the day progresses. It's never consistent, but overdoing it always makes my pain level skyrocket! I try not to compare my pain to others, but sometimes it's hard because I meet people who say they have back trouble and I would give anything to have their backs. When I first got injured, I did not understand why people who hurt less than I were more emotionally distraught. Eventually, I learned that my pain was my pain alone, my emotions were my emotions alone, and my confusion was my confusion alone, and the same rule applied to others living in chronic pain.

If I neglect Basic Functional Training, my back and hips tighten up and I hurt all the time, especially on the bottom of my feet. If I over-exercise, I hurt even more! My core is strong, but it's impossible to build my core strong enough to keep scar tissue from rubbing on the nerve roots and preventing the vertebrae sitting directly on top of my 4-level fusion from slipping out of place very easily because the natural alignment of my spine is gone. No form of core training can completely fix my back problem! I can no longer lift free weights. I am limited to certain machines and one exercise for my legs—ball squats. Some of the machines in the gym have done wonders for my chronic pain when used in a controlled fashion. People who say machines are not effective for building the core and overall body don't know what they are talking about. Weight machines are the best form of Functional Training for people like me who live in chronic pain. I can't do calisthenics without setting off my back, hip, leg, and foot pain. Getting on the floor and performing most body-weight exercises increases my pain. Suspension Training workouts (e.g., TRX straps) cause my L2-L-1 vertebrae to subluxate which accelerates wear and tear on the surrounding ligaments, discs, muscles, and other spinal tissues. It's very hard to accept these kinds of limitations. When I see people who have no chronic pain, but are too lazy to work out, I get frustrated because I would give anything to have their backs. The good news is that putting **Functional Training with a Fork** into practice has made my overall appearance and health better than most 49 year-old-males who have a good back!

Basic Functional Training helps provide my back with a deep myofascial release that can't be obtained by a mainstream massage. I have Kathy apply direct pressure to my back with her elbow to further alleviate tightness and inflammation (Rehabilitative Functional Training/Active Release Technique). Functional Training and Functional Hormone Replacement allows my pain medications to work better because they cause my body to release its own natural pain killers. I get an accumulative effect and don't have to take as many pain medications. I feel sorry for the people who are suffering more than they have to because they don't know about Basic Functional Training, Functional Hormone Replacement, and Rehabilitative Functional Training/Active Release Techniques. They have enabled me to become more active and experience less pain.

Regardless of how much I hurt at times, I push myself to keep working as a personal trainer. The word "quit" isn't in my vocabulary. There are a lot of people who need Functional Personal Trainers to make sure they don't hurt their lower backs and necks while exercising.

Did you know that chronic pain acts like a Dysfunctional Toxin inside the body? Chronic pain takes the term "adrenalize me" to a whole new level! Once your brain has decided you are in pain, it sends nerve signals down your spinal cord to your adrenal glands to have them release a hormone called epinephrine or adrenaline.[1] Then the hypothalamus of your brain sends signals to your pituitary gland that tell the outer part of your adrenal glands (adrenal cortex) to produce a stress hormone called cortisol.[2] There is a strong relationship between the nervous system and the immune system. As the stress from chronic pain continues, the nervous system causes the closing down of immune functions and dysfunction sets in.[3]

People like me who live in chronic pain have some degree of immune dysfunction, leaving us with less energy for daily activities.[4,5] The lack of sleep, emotional distress, and hormonal imbalances further compound the problem. Chronic pain causes stress that leads to adrenal gland insufficiency.[6] Adrenal gland disorders can cause hyperfunction or hypofunction. Chronic pain is a condition in which the adrenal glands don't produce the proper amounts of steroid hormones, primarily cortisol.

Cortisol levels can often become imbalanced during the different stages of adrenal insufficiency. Not only does chronic pain result in elevated cortisol, it causes epinephrine and norepinephrine to become elevated. Elevated epinephrine and norepinephrine levels start out as anxiety, but often lead to panic attacks![7] Anxiety and panic attacks cause a decrease in dopamine (a chemical in your brain that regulates important things such as emotional well-being, sex drive, impulsivity, and alertness).[8] Likewise, low dopamine levels lead to anxiety, panic attacks, and sexual dysfunction! Prescription medications, such as cabergoline, in addition to Functional Exercise, Functional Hormone Replacement, and Functional Sex, can be used to regulate dopamine levels. Testosterone levels also decrease when the adrenal gland and pituitary gland are thrown out of whack, which provides a double whammy.[9] This makes one's emotional state very complex when trying to learn how to cope with living in chronic pain!

Functional Alert: People suffering with chronic pain need adequate amounts of testosterone. When your body is lacking testosterone, your opioid system increases your perception of both acute pain and chronic pain. This leads to a decrease in pain tolerance!

One of cortisol's primary functions is to reduce inflammation and pain caused by tissue damage.[10] When cortisol levels increase, the body's immune defenses activate to try to heal the cause of pain and accelerate tissue recovery. If you are still in the early stages of living with chronic pain, your cortisol production will usually increase. This rise in cortisol has a side effect: lowered immunity. Chronically high cortisol levels can also destroy vital tissues, such as the tissues that line the GI tract, needed for proper immune functions.[11-12] They also destroy brain cells located in the hippocampus (the brain's memory center).[13] Elevated cortisol levels damage cells in the brain area responsible for both short-term and long-term memory. Fortunately, Functional Hormone Replacement, Functional Exercise, Functional Diet, Functional Sex, and narcotic pain medication can help reverse much of the damage being caused by chronic pain. The more extreme cases sometimes need drugs such as cabergoline to further enhance dopamine levels. Increasing dopamine levels helps control anger, depression, loss of libido, attention deficit disorder, and increases in appetite that can occur while living in chronic pain.[14]

Functional Alert: Pro-inflammatory cytokine activity is involved in the development and continuation of a variety of painful medical conditions.[15] Chronic pain causes the body to produce even more pro-inflammatory cytokines and free radicals!

If chronic pain continues long-term, the pendulum can swing, causing less cortisol to be released.[16] I have developed lower cortisol levels due to years of living in chronic pain! Here's how it works: At first, chronic pain overstimulates the three endocrine glands (hypothalamus, pituitary, and adrenal), but it eventually impairs them to the point that cortisol secretion stops or drops way below normal. Cortisol reduces inflammation in the body, which is good, but over time, these efforts wear down the three endocrine glands and immune system. Low cortisol levels can be just as damaging to the functions of the body as having levels that are too high. Chronically low levels of circulating cortisol, as seen in adrenal insufficiency, are associated with increased inflammation, which causes chronic pain to escalate. This lowers your immunity and makes you more prone to getting colds, viruses, chronic fatigue syndrome, and even cancer.[17]

Adrenal gland-related issues can be the root cause of asthma if you cannot produce enough hormones to control the inflammation inside the bronchial tubes and lungs.[18] Since my adrenal glands have been overworked from years of living in chronic pain, I now have exercised-induced asthma. You can see how that one problem with the human body leads to another!

Functional Alert: Those of you with exercised-induced asthma should never work out without having a rescue inhaler by your side. Seven thousand people die from asthma attacks each year in America. Don't be one of those statistics because you left your inhaler in the locker room or at home![19]

If you live in chronic pain, it's wise to use only enough pain medication to take the edge off. This helps the function of your immune system while still allowing you to function during daily activities. Functional Hormone Replacement, combined with Functional Training, Functional Sex, and a Functional Diet, also helps reduce pain and mental stress. Proper pain medicine also helps cortisol levels stay in balance so that your immune system can function better. Cortisol levels that are too high or too low from chronic pain dictate the need for pain management, Functional Hormone Replacement, and Functional Training to help bring cortisol levels back into normal range. Neglecting to seek pain management and to follow the principles found in this book can lead to developing cancer![20] I know that narcotics are unhealthy, but I believe that using them properly in very low doses is much healthier than suffering needlessly! In addition, I believe taking small amounts of narcotics on a daily basis has fewer side effects than taking small amounts of non-aspirin anti-inflammatory medications on a daily basis. There are approximately 20,000 deaths per year in the United States from taking nonsteroidal anti-inflammatory drugs such as ibuprofen![21] I used to take anti-inflammatories daily for my chronic back/leg pain until it caused permanent damage to the inner lining of my stomach. I now have acid reflux disease and a hiatal hernia. In the past, I have experienced a reduction in white blood cells and platelets from using anti-inflammatories. These are common side effects from using these pain killers.[22] I have also had stomach polyps removed during an endoscopy. Anti-inflammatories can cause life-threatening conditions such as heart attacks, stroke, and kidney failure, due to restricted blood flow to the blood-filtering components of the kidneys.[23] Other side effects include gastrointestinal bleeding and ulcers and a significant reduction in red blood cells, white blood cells, and platelets. They also can cause irritable bowel syndrome (heartburn, gas, nausea, and diarrhea), poor circulation, high blood pressure, lack of libido, Dysfunctional Toxin buildup, fluid buildup, congestion, and a loss of muscle, bone, and cartilage. I believe that non-aspirin nonsteroidal anti-inflammatory drugs can lead to kidney cancer. In fact, current research suggests that taking them increases the risk of developing the condition by 51%![24, 25] Now I take a low dose narcotic pain medicine daily instead of anti-inflammatories. My white blood cells and platelets have remained in normal range and my acid reflux disease has significantly lessened.

People like me hate cold weather with a passion because it intensifies our pain level. Cold weather and storms (snowstorms are the worst) cause a change in the barometric pressure (the weight of the atmosphere that surrounds us), and our already-damaged tissues expand (swell), causing even greater pain due to excessive pressure! Furthermore, those of us with neuropathy (nerve pain) experience an increased sensitivity of the nerve fibers in cold weather due to the nerve fibers swelling. This creates larger gaps that nerve impulses must jump in order to reach the nearby nerve and keep nerve impulses flowing in the right direction. Normal nerve signals are not powerful enough to jump the enlarged gap from the swollen nerves, so they build up and send out a very powerful signal across these enlarged gaps and the brain interprets them as intense pain! Using an ice pack on the damaged area reduces swelling of the nerves, which helps decrease nerve pain, whereas applying heat usually causes nerve tissue to swell and pain to worsen.

The Diagnostic and Statistical Manual of Mental Disorders estimates that only around 1-5% of Americans suffer from hypochondria (a mental, not physical, illness).[26] There are also a few fakers, malingerers, and drug seekers wanting medical attention. Sadly, the medical community is quick to lump way too many people into these categories simply because their problems don't show up on traditional medical tests, such as x-rays, CT scans, and MRIs. This seems to be particularly true of people with chronic pain from soft-tissue injuries. Unless doctors can find evidence of a ruptured tendon, torn piece of cartilage, or herniated disc, these patients are treated as if nothing is actually wrong with them.

Knowing what we know, Kathy and I would never judge anyone with chronic pain, regardless of their condition! A large percentage of soft-tissue injuries (injuries to tendons, ligaments, fasciae, nerves, and blood vessels) don't always show well with imaging techniques.[27, 28] The fact is, these are some of the most pain-sensitive tissues in your body, and, unfortunately, even if the injury is diagnosed, in many cases surgery can't be used to treat the chronic pain. Although we cannot always eliminate all the pain for our clients who have soft tissue injuries, we can provide a functional recovery through specific strengthening exercises in a Basic Functional Training format and Rehabilitative Functional Training.

A lot of people, especially females with fibromyalgia have had doctors tell them their pain and chronic fatigue were all in their heads. Why? It's because the results from the diagnostic tests that doctors currently have access to come back normal and the patients appear to be healthy. However, Kathy and I have worked with enough female clients who have had fibromyalgia to know their pain is real! For years, a lot of doctors considered fibromyalgia to be an imaginary disease of hypochondriacs. Current research proves they were wrong—the disease is real. Fibromyalgia patients have excessive amounts of nerve fiber called arteriole-venule (AV) shunts in their blood vessels. It was previously thought by the medical community that the blood vessels located in the nervous system were only responsible for regulating blood flow. However, they have recently learned that the nerve fibers in blood vessels bring about an increased sensitivity to the pain experienced by fibromyalgia sufferers! [29-34]

Functional Training with a Fork improves fibromyalgia symptoms by improving blood flow to the sensory nerve fibers in tiny muscular valves that open and close the blood vessels, which determine the rate and direction of blood flow. **Functional Training with a Fork** also helps counterbalance the secretion of hormonal imbalances in the brain by increasing endorphins (reduces pain sensitivity), and reducing substance P (increases pain sensitivity).[35, 36] **Functional Training with a Fork** helps the endocrine system secrete more of the mood enhancing hormones serotonin, testosterone, and dopamine. **Functional Training with a Fork** also helps reduce excess amounts of pro-inflammatory cytokines and free radicals that signal the white blood cells to make harmful autoantibodies. This allows for better blood flow and a reduction of nerve and muscle pain.[37]

Functional Alert: Three key factors to fibromyalgia pain control are Functional Hormone Replacement, Functional Training, and Functional Diet. These factors will lower the body's production of harmful autoantibodies and increase the body's natural pain killers! [38-40]

The older I get, the more I find I am not alone. Most people aren't going to tell you about how much they are suffering and, deep down, you probably don't want to hear about it anyway. Therefore, people living in chronic pain often keep it hidden from others to the best of their ability. You should never tell other people living in chronic pain how to live their lives. They are not lazy, just limited, and there is a huge difference! Their family members often have to take on more household and parenting responsibilities. Financial worries due to medical bills and decreased income often puts additional strain on relationships.

I have learned the importance of letting people in your life know how you are feeling. However, sharing too much information about your medical condition can cause them to feel overwhelmed, helpless, and depressed, which can turn into anxiety. Therefore, keep in mind that how much you share will be different for each person in your life.

You have to learn to accept your limitations instead of living in denial. Life is hard enough; there is no need to make it harder! If you're having trouble with a chore or activity, don't be too proud to ask them to lend a helping hand. There's a time to be determined and a time to be smart. Furthermore, it's not uncommon for those of us who live in chronic pain to be wrongfully judged by someone at some point in our lives. In other words, they think we are exaggerating the symptoms. People who wrongly judge others who live in chronic pain are showing their ignorance and inability to show compassion toward others who are suffering.

Functional Alert: Having a spouse who whines and complains constantly can make life extremely difficult. My wife married me "for better or for worse" and "in sickness and in health." I try to not complain in excess about my pain in order to give her the "better" side of me!

I know from past experiences that sitting around doing nothing and not employing Functional Training only made my pain worse. My core got weaker and my back stayed tight causing pain to run from my back all the way down into my feet. It would get so bad, I could barely walk on my feet at times. When living in chronic pain on a daily basis, there is no such thing as total acceptance. I have had to learn not to take my frustration and anger out on other people. It's sometimes easier said than done. I visit the gym to release my frustration. It also helps control my anxiety and any depression that tries to creep in when I feel a relapse coming on about accepting my permanent condition. I know I am always going to hurt (some days are much worse than others), so I will continue with my passion: Functional Training!

Functional Alert: I have taken responsibility to improve my situation. If I neglected to do so, it would only make my condition worse. Are you taking responsibility to improve your situation or are you making it worse by doing nothing?

      I have come to realize that having a positive attitude won't make all my pain disappear. However, it helps me overcome the challenges I have to face every single day of my life. Functional Training, Functional Hormone Replacement, Functional Diet, a good attitude, and helping others have helped me remain a productive member of society. I see a lot of people giving up, and I would like to encourage them to keep living their lives to the fullest because I believe God has a special purpose for each and every one of us. When it feels like everything around me is falling apart, I know it's time to get to the gym and it's one of the things I enjoy most! I hope this helps people to better understand why I am so against Dysfunctional Training such as CrossFit® for a lifestyle of fitness. I don't want to see them going through the chronic pain that I and many others have to endure.

Kathy: *I also live in chronic pain, but not to the degree that Ronnie does. I fell off a table hanging a light fixture. I broke my foot and have endured two painful surgeries. The last surgery involved cutting my foot completely in half and fusing it back together with screws and plates. I have to wear tennis shoes with special orthotics and still experience some nerve pain. I will always have limitations due to the fall. The table I fell off of was actually lower in height than a box used by CrossFitters to perform high box jumps. I believe box jumps over 24 inches in height are dangerous and overrated for all athletes trying to improve their vertical jump. Not only is it easy to fall off the high box while attempting to jump onto it or off of it, the tremendous impact puts wear and tear on the knees, ankles, feet, hips, and lower back. In addition, you should never jump off of a box, but rather step off it smoothly. The bottom line is, once you are injured you can't go back and change it!*

Ronnie and Kathy: *We would like to take this time to say God bless everyone who is living with some form of chronic pain. Please get your pain under control or it will decrease your life expectancy by approximately 10 years.[41] Never allow doctors, family members, and friends to dissuade you from using the appropriate pain medications, Functional Training, Functional Hormone Replacement, and Functional Diet to manage your chronic pain!*

CHAPTER 11

Hiring a Functional Personal Trainer

We believe a lot of people in today's society have the wrong mind-set and their priorities are not where they should be. We say this because when the time comes for them to make a decision on whether or not to hire or re-hire a Functional Personal Trainer, they seem to have time and money to spend on everything else except their looks and overall functionality. We understand that money and a lack of commitment are the primary reasons that many people stop training with us or never start in the first place. We also understand that not everyone can afford a trainer long-term. However, the thing we don't agree with is how some people have no problem wasting money on extravagant restaurants, vacations, new vehicles, clothes, etc., but are unwilling to make health and fitness a priority in their lives. Even worse, some of them are only in their 40s, but look much older and function as if they are as well.

Functional Alert: If you want to succeed in making exercise and diet work in your life, you must be committed. Hesitation and excuses will prevent you from accomplishing anything of great value!

We also understand that some of you perceive you don't have enough time for a trainer. We use the word "perceive" because we are firm believers that it's how you chose to organize your waking hours that matters most. People find or make time for things they perceive as important to them. We have worked with very busy surgeons, lawyers, and business owners who made the time to train with us because of its importance to their looks and overall functionality. You can always find a reason or excuse not to have time or money for your own well-being.

Here are three questions to ask yourself:

1. Do you believe that you can change and that your life will improve?
2. Are you doing what's healthiest or what's easiest?
3. Are you thinking short-term or long-term?

If you have been working out for three months and have yet to see significant results, it's time to hire a Functional Personal Trainer. Don't waste your time and money paying a personal trainer to hand out workouts that are never going to build muscle tone, improve functionality, and cause body-fat loss! When shopping for a personal trainer, don't always judge them by their looks alone. There are personal trainers who are built well, but lack knowledge. On the other hand, if someone is not built like a personal trainer, they are not setting a good example. In other words, a Functional Personal Trainer is going to look the part and have the knowledge to back it up! How can you as a client expect to follow a plan that your own personal trainer ignores? Where is the motivation in that?

Functional Alert: When interviewing a personal trainer, always ask them for their opinion on CrossFit®. If they think it's a good way to get into shape, then we believe they are the wrong trainer for you!

A Functional Personal Trainer will tell you upfront that you must commit to making a lifestyle change and that dietary habits make up approximately 70% of your success. They present things in a realistic manner. They treat you with respect and have your best interest in mind. If they train you well, they realize you will come back. They understand that the "one-size-fits all" cookie-cutter approach won't work. Instead, they will perform a functional evaluation and customize their Functional Training methods to motivate you as an individual. A Functional Personal Trainer will inspire you; they don't use pressure tactics! They realize that trying to pressure you to lose weight/body fat actually makes you feel helpless, which could lead to you giving up. A Functional Personal Trainer learns about your interests so that you and they can build an emotional connection.

Functional Alert: Our clients become our friends and then they become like family!

There are some personal trainers who are great at their jobs; the rest are mediocre or downright pitiful. A reputable gym won't intentionally hire Dysfunctional Personal Trainers. You should feel comfortable with your personal trainer. In some cases, personalities don't match and you may have to find another personal trainer. As a client you are paying for interaction and results! A Functional Personal Trainer will design your program so that you will improve overall muscle tone, body-fat loss, and functional abilities. If your body isn't changing, you have a Dysfunctional Personal Trainer and/or you are not following their instructions. It's not uncommon for some people to perceive they are not achieving results because they have unrealistic expectations. Getting into shape doesn't happen overnight. Even the best personal trainers can't deliver overnight results such as losing 30 pounds of body fat or dropping 6 pant sizes in a month. They really can't help you reach your goals if you are overeating, drinking too much alcohol, or not exercising outside of your appointments. Be reasonable about your goals and take responsibility for your part of the program.

Personal trainers often hear clients complaining that they aren't losing body fat. The problem is, they continue to consume high-calorie meals from a fast-food restaurant or somewhere else. Don't hesitate to ask your personal trainer for further guidance if you are not making the progress you desire. Sometimes it can be as simple as adding an extra day of training and/or taking away 250 calories per day.

Functional Alert: The vast majority of people quit working out once they stop using a personal trainer. They often return to the very things in life that got them into trouble to begin with. The small percentage that continue training on their own usually get lazy and lose some of their results because they no longer have anyone pushing them in a safe manner!

Never allow a personal trainer to discourage you! A Functional Personal Trainer always shows up for their appointments. They will not allow you to pay them under the table behind the management's back. If they will cheat the gym, they will also cheat you! Drop a Dysfunctional Trainer and find yourself a Functional Personal Trainer. A Dysfunctional Personal Trainer won't seem interested in hearing about your medical conditions. They are also notorious for not taking you seriously when you tell them a particular exercise causes you joint pain. They often say, "No pain, no gain!" A Functional Personal Trainer will know the difference between good muscular pain during and after a workout versus bad pain that signals injury. Stay away from Dysfunctional Personal Trainers on a power trip who yell at you in a rude way or use pressure tactics to get you to lose weight, perform exercises that cause you joint pain, or lift weights that are beyond your capabilities! These same trainers usually don't have the ability to assess your level of fitness without making you feel extremely nauseated or making you throw up. A Functional Personal Trainer will be able to gauge your tolerance for exercises, stamina, strength, and flexibility.

Functional Alert: Hiring a Functional Personal Trainer is fun like small group training, but more productive for improving faithfulness to exercise!

A Functional Personal Trainer will be there to support you during your lifestyle change. They understand that the primary reason most people join a gym is to lose body fat, tone up, and improve functionality, while using the greatest and latest exercise equipment. A Functional Personal Trainer incorporates efficient ways to use equipment to make working out faster, more enjoyable, and effective, while keeping it safe. They will show you some exercises to do away from the gym, if requested. However, they won't usually have you performing exercises at the gym that you could be doing at home.

Functional Alert: Dysfunctional Personal Trainers will often avoid teaching clients how to properly use the most productive muscle toning equipment: basic exercises with free weights, machines, and cables!

Dysfunctional Personal Trainers learn the bare minimum and are perfectly content. They are easily bored and want to be original. They often use you as a guinea pig to try out a bizarre exercise they saw on the Internet or read about in a magazine or book. We refer to this as "Look at me!" Some have memorized a great deal about exercise and nutrition, but don't know how to apply it in real-life situations. They have years of experience, which, unfortunately, consists of doing the wrong things over and over again! These are the types of personal trainers you need to avoid. We've seen them give out very bad advice because they read it in a magazine or watched something on YouTube and believed it was based on facts. Some learn faulty information through certifications or continuing educational requirements. Even professions requiring extensive education and hours of hands-on training have their share of incompetents. The bottom line is, personal training is just like any other job. You have some who love their job and know what they are doing, and others who are there for a paycheck and don't really seem to care about their clients or know what they are doing.

Functional Alert: We have great respect for parents who care enough about their toddlers to put them on a Functional Diet and then hire a Functional Personal Trainer for them when they reach adolescence. It's great to see parents who want their children to be responsible, healthy, and attractive so they can succeed in life!

CHAPTER 12

How to Become a Functional Personal Trainer

People want results without getting injured. Unfortunately, throughout the years we have seen people getting injured without getting results. We also have seen people who have gotten neither injuries nor results. A Functional Personal Trainer provides the type of Functional Training that is best for each individual. They will work with their clients, not against them, in order to help them overcome any obstacles they may face while taking their limitations, age, and overall health into account.

Ronnie: *I have been through a vast number of personal training certifications throughout the years. One thing that I have learned is that even the most recognized certifications provide conflicting and inaccurate information. Learning to think for myself and question everything was by far the most important thing I learned in college. When you learn to apply deductive logic, inconsistencies involving beliefs and instructions will disappear. The bottom line is, book knowledge is a must, but so is knowing what to discard as inaccurate information and knowing how to take the accurate information and apply it in real life.*

As Functional Personal Trainers, our decisions not to prescribe certain exercises for our clients is based solely on personal experience and what our clients tell us. It's important for clients to listen to their bodies and it's equally important for us to listen to our clients. A sign of incredible self-confidence is being a good listener and doing what's in the best interest of the client! The first thing we ask them is whether they have any injuries, or if there is anything else we should know about their health. Next, we find out about their goals and work-out history. Your clients and other gym members around you will greatly respect the fact that you value safety first.

Functional Alert: People are drawn to personal trainers who are easy to connect with and make a good first impression!

As Functional Personal Trainers, we use time-tested and proven methods and avoid using exercises that are of little to no value. There is such a thing as being too creative in order to make yourself look original or set yourself apart from other trainers. This gets you away from the basics that work and are safe! Serious clients are not interested in stringing together exotic looking moves that are mere child's play or can be dangerous. They want maximum results without becoming injured! You can't get maximum results if you're constantly trying to reinvent the wheel or get away from the basics. Dysfunctional Personal Trainers use their clients as guinea pigs for every new fitness trend that appears. Some trainers simply don't know any better because they've never been taught about the 7 types of Functional Training. Others do this in attempt to draw attention to themselves hoping that the naive will fall for their circus acts. They give the term "Functional Training" a bad rap!

Functional Alert: As a Functional Personal Trainer, taking a strong stance against Dysfunctional Training is the beginning of wisdom! You must remember to stay true to what works and not be at the mercy of the fads that come and go in the industry. You must also put aside your personal likes and training biases and place your client's results and safety first!

There are misguided personal trainers who believe that new ideas are better than older ones. This is not true! In fact, anytime you get away from basic exercises, your results will suffer and the risk of injury increases. There is rarely anything new of any value when it comes to exercise other than tweaking the exercises that have been used for many years. For example, people have done squats for longer than we have been alive. We don't know who invented them and it doesn't matter. All we care is that they produce results for our clients! We know that in order to obtain maximum results, those who are capable of doing squats and lunges must keep squats and lunges in their routine on a regular basis, while sometimes changing to other exercises that are similar to prevent overuse and boredom.

Functional Alert: You cannot re-invent basic movements, but you can apply them in a different manner by changing how they are implemented (e.g., straight sets, supersets, or single-drop sets). These are by far the most effective Functional Training methods and they prevent your client from getting bored. In addition, you can change things up by training each muscle group once, twice, or three times per week. Another way to seek progress is by changing the exercise routinely used for a particular muscle group. Muscle Confusion is a myth. Constantly changing up your exercises will actually slow down your progress in the gym! In order to gain maximum muscle size, it's best to perform a lot of sets using "the most bang for your buck exercises" most of the time. You'll get a better training effect from the law of repeated efforts. However, changing exercises can help prevent boredom and over use injuries!

A personal trainer needs to be taught how the body works biomechanically. Learning how to properly use each piece of exercise equipment in accordance with each person's biomechanics and pre-existing injuries is priceless! Performing the wrong exercises, stretches, or type of Functional Training for an individual can do more harm than good. For example, if someone has a chronic lower-back condition involving a disc, performing exercises that directly target the lower back and abdominals can be the worst movements a personal trainer could prescribe!

There are some personal trainers who don't pay any attention to joint protection, especially if they are inexperienced and training younger people. Young joints still need as much attention as older ones, even though some trainers ignore them in the short-term, thinking their clients' joints can take it. This kind of attitude is wrong! If you don't take good care of young joints, they will get old fast and will start hurting. Keep in mind, there will always be a few genetically gifted individuals who can take an enormous amount of impact on their joints and still be okay for most of their lives, but chances are great your client isn't one of them. Some personal trainers have convinced themselves that using certain training methods is okay because they don't want to go against their whole belief system. For example, lifting weights on a Swiss ball® or stability ball while in a lying or seated position is dangerous because the ball can pop and cause serious injury or even death! Several people have been severely injured while lifting weights on stability balls and some hefty law suits followed.[1-4] One of these people was the starting forward of the Sacramento Kings. A stability ball that was supposed to be able to withstand 600 pounds burst while this 195-pound man was lying on it performing dumbbell chest presses.[5]

These balls often become weakened from nicks, overuse, and over-inflation. Furthermore, you can't lift as much weight while lying or sitting on a Swiss ball® or stability ball, which significantly decreases your ability to build muscle tone, strength, and overall functionality. There's a very good reason people have been lifting on stable surfaces such as benches for years. It's by far the safest and most effective way to build muscle tone and strength, which enhances overall functionality. Swiss balls®/stability balls are excellent tools for exercises such as squats and lunges (given the surface that the ball rolls on is smooth during exercise) because they offer lower-back support and take strain off the knees. But Functional Personal Trainers won't have their clients lift weights on these inflatable balls.

Functional Alert: Personal Trainers shouldn't have their clients lift weights on BOSU®balls, Swiss balls®/stability balls, or performing high-impact circuits to lose body fat and tone up!

As a personal trainer, you will struggle in the workforce if your foundation is laid poorly. A large percentage of your education needs to be spent in a gym setting under the guidance of a highly experienced Functional Personal Trainer. This will enable you to properly teach your clients how to use free weights, machines, cables, and body-weight exercises while applying the 7 types of Functional Training.

In order to build a strong foundation, you must work one on one with a Functional Personal Trainer, so you can ask technical questions and learn from their knowledge and experience. Don't be afraid to ask questions in fear of looking ignorant. You will never learn to excel as a personal trainer if you don't ask a lot of questions! Simply shadowing another Functional Personal Training while they are working with a client is only a small part of what you need to learn.

There is no room in the fitness industry for personal trainers who are disengaged from their clients because they are constantly looking at themselves in the mirror, watching others, or playing on their cell phones. As a personal trainer, if you are not watching your client's form, then there is no point for them to be paying you! In order to be a Functional Personal Trainer you have to be able to multi-task. This means being able to communicate with them while simultaneously watching their exercise form.

We would like to point out that some people feel self-conscious in the gym, especially beginners. It generally goes something like: "I'm too old, fat, inexperienced, or disabled." Never forget that most people want to blend in with the crowd, not be put on display. Therefore, we ask that all personal trainers understand that others in the gym are watching. It's also important to understand that working out in a gym can be very intimidating at first for a lot of people. We think it's easy for some of us to forget this because we are so accustomed to being in the gym.

Functional Alert: The only time a person should feel intimidated in the gym is when they don't have a clue as to what they are doing. That's why gyms offer personal training!

If your clients don't feel comfortable with you, they won't be around for long. In other words, you are not only hurting them, but you are hurting yourself as well. Give your clients every reason to stay in the gym. Encourage their desire to have a functional body and get back their energy and confidence. Clients don't want to be taken through fatiguing workouts that don't produce optimal results. They want to be taken through methodical workouts that do bring forth maximum results. Who wants to put forth the effort, hard work, and dedication and get little in return? The answer is no one!

HOW TO BECOME A FUNCTIONAL PERSONAL TRAINER

Functional Alert: Clients who enjoy how Functional Training and diet improves their quality and quantity of life is a major motivating factor!

We understand that a lot of clients are just not committed and find excuses to quit even though a lot of Functional Personal Trainers have gone above and beyond their duties. However, there are also trainers who have caused their clients to leave. We have seen Dysfunctional Personal Trainers try to force their clients to learn only one way of training (regardless of their age or limitations) because it was the only one they knew. Their clients leave and they don't even know why. Think of all the clients who have disappeared over the years. Did they or someone else come back to the gym and tell the trainers why they stopped coming? No, they probably did not! There have been countless clients who complained about being injured or not getting results. What happened to those clients? For every client who sticks around to tell their tale, we bet twice as many leave and slip into oblivion, unsatisfied or tending to their injuries.

Functional Alert: To other personal trainers who care about their clientele, we owe respect. To everyone else in the fitness industry we owe the truth!

People wanting to lose weight, tone their muscles, and improve overall functionality need to avoid useless and/or dangerous exercises! For example, the vast majority of people shouldn't be doing heavy deadlifts and clean and jerks because they put them at risk of herniating a disc. These types of things need to be fixed in the fitness industry!
On a personal level, we feel as if we are doing all the things we should, and we are staying the course. As a personal trainer ask yourself this, Do I train myself the same way as I would train a client if I were in their situation?

Functional Alert: A gym without personal trainers incorporating the proper types of Functional Training is a dangerous gym!

Having an attitude of "I love my profession and want to learn more" says a lot about a person. Learning the 7 types of Functional Training is going to help make your job so much easier! If being a personal trainer isn't something you absolutely love, then we believe you should find a different career. It's not uncommon for a person just getting involved in this profession to be extremely excited about learning more and being the best they can be. However, some eventually burn out and lose interest, which causes them to start regressing. They become indifferent about their clients' results. It takes only one Dysfunctional Personal Trainer or one Dysfunctional Manager to make the entire gym look bad.

There are three underlying factors that are the root cause of most personal trainers losing their motivation:

1. Long work hours. Personal trainers have to work a lot of hours. You can't expect to work long hours every day and not get burned out. You have to decide whether you are going to work more days and fewer hours or fewer days and longer hours. If possible, lock your consistent clients into the same spots every week.

2. Inability to obtain a large enough clientele base to make it in the fitness industry. Beginning personal trainers often struggle getting their clientele built up because they don't have a good foundation laid regarding the 7 types of Functional Training and how to apply them properly. Personality also plays a role. One of the best marketing strategies is word-of-mouth and it's hard to make a name for yourself as a newbie unless you know what you are doing. If your clients are impressed by you teaching them how to use the proper types of Functional Training and the state-of-the-art equipment at your gym, chances are great they will tell others how much they like the training and the results they are getting. Functional Personal Trainers incorporate safe ways to use the most effective equipment to make working out safer, faster, and more enjoyable for their clients. One example is a 30-minute workout session based mostly around machines to make working out safe, fast, and enjoyable!

3. Dysfunctional Management. Personal trainers take jobs because they believe in a particular gym or the personal training company contracted by the gym. If the management is not good, personal trainers will become dissatisfied and less productive.

CHAPTER 13

Functional Managers in the Fitness Industry

The demand for gyms will continue to rise as the general public becomes more health conscious and the population places a greater emphasis on staying fit. Being a manager in this growing fitness industry can be a very rewarding job, but it can also be a very difficult job. Managers are constantly having to put out fires. They get cursed at by gym members who are unaware of stipulations plainly stated on their contracts; they have to listen to unrealistic demands; and they have to confront members and employees who refuse to follow the rules. Experienced managers will tell you, "It's always something!"

If you are a manager, we offer some suggestions, based on our experience, so that you can help protect the growing fitness industry, yourself, and the people involved. We know that the fitness industry is a business and your primary objectives over the long haul are making money for the company, providing excellent customer service, and keeping work-related drama to a minimum!

Functional Alert: Good customer service is of the utmost importance because the reputation of the business and employees means everything in the long run!

Team members appreciate it when you show empathy, trust, and openness. Our experience at working in various gyms has taught us that the business is only as good as the Functional Employees and Functional Gym Members it keeps! Team members enjoy being asked for their ideas on how to improve the fitness industry and if there are any problems that concern them. You can't have good leadership skills without listening to what others have to say! A Functional Manager publicly gives credit to employees who come up with good ideas. Dysfunctional Managers take credit for their employee's ideas and are disliked by staff.

A poor staff can make any Functional Manager look dysfunctional. Some employees show little concern for the success of their employer and their own careers. In the fitness industry, Dysfunctional Employees often undermine what Functional Managers and other employees accomplish.

Functional Alert: Firing Dysfunctional Employees can actually be a motivational tool because it shows the rest of the staff that good performance is recognized!

Employees respect managers who lead by example. They appreciate it when you keep your door open. Employees will go the extra mile for you if you make them feel needed, respected, and appreciated. They don't like inner-work-force competition among departments because it makes them feel powerless, bitter, and insecure about their jobs. We have seen employees getting turned off and not working as hard for the company when management doesn't make them feel a part of the team. Functional Employees want to do well at work, but they need their time away to enjoy hobbies and spend time with their families. We have seen Functional Employees quit because they have been made to feel guilty for taking a little time off work.

We believe it's beneficial for managers to have employees they trust, respect, and would listen to so that they can make the business function better. We've noticed this makes both managers and employees feel good about themselves and proud to be working for the company. Once you have established a good relationship with your employees by treating them with respect, they will value you as their leader and work hard to make the business a success. Before you know it, the business begins to make more money and everyone looks good!

Ronnie: *A gym owner once asked me, "Why are you going out of your way to help make my business grow?" I replied, "Because you believe in me!"*

We've noticed that staff members and customers who have legitimate complaints really appreciate a prompt and respectful response. Management plays a huge role in employee performance and the amount of money customers are willing to spend over the long haul.

Functional Alert: As a manager, you should be aware that it's very difficult for people to leave a gym or personal training company they love. It's even harder for them to leave a job with a manager they love!

CHAPTER 14

Be a Functional Gym Member

Functional Gym Members go to the gym to stay in shape. They don't like it when they can't focus on the task at hand. Dysfunctional Gym Members create a bad environment for Functional Gym Members and often whine to management about anything and everything. Here are some tips to help ensure you are a Functional Gym Member:

- Follow the gym rules.

- Avoid texting on the cell phone while taking up more than your share of time on a piece of exercise equipment. In today's society there's too much "texting" and not enough "flexing"!

- Re-rack your weights.

- Wipe off your sweat with a cloth towel or paper towel after using a piece of exercise equipment.

- Do not move big, heavy machines, and if you move smaller pieces of exercise equipment (e.g., benches, barbells, and dumbbells) put them back where they belong when you are finished. Leaving equipment scattered prevents handicapped access (e.g., people in wheelchairs) and is a trip hazard for everyone.

- Do not slam or drop the weights at the end of your work set. It tears up the gym's expensive equipment. It also puts you and the next person at risk of becoming injured from damaged equipment (e.g., a cable breaking).

- Avoid swinging kettlebells or performing overhead presses in close proximity to other gym members. Doing so could cause a fatal injury.

- Avoid doing CrossFit® in mainstream gyms. Join a CrossFit® gym if you are preparing for a CrossFit® sporting event.

- Avoid shadow boxing, martial arts movements, and pretending you are swinging an invisible golf club, etc., in the gym area. It's a good way to accidently hurt another gym member.

- Learn how to properly exhale air during heavy and intense lifts in order to avoid yelling or making excessively loud grunting noises. This will ensure you are not annoying other gym members and breaking their concentration.

- Work on form instead of trying to lift too much weight. People who lift too heavy often find themselves trapped underneath a bar or dropping weights on their toes or other gym members.

- Avoid taking over several sets of dumbbells or pre-loaded barbells.

- Do not gather in groups around weight machines with one person resting on it, making it a social event.

- Use deodorant so everyone around you doesn't become nauseated from unacceptable body odor. Don't try to cover up body odor with cologne and perfume because they restrict others' ability to breathe, especially those with allergies and asthma.

- Avoid making a mess in the bathrooms and changing areas.

- Do not needlessly walk around naked in the changing room. You may end up on YouTube or FaceTime and never find out.

- Don't train other gym members and take money under the table without the gym owner's permission. If you want to become a personal trainer, then apply for the position.

- Show respect to other gym members and the staff.

- Respect people's privacy.

- If you find someone's personal belongings lying around, return them to the front desk.

BE A FUNCTIONAL GYM MEMBER

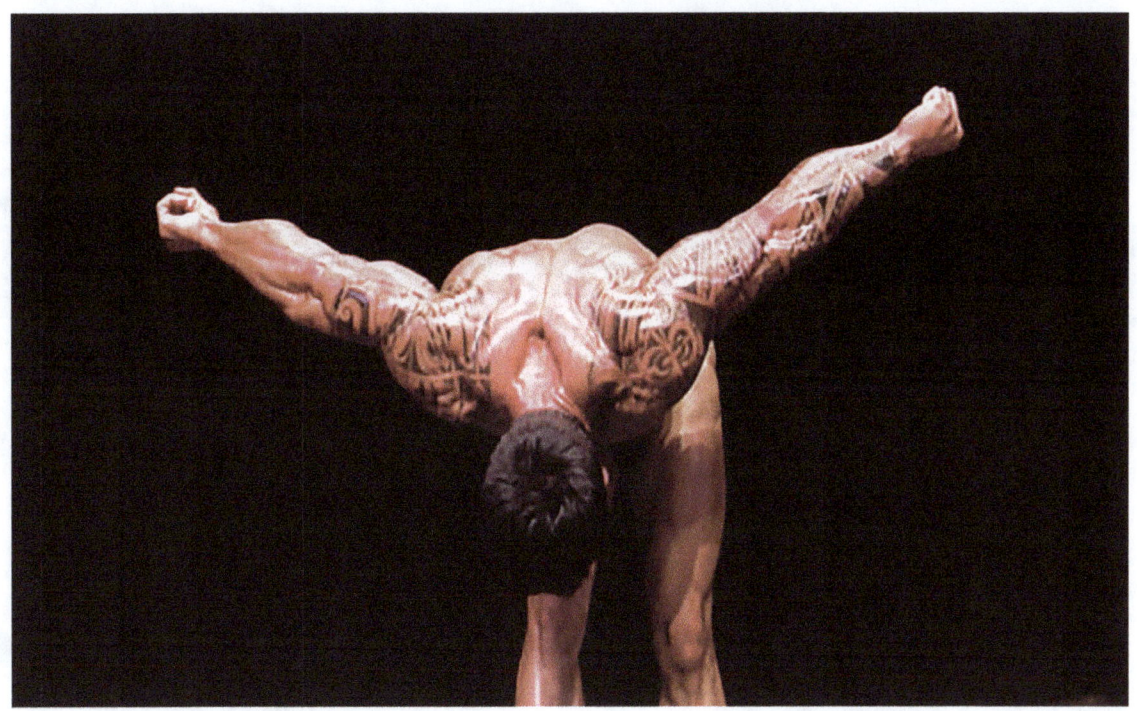

Authors' Final Note: *We want you to be happy and live a long life.*
Functional Training with a Fork *teaches you how to invest in yourself. The things you have learned in this book are useless if you don't start applying them now. There are things written in this book that we "know" and things written that we "believe." We know God's divine power has given us the tools we need to live a functional life! We believe* ***Functional Training with a Fork*** *is the key that unlocks the door to living a longer and happier life. We would like to thank everyone for their support in promoting* ***Functional Training with a Fork****.*

REFERENCES

Introduction

1. Statistics related to overweight and obesity: Economic costs related to overweight and obesity, Weight-control Information Network, 2006, retrieved 2009

2. Blackburn, G L; Walker, W A (July 1, 2005), Science-based solutions to obesity: What are the roles of academia, government, industry, and health care? The American journal of clinical nutrition (American Society for Clinical Nutrition) 82 (1): 207–210

3. U.S. National Center for Health Statistics, National Vital Statistics Reports (NVSR), Deaths: Preliminary Data for 2008 Vol. 59, No. 2, December 9, 2010

4. Amber L. Howard, Monique Robinson, Grant J. Smith, Gina L. Ambrosini, Jan P. Piek, and Wendy H. Oddy. ADHD Is Associated With a 'Western' Dietary Pattern in Adolescents. Journal of Attention Disorders, 2010

5. http://www.heart.org/HEARTORG/Conditions/HighBloodPressure/PreventionTreatmentofHighBloodPressure/Stress-and-Blood-Pressure_UCM_301883_Article.jsp

6. Br Heart J. 1957 Jan; 19(1): 45–52. PMCID: PMC503361 ADRENALINE SENSITIVITY OF PERIPHERAL BLOOD VESSELS IN HUMAN HYPERTENSION Robert S. Duff Cardiological Department, St. Bartholomew's Hospital

7. Palacios R, Sugawara I (January 1982). "Hydrocortisone abrogates proliferation of T cells in autologous mixed lymphocyte reaction by rendering the interleukin-2 Producer T cells unresponsive to interleukin-1 and unable to synthesize the T-cell growth factor". Scand. Journal of Immunology 15 (1): 25–31

8. Padgett, David; Glaser, R (August 2003). "How stress influences the immune response". Trends in Immunology 24 (8): 444–448

9. Katherine M. Flegal, PhD; Margaret D. Carroll, MS; Cynthia L. Ogden, PhD; Clifford L. Johnson, MSPH (2002). Prevalence and Trends in Obesity among US Adults, 1999–2000". JAMA 288 (14): 1723–1727

10. Ng, M.; Fleming, T.; Robinson, M.; Thomson, B.; Graetz, N.; Margono, C. et al. (29 May 2014). "Global, regional, and national prevalence of overweight and obesity in children and adults during 1980–2013: A systematic analysis for the Global Burden of Disease Study 2013". The Lancet

11. John LaRosa of MarketData; National Weight Control Registry; American Society for Metabolic and Bariatric Surgery; Jo Piazza, author of "Celebrity Inc.: How Famous People Make Money.

12. http://www.ncbi.nlm.nih.gov/m/pubmed/8527285/

13. http://archive.argusleader.com/usatoday/article/26898487

14. Epidemiology of Weight Training-Related Injuries Presenting to United States Emergency Departments, 1990 to 2007 Zachary Y. Kerr, MA*, Christy L. Collins, MA‡† and R. Dawn Comstock, PhD*‡§

15. http://archive.argusleader.com/usatoday/article/26898487

CHAPTER 1

The Functional Food Spectrum

1. Dietary Reference Intakes for Energy, Carbohydrate, fibre, Fat, Fatty Acids, Cholesterol, Protein, and Amino Acids (Macronutrients) (2005), Chapter 7: Dietary, Functional and Total fibre.US Department of Agriculture, National Agricultural Library and National Academy of Sciences, Institute of Medicine, Food and Nutrition Board

2. Sies, Helmut (1997). "Oxidative stress: Oxidants and antioxidants". Experimental physiology 82 (2): 291–5

3. Ghaffar, Abdul (2006). Microbiology and Immunology On-Line Textbook. USC School of Medicine. Retrieved 1 January 2007

Exercise Is Not Enough

1. http://us.wow.com/wiki/Weight_gain

2. Beth Israel Deaconess Medical Center. "Fundamental Process Of Tumor Growth Explained." Science Daily, 13 March 2008

Macronutrients

1. McNab, B. K. 1997. On the Utility of Uniformity in the Definition of Basal Rate of Metabolism. Physiol. Zool. Vol.70; 718–720

2. Workers taking the most sick days. Michael B. Sauter, Samuel Weigley and Alexander E.M. Hess. Retrieved May 9, 2013

3. Tom W. Smith, Paid Sick Days: A Basic Labor Standard for the 21st Century, National Opinion Research Center at the University of Chicago, August 2008

4. Curr Opin Endocrinol Diabetes Obes. Authors manuscript; available in PMC 2010 Feb. 1

5. http://www.ncbi.nlm.nih.gov/pmc/articles/PMC3649463/

6. Curr Opin Endocrinol Diabetes Obes. Authors manuscript; available in PMC 2010 Feb. 1

7. King MW. "Serotonin". The Medical Biochemistry Page. Indiana University School of Medicine. Retrieved 1 December 2009

8. http://en.wikipedia.org/wiki/Specific_dynamic_action

9. Pan H, Guo J, Su Z (May 2014). "Advances in understanding the interrelations between leptin resistance and obesity". Physiology & Behavior 130: 157–169

10. High Protein Diets Improve Your Brain's Leptin Function Am J Clin Nutr. Weigle DS, Breen PA, Matthys CC, Callahan HS, Meeuws KE, Burden VR, Purnell JQ

11. Whey Protein Improves Leptin and Insulin Function Br J Nutr. Pichon L, Potier M, Tome D, Mikogami T, Laplaize B, Martin-Rouas C, Fromentin G

12. The Journal of Clinical Endocrinology & Metabolism, Sep 1 1998, 83(9):3243-3246, "Inverse Correlation between Serum Testosterone and Leptin in Men"

Refined Sugar and Artificial Sweeteners

1. http://www.scienceworldreport.com/articles/17248/20140918/artificial-sweeteners-cause-gut-bacteria-change-glucose-intolerance-isnt-sweet.htmhttp://wiki-fitness.com/truvia-vs-splenda/J Toxicol Environ Health A. 2008; 71(21):1415-29. Splenda alters gut microflora and increases intestinal p-glycoprotein and cytochrome p-450 in male rats. Abou-Donia MB[1], El-Masry EM, Abdel-Rahman AA, McLendon RE, Schiffman SS.

2. Diabetes Metab Syndr Obes. 2012; 5: 175–189. Published online 2012 Jul 6. Comparison with ancestral diets suggests dense acellular carbohydrates promote an inflammatory microbiota, and may be the primary dietary cause of leptin resistance and obesity. Ian Spreadbury

3. Effects of carbohydrate sugars and artificial sweeteners on appetite and the secretion of gastrointestinal satiety peptides. Br J Nutr. 2011 May; 105(9):1320-8. doi: 10.1017/S000711451000512X. Epub 2011 Jan 24. Steinert RE[1], Frey F, Töpfer A, Drewe J, Beglinger C.

4. http://www.ncbi.nlm.nih.gov/pubmed/22252107

5. Shapiro A, Mu W, Roncal C, Cheng K, Johnson R, Scarpace P (November 2008). Fructose-induced leptin resistance exacerbates weight gain in response to subsequent high-fat feeding. Am. J. Physiol. Regul. Integr. Comp. Physiol. 295 (5): R1370–R1375. doi:10.1152/ajpregu.00195.2008

6. Am J Ind Med. 2014 Apr; 57(4):383-97. Epub 2014 Jan 16.The carcinogenic effects of aspartame: The urgent need for regulatory re-evaluation. Soffritti M[1], Padovani M, Tibaldi E, Falcioni L, Manservisi F, Belpoggi F

7. Artificial sweeteners: okay in moderation. Harvard women's health watch 11:11 2004 Jul pg.23

8. Pan A, Hu FB. Effects of carbohydrates on satiety: differences between liquid and solid food. Curr Opin Clin Nutr Metab Care. 2011; 14:385-90

9. Mozaffarian D, Hao T, Rimm EB, Willett WC, Hu FB. Changes in diet and lifestyle and long-term weight gain in women and men. N Engl J Med. 2011; 364:2392-404.

Sugar Alcohols

1. Sugar alcohols. (2005, April 27). In Wikipedia, the Free Encyclopedia. Retrieved March 21, 2015

Alcohol

1. Alcohol. Author manuscript; available in PMC 2009 Oct 7. Published in final edited form as: Alcohol. 2009 Sep; 43(6): 433–441.

2. http://www.reducetriglycerides.com/alcohol_beer_wine_template.htm

3. Alcohol Clin Exp Res. 2013 Apr; 37(4):539-49. Epub 2013 Jan 24. Alcohol and sleep I: effects on normal sleep. Ebrahim IO[1], Shapiro CM, Williams AJ, Fenwick PB.

4. The Effect of Evening Alcohol Consumption on Next-Morning Glucose Control in Type 1 Diabetes Benjamin C. Turner, MRCP1, Emma Jenkins, BSC1, David Kerr, MD, FRCP1, Robert S. Sherwin, MD2 and David A. Cavan, MD, FRCP1

Mixing Carbs and Fats

1. http://www.renalandurologynews.com/high-fiber-intake-reduces-inflammation-death-risk-in-ckd-patients/article/217935/

2. 2007 American Society for Clinical Nutrition. High-glycemic-index carbohydrate meals shorten sleep onset [1,2,3] Ahmad Afaghi, Helen O'Connor, and Chin Moi Chow

3. J Biol Chem. 2013 Jul 19; 288(29):21074-81. Epub 2013 Jun 6.Differential contribution of insulin and amino acids to the mTORC1-autophagy pathway in the liver and muscle. Naito T[1], Kuma A, Mizushima N

4. J Am Coll Nutr. 2013; 32(1):66-74. The effects of soy and whey protein supplementation on acute hormonal reponses to resistance exercise in men. Kraemer WJ[1], Solomon-Hill G, Volk BM, Kupchak BR, Looney DP, Dunn-Lewis C, Comstock BA, Szivak TK, Hooper DR, Flanagan SD, Maresh CM, Volek JS

Timing Carbs

1. Stedman, Thomas Lathrop (December 2005) [1911]. "Stedman's Medical Dictionary" (28th Ed.). Baltimore: Lippincott Williams & Wilkins. p. 2100. ISBN 0-7817-3390-1

2. Crohn's Disease-Associated Adherent-Invasive Escherichia coli Adhesion Is Enhanced by Exposure to the Ubiquitous Dietary Polysaccharide Maltodextrin Kourtney P. Nickerson[1,2] and Christine McDonald[1,2,*] Emiko Mizoguchi, Editor

3. Semrad CE. Approach to the patient with diarrhea and malabsorption. In: Goldman L, Schafer AI, eds. Goldman's Cecil Medicine. 24th ed. Philadelphia, PA: Saunders Elsevier; 2011: chap 142.

Timing Fats

1. Van Cauter E, Leproult R, Plat L (2000). "Age-related changes in slow-wave sleep and REM sleep and relationship with growth hormone and cortisol levels in healthy men". Journal of the American Medical Association 284 (7): 861–868

2. Colorado State Edu. Growth Hormone (Somatotropin). Available from: http://www.vivo.colostate.edu/hbooks/pathphys/endocrine/hypopit/gh.html

3. Men'sHealth. Why You Should Avoid Carbs at Bedtime. A midnight snack may stifle muscle growth. By Florence Comite, MD, November 21, 2013

4. Informed Health Online [Internet]. Type 1 diabetes: Measuring sugar levels in blood and urine yourself. Last Update: October 23, 2013

5. http://www.snac.ucla.edu/documents/Calories2010_000.pdf

6. Perello M, Scott MM, Sakata I, Lee CE, Chuang JC, Osborne-Lawrence S et al. (Feb 2012). Functional implications of limited leptin receptor and ghrelin receptor coexpression in the brain. The Journal of Comparative Neurology 520 (2): 281–94

7. Inui A, Asakawa A, Bowers CY, Mantovani G, Laviano A, Meguid MM et al. (Mar 2004). Ghrelin, appetite, and gastric motility: the emerging role of the stomach as an endocrine organ. FASEB Journal: Official Publication of the Federation of American Societies for Experimental Biology 18 (3): 439–56

8. Trends Endocrinol Metab. 2010 Feb; 21(2):68-74. Epub 2009 Oct Insulin, leptin and reward. Davis[1], Choi DL, Benoit SC

9. Psychosom Med. 2004 Nov-Dec; 66(6):876-81.Cortisol, hunger, and desire to binge eat following a cold stress test in obese women with binge eating disorder. Gluck ME[1], Geliebter A, Hung J, Yahav E

10. Ann Med. 2000 Apr; 32(3):222-32.Separate systems for serotonin and leptin in appetite control. Halford JC[1], Blundell JE

11. Physiol Behav. 2012 Mar 20; 105(5):1202-7. Epub 2011 Dec 30.Dopamine and food reward: effects of acute tyrosine/phenylalanine depletion on appetite. Hardman CA[1], Herbert VM, Brunstrom JM, Munafò MR, Rogers PJ

12. The Journal of Clinical Endocrinology & Metabolism, Sep 1 1998, 83(9):3243-3246, Inverse Correlation between Serum Testosterone and Leptin in Men

13. Dhindsa SS, et al. "Testosterone replacement decreases insulin resistance in hypogonadal men with type 2 diabetes" [Abstract OR22-1.] Presented at ENDO 2013 (Annual Meeting of The Endocrine Society), June 19, 201

14. http://www.cdc.gov/nutrition/everyone/basics/fat/unsaturatedfat.html

15. http://culinaryarts.about.com/od/culinaryreference/a/fattable.htm

16. http://www.macnutoil.com/professional.htm

17. http://www.oliveoilsource.com/page/heating-olive-oil

18. http://www.whyoliveoil.com/oxidation-of-fatty-acids/

19. http://www.marksdailyapple.com/nuts-omega-6-fats/#axzz3V4xt7zkE

20. http://whatscookingamerica.net/Information/CookingOilTypes.htm

21. http://drbenkim.com/articles-oils.html

22. http://articles.mercola.com/sites/articles/archive/2003/10/15/cooking-oil.aspx

23. http://drbenkim.com/articles-oils.html

24. http://cholesterol.about.com/od/cholesterolnutrition101/f/hightransfats.htm?utm_term=foods%20that%20contain%20trans%20fats&utm_content=p1-main-1-title&utm_medium=sem&utm_source=msn&utm_campaign=adid-aab09a96-399f-4d13-896e-0d7809f14b60-0-ab_mse_ocode-22880&ad=semD&an=msn_s&am=exact&q=foods%20that%20contain%20trans%20fats&dqi=foods%2Bthat%2Bcontian%2Btrans%2Bfats&o=22880&l=sem&qsrc=999&askid=aab09a96-399f-4d13-896e-0d7809f14b60-0-ab_mse

25. http://articles.mercola.com/sites/articles/archive/2003/10/15/cooking-oil.aspx

26. Dolecek, T.A. "Epidemiological evidence of relationships between dietary polyunsaturated fatty acids and mortality in the Multiple Risk Factor Intervention Trial." PSEBM. 200:177-182, 1992

27. Lands, William E.M. (December 2005). "Dietary fat and health: the evidence and the politics of prevention: careful use of dietary fats can improve life and prevent disease." Annals of the New York Academy of Sciences 1055: 179-192. Blackwell.

28. Okuyama, Hirohmi; Ichikawa, Yuko; Sun, Yueji; Hamazaki, Tomohito; Lands, William E.M. (2007). "3 fatty acids effectively prevent coronary heart disease and other late-onset diseases: the excessive linoleic acid syndrome." World Review of Nutritional Dietetics 96 (Prevention of Coronary Heart Disease): 83-103. Karger

29. Hibbeln, Joseph R. (June 2006). "Healthy intakes of n-3 and n-6 fatty acids: estimations considering worldwide diversity." American Journal of Clinical Nutrition 83 (6, supplement): 1483S-1493S. American Society for Nutrition.

30. Gillingham LG, Harris-Janz S, Jones PJ. Dietary monounsaturated fatty acids are protective against metabolic syndrome and cardiovascular disease risk factors. Lipids. 2011; 46(3):209-228.

31. https://www.healthbeyondhype.com/info/are-you-balancing-your-omega-3-and-omega-6-fatty-acids

32. Plasma Phospholipid Fatty Acids and Prostate Cancer Risk in the SELECT Trial Theodore M. Brasky, Amy K. Darke, Xiaoling Song, Catherine M. Tangen, Phyllis J. Goodman, Ian M. Thompson, Frank L. Meyskens Jr, Gary E. Goodman, Lori M. Minasian, Howard L. Parnes, Eric A. Klein and Alan R. Kristal

33. Diabetes Sci Technol. 2007 May; 1(3): 415–422. Published online 2007 May. PMCID: PMC2769584 Replacements for Trans Fats—Will There Be an Oil Shortage? David C. Klonoff, M.D., FACP

34. May Formation of genotoxic dicarbonyl compounds in dietary oils upon oxidation. Lipids 2004 May;39(5):481-6 Kazutoshi Fujioka, Takayuki Shibamoto

35. http://www.countdowntofitness.com/fitnessblog/2011/03/23/is-your-fish-oil-rancid-and-causing-disease/ Is Your Fish Oil Rancid and Causing Disease? March 23, 2011 by Doreen

36. http://www.liveinthenow.com/article/beware-rancid-fish-oil-capsulesomega 3 s safer than omega 6- http://ebm.sagepub.com/content/200/2/177.short

Basic Concepts of Losing Body Fat

1. http://livewell.jillianmichaels.com/carbohydrates-burned-during-exercises-4302.html

2. Seale JL, Conway JM. Relationship between overnight energy expenditure and BMR measured in a room-sized calorimeter. Eur J Clin Nutr. 1999 Feb; 53(2):107-11

3. Zhang K, Sun M, Werner P, Kovera AJ, Albu J, Pi-Sunyer FX, Boozer CN. Sleeping metabolic rate in relation to body mass index and body

composition. Int J Obes Relat Metab Disord. 2002 Mar; 26(3):376-83

4. Blackwell Publishing Ltd. "Burning Fat and Carbohydrate during Exercise." ScienceDaily. ScienceDaily, 19 June 2007

5. http://www.dummies.com/how-to/content/busting-the-great-myths-of-fat-burning.html

6. J Appl Physiol (1985). 2005 Jan; 98(1):160-7. Epub 2004 Aug 27. Determinants of fat oxidation during exercise in healthy men and women: a cross-sectional study. Venables MC[1], Achten J, Jeukendrup AE

7. Urban LE, MCrory MA, Dallal GE, Das SK, Saltzman E, Weber JL, and Roberts SB. "Accuracy of Stated Energy Contents of Restaurant Foods." JAMA. 2011; 306[3]287-293. - See more at: http://now.tufts.edu/news-releases/nutrition-researchers-examine-restaurants-cal#sthash.96nEHkLJ.dpuf

8. http://www.msgtruth.org/whywe.htm

9. Genes and biochemical pathways in human skeletal muscle affecting resting energy expenditure and fuel partitioning Xuxia Wu , Amit Patki , Cristina Lara-Castro , Xiangqin Cui , Kui Zhang , R. Grace Walton , Michael V. Osier , Gary L. Gadbury , David B. Allison , Mitchell Martin , W. Timothy Garvey Journal of Applied Physiology Published 1 March 2011 Vol. 110 no. 3, 746-755 D 10.1152/japplphysiol.00293.2010

10. Clin Endocrinol (Oxf). 1999 Feb; 50(2):229-35.Functional hypothalamic amenorrhoea: a partial and reversible gonadotrophin deficiency of nutritional origin.Couzinet B[1], Young J, Brailly S, Le Bouc Y, Chanson P, Schaison G

11. Androgens in Women with Anorexia Nervosa and Normal-Weight Women with Hypothalamic Amenorrhea K.K. Miller, E.A. Lawson, V.Mathur, T.L. Wexler, E. Meenaghan, M.Misra, D.B. Herzog, and A. Klibanski

12. Nature Reviews Endocrinology 4, 407-414 (July 2008) Endocrine abnormalities in anorexia nervosa. Elizabeth A Lawson & Anne Klibanski

13. http://www.t-nation.com/readArticle.do?id=460285

14. Psychoneuroendocrinology. 2014 Jul; 45:96-107. Epub 2014 Mar 21.Effect of sub chronic tryptophan supplementation on stress-induced cortisol and appetite in subjects differing in 5-HTTLPR genotype and trait neuroticism. Capello AE[1], Markus CR[2]

15. J Clin Endocrinol Metab. 2002 Dec; 87(12):5587-93.Abnormal cortisol metabolism and tissue sensitivity to cortisol in patients with glucose intolerance. Andrews RC[1], Herlihy O, Livingstone DE, Andrew R, Walker BR

16. Journal of Clinical Endocrinology & Metabolism"; Leptin Levels Are Dependent on Sleep Duration: Relationships with Sympathovagal Balance, Carbohydrate Regulation, Cortisol, and Thyrotropin; Karine Spiegel, et al.; November 2004

17. J Pers Soc Psychol. 2008 Jun; 94(6):1078-93. The social endocrinology of dominance: basal testosterone predicts cortisol changes and behavior following victory and defeat. Mehta PH[1], Jones AC, Josephs RA

18. J Clin Psychiatry. 2005 Jan; 66(1):7-14.Low testosterone levels predict incident depressive illness in older men: effects of age and medical morbidity. Shores MM[1], Moceri VM, Sloan KL, Matsumoto AM, Kivlahan DR

19. Schwartz MW, Woods SC, Porte D, Seeley RJ, Baskin DG (Apr 2000). "Central nervous system control of food intake". Nature 404 (6778): 661–71. (Inactive 2015-02-01)

20. Taheri S, Lin L, Austin D, Young T, Mignot E (Dec 2004). "Short sleep duration is associated with reduced leptin, elevated ghrelin, and increased body mass index". PLoS Medicine 1 (3)

21. Bennett MP, Zeller JM, Rosenberg L, et al. The effect of mirthful laughter on stress and natural killer cell activity.

22. http://www.livestrong.com/article/170399-effects-of-laughter-on-the-human-brain/

23. Harris, W., Schoenfeld, C. D., Gwynne, P. W., Weissler, A. M.,Circulatory and humoral responses to fear and anger, The Physiologist, 1964, 7, 155

24. Raymond W. Novaco, Anger, Encyclopedia of Psychology, Oxford University Press, 2000

25. http://www.npr.org/blogs/thesalt/2014/01/15/262741403/why-sugar-makes-us-feel-so-good

26. http://www.sciencedaily.com/releases/2010/07/100713011053.htm

27. (2009). Food and beverage industry profile. Center for Responsive Politics.

28. http://preventioninstitute.org/focus-areas/supporting-healthy-food-a-activity/supporting-healthy-food-and-activity-environments-

advocacy/get-involved-were-not-buying-it/735-were-not-buying-it-the-facts-on-junk-food-marketing-and-kids.html

29. Over 95% of food and beverage ads on children's programming are unhealthy products: Study By Stephen DANIELLS, 20-Dec-2013 http://www.foodnavigator-usa.com/Manufacturers/Over-95-of-food-and-beverage-ads-on-children-s-programming-are-unhealthy-products-Study

30. Healthy Kids. Do junk food ads contribute to childhood obesity? Beth Wallace Smith, RD. Read more at http://www.philly.com/philly/blogs/healthy_kids/Do-junk-food-ads-contribute-to-childhood-obesity.html#BHZk5Beb2pUkETIT.99

31. http://www.msgtruth.org/avoid.htm

32. Why you shouldn't buy supermarket birthday cakes. Retrieved June 4,2012, from http://foodbabe.com

33. http://fivehundredpoundpeeps.blogspot.com/2011/10/msg-is-used-to-make-lab-rats-fat-how.html

34. http://www.livingwithrheumatoidarthritis.com/MSG.html

35. Warshaw, Hope. "High-fructose corn syrup vs. sugar". The Washington Post. Retrieved 5 June 2014

36. http://www.highfructosecornsyrup.org/2009/02/guess-whats-lurking-in-your-food.html

37. http://articles.mercola.com/sites/articles/archive/2010/01/02/highfructose-corn-syrup-alters-human-metabolism.aspx

38. Cole LA (2009). "New discoveries on the biology and detection of human chorionic gonadotropin". Reprod. Biol. Endocrinol. 7: 8

CHAPTER 2

Functional Training

1. How Fast is CrossFit Growing? The Chart Tells The Story. http://www.tabatatimes.com/how-fast-is-crossfit-growing-the-chart-tells-the-story/

2. Clin Orthop Relat Res. 1975 ;(107):11-24.Synovial fluid analysis. Yehia SR, Duncan H

3. http://iphysioperth.com.au/news/the-five-most-common-crossfit-injuries-part-1/

4. http://www.examiner.com/article/rise-crossfit-injuries-a-boon-for-chiropractors

Functionally Fit

1. Can Exercise Training With Weight Loss Lower Serum C - reactive protein Levels? Koichi Okita, Hirotaka Nishijima, Takeshi Murakami, Tatsuya Nagai, Noriteru Morita, Kazuya Yonezawa, Kenji Iizuka, Hideaki Kawaguchi, Akira Kitabatake Accepted July 2, 2004

2. Cakir Atabek H., Demir, S., Pinarbasill, R., Gunduz, N., Effects of Different Training Intensity on Indices of Oxidative Stress. Journal of Strength and Conditioning. Retrieved September, 2010. 24 (9) 2491-2497

3. Beavers, K., Binkley, T., Nicklas, B., Effect of Exercise Training on Chronic Inflammation. Clinica Chimica Acta. 2010. 411, 785-793

4. http://www.ncbi.nlm.nih.gov/pubmed/22978553?dopt=AbstractPlus%20

5. Effect of muscular exercise on the plasma level of cortisol in man. European Journal of

6. http://link.springer.com/article/10.1007/s00018-014-1575-6

7. Elwood P, Galante J, Pickering J, et al. Healthy Lifestyles Reduce the Incidence of Chronic Diseases and Dementia: Evidence from the Caerphilly Cohort Study. PLOS ONE. Retrieved 2013; 8(12) e81877.http://www.plosone.org/article/info%3Adoi%2F10.1371%2Fjournal.pone.0081877

8. Is the gut an athletic organ? Digestion, absorption and exercise. Brouns F[1], Beckers E

9. Sports Med. Retreived 1993 Apr; 15(4):242-57

10. Endocrinology. A. Cornil, A. De Coster, G. Copinschi, J. R. M. Franckson. Retrieved (1965)

11. "Exercise for depression". Cochrane Database Syst Rev 9: Cooney GM, Dwan K, Greig CA, Lawlor DA, Rimer J, Waugh FR et al. Retreived (2013). CD004366

12. Massages Boost the Immune System by Live Science Staff. Retreived September 08, 2010. http://www.livescience.com/34910-massage-benefits-immune-system-100908.html

13. Stress causes release of white blood cells count- http://www.livestrong.com/article/100754-causes-elevated-white-blood-count/

14. Diabetes and exercise. Br J Sports Med. N. S. Peirce. Retreived 1999 Jun; 33(3): 161–173

15. Physical activity, fitness, and gray matter volume. Neurobiology. Aging. 35 Suppl 2: S20–528.Erickson KI, Leckie RL, Weinstein AM Retreived September 2014

16. Fiziol Cheloveka; Acute Testosterone and Cortisol Responses to High Power Resistance Exercise; Andrew Fry & Charles Lohnes; July-Aug. 2010

17. Journal of Applied Physiology; Changes in Hormonal Concentrations After Different Heavy-resistance Exercise Protocols in Women; William J. Kraemer, et al., Aug. 1993

18. Parker-Pope, T. (2001). For a Healthy Brain You really need to use your Head -- Physical and Mental Exercise Can Stave off Mental Decline. The Wall Street Journal Europe, November 26, 2001, 8. Retrieved October 5, 2006, from ProQuest database

19. The effects of a 9-week program of aerobic and upper body exercise on the maximal voluntary ventilation of chronic obstructive pulmonary disease patients J Cardiopulm Rehabil. Retreived 1995 Mar-Apr; 15(2):130-3.Dugan D[1], Walker R, Monroe DA

20. Changes in arterial dispensability and flow-mediated dilation after acute resistance vs. aerobic exercise J Strength Cond Res. 2010 Oct; 24(10):2846-52. Collier SR[1], Diggle MD, Heffernan KS, Kelly EE, Tobin MM, Fernhall B

21. July issue of Hepatology, a journal published by John Wiley & Sons on behalf of the American Association for the Study of Liver Diseases (AASLD. Retreived July 1, 2009 Eurekalert

22. The Independent Effects of Physical Activity in Patients with Non-Alcoholic Fatty Liver Disease. St. George, Alexis; Bauman, Adrian; Johnston, Amanda; Farrell, Geoff; Chey, Tien; George, Jacob. Hepatology; July 2009. Volume 50 Issue 1, Pages 68-76

23. The Effect of Exercise on Visceral Adipose Tissue in Overweight Adults: A Systematic Review and Meta-Analysis. Dirk Vissers,* E-mail: dirk.vissers@ua.ac.beAffiliation: Faculty of Medicine and Health Sciences, University of Antwerp, Antwerp, Belgium ☐ Wendy Hens, Jan Taeymans, Jean-Pierre Baeyens, Jacques Poortmans, Jacques Poortmans, Luc Van Gaal. Published: February 8, 2013

24. A Philp, A L Macdonald and P W Watt. Lactate a signal coordinating cell and systemic function. J Exp Biol 2005; 208: 4561-4575

25. http://benefitof.net/benefits-of-lactic-acid. C Kapoor retrieved on September 5, 2011

26. Textbook of Medical Physiology", by Arthur C. Guyton and John E. Hall, 11th Edition. Published 2006

27. Exercise beyond menopause: Dos and Don'ts. Nalini Mishra, V. N. Mishra,[1] and Devanshi[2] J Midlife Health. 2011 Jul-Dec; 2(2): 51–56

28. Exercise to improve spinal flexibility and function for people with Parkinson's disease: a randomized, controlled trial. Schenkman M[1], Cutson TM, Kuchibhatla M, Chandler J, Pieper CF, Ray L, Laub KC. J Am Geriatr Soc. 1998 Oct; 46(10):1207-16

29. Weight Training - Protecting You Against Free Radical Damage. http://www.preventdisease.com/fitness/fitadults/ARTICLES/weighttraining_freeradicals.html

30. Is Exercise the Best Antioxidant Supplement? Len Kravitz, Ph.D. program coordinator of exercise science and a researcher at the University of New Mexico, Albuquerque. Ristow, M., Zarse, K., Oberbach, A., Kloting, N., Birringer, M., Kiehntopt, M. et al. (2009)

31. Gray H, Clemente CD, ed. Gray's Anatomy. 13th ed. Philadelphia, Pa: Lea & Febiger; 1985. 44. Robinson J. Beyond Legendary Abs. Los Angeles, Calif: Health for Life; 1986

32. http://www.mayoclinic.org/diseases-conditions/enlarged-heart/basics/prevention/CON-20034346

33. Effects of caffeine on human behavior. Food Chem Toxicol. 2002 Sep; 40(9):1243-55. Smith A[1].

Free Weights vs. Machines

1. Garhammer, J. Free weight equipment for the development of athletic strength and power—part I.Natl. Strength Cond. Assoc. J. 3(6):24–26, 33. 1981

2. Silvester, L.J., C. Stiggins, C.McGawen, and G.R. Bryce.The effect of variable resistance and free-weight training programs on strength selected isotonic and isokinetic exercises, modalities and programs on the acquisition of strength and power in collegiate football players. Natl. Strength Cond. Assoc. J. 4(1):40–42. 1982

3. O'Shea, P. Scientific Principles Methods of Strength Fitness. Reading, MA: Addison Wesley, 1969

4. O'Shea, P. Quantum Strength & Power Training. Corvallis, OR: Patrick's Books, 1995

5. O'Shea, P. Toward an understanding of power Strength Cond. J.1:34–35. 1999

Lower-Back Injuries

1. Gray H, Clemente CD, ed. Gray's Anatomy. 13th ed. Philadelphia, Pa: Lea & Febiger; 1985. 44 Robinson J. Beyond Legendary Abs. Los Angeles, Calif: Health for Life; 1986

2. 45. Bogduk N, Pearcy M, Hadfield G. Anatomy and biomechanics of psoas major. Clin Biomech. 1992; 7:109-119

3. 45. Bogduk N, Pearcy M, Hadfield G. Anatomy and biomechanics of psoas major. Clin Biomech. 1992; 7:109-119

4. http://qa.1napsgear.org/index.php?question_id=166

5. Intervertebral Disc Disorders. MDGuidelines. Reed Group. 1 December 2012

Transverse Abdominis

1. http://bamboocorefitness.com/the-transverse-abdominis-the-spanx-of-your-abdominal-muscles/

Building Up the Glutes

1. Fact sheet 344: Falls. World Health Organization. October 2012. Retrieved 3 December 2012

Functional Sets, Active Release Techniques, and Gentle Static Stretching

1. http://en.wikipedia.org/wiki/Active_Release_Technique Principles of Anatomy & Physiology, 12th Edition, Tortora & Derrickson, Pub: Wiley & Sons

2. Clin Orthop Relat Res. 1975 ;(107):11-24.Synovial fluid analysis. Yehia SR, Duncan H

Overtraining

1. Physiology of Behavior Carlson, Neil (2013). Pearson. pp. 602–606. ISBN 9780205239399

2. The Influence of Exercise on Cognitive Abilities Compr Physiol. Fernando Gomez-Pinilla[1,*] and Charles Hillman[2] Retrieved 2013 Jan; 3(1): 403–428

Stress Kills

1. Resistance Training Improves Generalized Anxiety Disorder. Nancy A. Melville. June 02, 2011. American College of Sports Medicine (ACSM) 58th Annual Meeting: Abstract 601

2. Dunn AL, Trivedi MH, Kampert JB, Clark CG, Chambliss HO (2005) Exercise treatment for depression: Efficacy and dose response. American Journal of Preventive Medicine 28(1): 1–8

3. Elwood P, Galante J, Pickering J, et al. Healthy Lifestyles Reduce the Incidence of Chronic Diseases and Dementia: Evidence from the Caerphilly Cohort Study. PLOS ONE 2013; 8(12) e81877.http://www.plosone.org/article/info%3Adoi%2F10.1371%2Fjournal.pone.0081877

4. How does stress affect the skin? http://www.sharecare.com/health/skin-and-beauty/how-does-stress-affect-skin

5. http://www.livestrong.com/article/100754-causes-elevated-white-blood-count/

6. How Chronic Stress Leads To Heart Attack And Stroke. Posted: 06/23/2014 10:43 am. http://www.huffingtonpost.ca/2014/06/23/stress-heart-attack_n_5521861.html

7. The journal of Clinical Endocrinology and Metabolism, Retrieved April 2013

8. Atrophy and impaired muscle protein synthesis during prolonged inactivity and stress. Paddon-Jones D[1], Sheffield-Moore M, Cree MG, Hewlings SJ, Aarsland A, Wolfe RR, Ferrando AA. J Clin Endocrinol Metab. 2006 Dec; 91(12):4836-41. Epub 2006 Sep 19

9. Nicotine Promotes Insulin Resistance. Retrieved June 13, 2009 http://www.newsmedical.net/news/20090613/Nicotine-promotes-insulin-resistance.aspx

10. http://www.intelegen.com/nutrients/weight_loss_cortisol_and_insulin.htm

11. HOW CELLS COMMUNICATE DURING THE FIGHT OR FLIGHT RESPONSE. University of Utah. Retrieved 18 April 2013

12. http://www.sciencedaily.com/releases/2010/09/100907163313.htm

13. https://books.google.com/books?id=QW1qkEbzligC&pg=PA152&lpg=PA152&dq=alcohol+increased+proinflammatory+cytokines&source=bl&ots=SGlbVCLZaQ&sig=2a0gIbZk8qybyEnpRhBza2IHPsQ&hl=en&sa=X&ei=t5EuVf6qKIukNqz1gpgP&ved=0CDAQ6AEwAg#v=onepage&q=alcohol%20increased%20proinflammatory%20cytokines&f=false

14. McAuley MT, Kenny RA, Kirkwood TB, Wilkinson DJ, Jones JJ, Miller VM (2009). A mathematical model of aging-related and cortisol induced hippocampal dysfunction. BMC Neurosci 10: 26

15. Falls in cognitive impairment and dementia. Shaw FE[1].Clin Geriatr Med. 2002 May; 18(2):15973

16. http://www.seattletimes.com/lifestyle/the-most-dangerous-activity-driving/

17. http://www.researchgate.net/publication/236968467_The_Influence_of_Exercise_on_Cognitive_Abilitie

Healing the Brain with Functional Training

1. American Psychiatric Association (2013). Diagnostic and Statistical Manual of Mental Disorders (5th ed.). Arlington, VA: American Psychiatric Publishing. pp. 271–280

2. http://www.livestrong.com/article/39012-working-weights-relieve-stress/

3. Nauert PhD, R. (2006). Depression's Chemical Imbalance Explained. Psych Central. Retrieved on April 16, 2015, from http://psychcentral.com/news/2006/11/09/depressions-chemical-imbalance-explained/398.html

4. Tipton KF, Boyce S, O'Sullivan J, Davey GP, Healy J; Boyce; O'Sullivan; Davey; Healy (August 2004). "Monoamine oxidases: certainties and uncertainties". Curr. Med. Chem. 11 (15): 1965-82

5. http://www.ncbi.nlm.nih.gov/m/pubmed/16421512/

6. http://www.ncbi.nlm.nih.gov/pmc/articles/PMC2077351/

7. http://usatoday30.usatoday.com/news/health/painter/2010-04-26-yourhealth26_ST_N.htm

8. Attrition: PTSD and Chemical Imbalance. http://www.strategypage.com/htmw/htatrit/20091230.aspx

9. Brain Chemicals and Exercise. Ashley Miller, Demand Media. http://healthyliving.azcentral.com/brain-chemicals-exercise-4416.html

10. Therapist using horses in treating PTSD. By BEN BAUGH. Feb 1 2009 12. http://www.aikenstandard.com/article/20090201/AIK0101/302019974

11. http://morallowground.com/2011/11/03/every-80-seconds-a-u-s-military-veteran-dies-by-suicide/

12. http://veteransforcommonsense.org/2012/05/09/us-army-examines-why-some-soldiers-avoid-ptsd-care-strategies-to-keep-them-in-treatment

13. Saratoga War Horse Project bonds vets, horses. By Susan Salk on July 1, 2013. http://offtrackthoroughbreds.com/2013/07/01/saratoga-war-horse-project-bonds-vets-horses

14. http://ptsd.about.com/od/selfhelp/qt/Slip.htm

15. http://usnews.nbcnews.com/_news/2012/11/26/15395330-ptsd-may-be-overdiagnosed-but-ptsd-deniers-are-wrong-psychologists-say?lite

CHAPTER 3

The 7 Types of Functional Training

1. The growth of tendon strength D. H. Elliott. Bull Br Assoc Sport Med. 1968; 3(2): 46–51. PMCID: PMC1435587

2. Edgerton, V.R. Mammalian muscle fiber types and their adaptability. Amer. Zool. Vol?: 113-125, 1978

3. Fahey, T.D. Basic Weight Training for Men and Women. Mt. View, CA: Mayfield Publishing, 1994

4. Komi, P.V. (ed.) Strength and Power in Sport. London: Blackwell Scientific Publications, 1992

5. Komi, P.V. Physiological and biomechanical correlates of muscle function: effects of muscle structure and stretch-shortening cycle on force and speed. Exercise Sci. Sports Rev. 12: 81-121, 1984

6. Mastropaolo, J.A. A test of the maximum-power theory for strength. Eur. J. Appl. Physiol. 65: 415-420, 1992

7. Sale, D.G. Neural adaptation to resistance training. Med. Sci. Sports Exerc. 20 (suppl.): S135-S145, 1988

8. Paton CD, Hopkins WG., Combining explosive and high-resistance training improves performance in competitive cyclists. Journal of Strength and Conditioning Research, vol. 19, no. 4, pg. 826-30, 2005

9. Quinn, Elizabeth (n.d.). Exercise Science - The Science Behind Your Workout. Sportsmedicine.about.com. Retrieved on 2008-10-01

10. http://www.sportsci.org/encyc/adaptex/adaptex.html

11. http://www.animal-mrt.com/delayed-onset-muscle-soreness-doms-lactic-acid/

12. http://en.wikipedia.org/wiki/BodyPump

13. http://en.wikipedia.org/wiki/Proprioception

14. http://en.wikipedia.org/wiki/Scar

15. Mobility Device Use in the United States. H. Stephen Kaye, Ph.D. Taewoon Kang, Ph.D. Mitchell P. LaPlante, Ph.D. Disability Statistics Center Institute for Health and Aging University of California San Francisco, California June 2000

CHAPTER 4

Dysfunctional Training (DFT)

1. http://en.wikipedia.org/wiki/CrossFit

2. http://thestatetimes.com/2015/02/25/what-is-crossfit/

3. http://crossfitsoutharlington.com/competing-against-others/

4. http://www.ncbi.nlm.nih.gov/pubmed/24276294

5. http://www.ncbi.nlm.nih.gov/pubmed/24276294

6. http://ask.metafilter.com/154545/How-to-CrossFit-while-recovering-from-injury

7. http://marathonandbeyond.com/choices/latta.html

8. Special Feature for the Olympics: Effects of Exercise on the Immune System. Immunology and Cell Biology (2000) 78, 532–535; doi:10.1111/j.1440-1711.2000.t01-11-.xExercise and cytokines. Bente Klarlund Pedersen[1, 1]The Copenhagen Muscle Research Centre, Department of Infectious Diseases, University of Copenhagen, Copenhagen, Denmark

9. http://www.bioportfolio.com/resources/pmarticle/11145/Lower-White-Blood-Cell-Counts-In-Elite-Athletes-Training-For-Highly-Aerobic.htmlDavies KJA, Quintanilha AT, Brooks GA & Packer L (1982). Free radicals and tissue damage produced by exercise. Biochem Biophy Res Commun 107, 1198–1205.

10. Essig DA & Nosek TM (1997). Muscle fatigue and induction of stress protein genes: a dual function of reactive oxygen species? Can J Appl Physiol 22, 409–428

11. Leeuwenburgh C, Fiebig R, Chandwaney R & Ji LL (1994). Aging and exercise training in skeletal muscle: responses of glutathione and antioxidant enzyme systems. Am J Physiol 267, 439–445

12. Salminen A & Vihko V (1983). Endurance training reduces the susceptibility of mouse skeletal muscle to lipid peroxidation in vitro. Acta Physiol Scand 117, 109–113

13. Sastre J, Asensi N, Gascó E, Pallardó FV, Ferrero JA, Furukawa T et al. (1992). Exhaustive physical exercise causes oxidation of glutathione status in blood: Prevention by antioxidant administration. Am J Physiol 32, 992–995

14. Viña J, Gimeno A, Sastre J, Desco C, Asensi M, Pallardo FV et al. (2000a). Mechanism of free radical production in exhaustive exercise in humans and rats; role of xanthine oxidase and protection by allopurinol. IUBMB Life 49, 539–544

15. Viña J, Gomez-Cabrera MC, Lloret A, Marquez R, Minana JB, Pallardo FV et al. (2000b). Free radicals in exhaustive physical exercise: mechanism of production, and protection by antioxidants. IUBMB Life 50, 271–277

16. Biology of Sport. Biology of Sport, Vol. 23 N. EFFECTS OF BRIEF MAXIMAL EXERCISE ON INTERLEUKIN-6 AND TUMOR NECROSIS FACTOR-ALPHA. M. Denguezli-Bouzgarrou, M. Ben Jabrallah , S. Gaid , F. Slama , H. Ben Saad , Z. Tabka

17. http://www.ncbi.nlm.nih.gov/pubmed/21584686

18. http://onlinelibrary.wiley.com/doi/10.1113/jphysiol.2004.080564/full#b26

19. http://www.ask.com/sports-active-lifestyle/static-balance-dcdd696e1db32ba6

Exercises Performed on Unstable Devices Such as a BOSU®ball

1. Behm DG, Anderson K, Curnew RS (2002). Muscle force and activation under stable and unstable conditions. J Str Cond Res. 16: 416-422

2. http://www.ask.com/science/difference-between-static-dynamic-balance-394399048ddebad

3. Proprioception and muscle torque deficits in children with hypermobility syndrome. 2009 Feb; 48(2):152-7. Doi: 10.1093/rheumatology/ken435. Epub 2008 Dec 16.Fatoye F[1], Palmer S, Macmillan F, Rowe P, van der Linden M

4. http://www.ncbi.nlm.nih.gov/pubmed/19417231

5. http://thekeep.eiu.edu/cgi/viewcontent.cgi?article=1014&context=kss_fac

6. Willardson JM, Fontana FE, Bressel E (2009). Effect of surface stability on core muscle activity for dynamic resistance exercises. Int J Sports Physiol Perform. 4(1), 97-109

7. Soderman, K. et al. Balance board training: prevention of traumatic injuries of the lower extremities in female soccer players? A prospective randomized intervention study. Knee Surg Sports Traumatol Arthrosc. 8(6):356-63. 2000

8. http://breakingmuscle.com/strength-conditioning/science-says-you-should-ditch-the-unstable-surface-training

9. http://www.menshealth.com/fitness/

10. http://www.ctlawtribune.com/id=1202721254174/Woman-Injured-On-Gyms-Exercise-Device-Collects-750000-Settlement

11. http://foxct.com/2015/03/20/62-year-old-awarded-750000-in-suit-against-branford-gym/

12. http://lawsuitssettlementfunding.com/press-releases.php

CHAPTER 5

Functional Muscle Fiber Training

1. Elizabeth Quinn (October 30, 2007). Fast and Slow Twitch Muscle Fibers. About.com. Retrieved on 2008-05-13

2. Karp, Jason R. Muscle Fiber Types and Training. Coachr.org. Retrieved on 2008-10-17

3. Baggett, Kelly (n.d.). Understanding Muscle Fiber Types. Bodybuilding.com. Retrieved on 2008-10-17

4. Andersen, JL; Schjerling, P; Saltin, B. Muscle, Genes and Athletic Performance. Scientific American. 9/2000

5. http://www.ncbi.nlm.nih.gov/pmc/articles/PMC1479884/

6. http://quizlet.com/10102247/twitch-fiber-types-flash-cards/

7. Gabriel DA, Kamen G, Frost G. Neural adaptations to resistive exercise: mechanisms and recommendations for training practices. Sports Med. 2006; 36(2): 133-49

8. Exercise training increases oxidative capacity and attenuates exercise-induced ultrastructural damage in skeletal muscle of aged horses. Jeong-su Kim , Kenneth W. Hinchcliff , Mamoru Yamaguchi , Laurie A. Beard , Chad D. Markert , Steven T. Devor. Journal of Applied Physiology Published 1 January 2005 Vol. 98 no. 1, 334-342

9. The Weight Trainer. Muscle Growth Part I: Why, And How, Does A Muscle Grow and Get Stronger? By Casey Butt, Ph.D.

10. Human Skeletal Muscle Fiber Type Classifications. Wayne Scott, Jennifer Stevens and Stuart A Binder–Macleod

11. Henneman, et al., 1974

12. Bielinski R, Schutz Y, Jéquier E. Energy metabolism during the post exercise recovery in man. Am J Clin Nutr. 1985; 42:69-82

13. http://athletics.wikia.com/wiki/Type_II_Muscle_Fiber#cite_note-NickH-3

14. http://www.ncbi.nlm.nih.gov/pmc/articles/PMC2957584/

15. Loss of type-2 in elderly-Differential features of muscle fiber atrophy in osteoporosis and osteoarthritis C. Terracciano, M. Celi, D. Lecce, J. Baldi, E. Rastelli, E. Lena, R. Massa, and U. Tarantino http://www.ncbi.nlm.nih.gov/pmc/articles/PMC3572370/

16. http://www.ncbi.nlm.nih.gov/pmc/articles/PMC2828690/

17. Baggett, Kelly (n.d.). Understanding Muscle Fiber Types. Bodybuilding.com. Retrieved on 2008-10-17

18. http://en.wikipedia.org/wiki/Progressive_overload#cite_note-1

19. http://www.nytimes.com/2008/11/02/sports/playmagazine/112pewarm.html

20. Muscle fiber recruitment- Henneman, et al., 1974

21. J Strength Cond Res. 2007 Feb; 21(1):223-6. The effect of static, ballistic, and proprioceptive neuromuscular facilitation stretching on vertical jump performance. Bradley PS[1,] Olsen PD, Portas MD.

22. J Strength Cond Res. 2004 Nov; 18(4):885-8. The effect of different warm-up stretch protocols on 20 meter sprint performance in trained rugby union players. Fletcher IM[1], Jones B

23. http://www.cleveland.com/healthfit/index.ssf/2010/04/static_stretching_before_worko.html\

24. http://well.blogs.nytimes.com/2013/04/03/reasons-not-to-stretch/

25. http://www.health101.org/art_Why_Not_Pilates.htm

26. http://natajournals.org/doi/pdf/10.4085/1062-6050-50.1.01

27. http://www.yogatuneup.com/blog/2011/03/16/overstretching/

28. http://www.nytimes.com/2012/01/08/magazine/how-yoga-can-wreck-your-body.html?_r=0

29. http://www.livestrong.com/article/466508-joint-hypermobility-syndrome-and-yoga-pilates/

30. http://www.theyogablog.com/yoga-butt/

31. http://www.dailymail.co.uk/health/article-2161301/Pilates-make-bad-worse-Experts-agree-help-reduce-pain-improve-posture-hidden-dangers.html

32. http://www.city-data.com/forum/exercise-fitness/1679227-back-pain-pilates.html

33. http://www.livestrong.com/article/324919-yoga-increased-si-joint-pain/

34. http://tenniselbowclassroom.com/tennis-elbow-posts/yoga-elbow-hypermobility-tennis-elbow/

35. http://www.dailymail.co.uk/health/article-2161301/Pilates-make-bad-worse-Experts-agree-help-reduce-pain-improve-posture-hidden-dangers.html

CHAPTER 6

Muscle Toning vs. Bulking

1. University of Oregon (n.d.). Muscle Physiology. UOregon.edu. Retrieved on 2008-05-1
2. http://www.ncbi.nlm.nih.gov/pmc/articles/PMC2957584/
3. http://www.healthline.com/health/low-testosterone/testosterone-levels-by-age#Adolescence3
4. http://www.muscleandstrength.com/articles/losing-muscle-cortisol.html
5. DOE/Lawrence Livermore National Laboratory. "Number of Fat Cells Remains Constant from Teenhood in All Body Types." ScienceDaily. ScienceDaily, 12 May 2008. www.sciencedaily.com/releases/2008/05/080509133100.htm
6. http://www.livestrong.com/article/310070-how-many-calories-does-a-pound-of-muscle-burn-per-day
7. Westcott and Guy 1996
8. http://www.ohio.edu/people/schwiria/bios446/L11Exercise%20Metabolism&Thermal%20Stress.htm
9. http://www.ohio.edu/people/schwiria/bios446/L11Exercise%20Metabolism&Thermal%20Stress.htm

CHAPTER 7

Functional Cardio

1. DIABETES-http://www.huffingtonpost.com/dr-mark-hyman/skinny-fat_b_1799797.html
2. http://coachmikeblogs.com/chronic-cardio-excess-free-radicals/
3. http://jap.physiology.org/content/73/5/1805
4. http://www.ncbi.nlm.nih.gov/pmc/articles/PMC1474177/
5. http://www.ncbi.nlm.nih.gov/pmc/articles/PMC1474177/
6. Radak Z, Chung HY, Koltai E, et al. Exercise, oxidative stress and hormesis. Ageing Res Rev. 2008 Jan; 7(1):34-42. Epub 2007 Aug 2
7. Neubauer O, Reichhold S, Nersesyan A, et al. Exercise-induced DNA damage: is there a relationship with inflammatory responses? Exerc Immunol Rev. 2008;14:51-72
8. Fisher-Wellman K, Bloomer RJ. Acute exercise and oxidative stress: a 30 year history. Dyn Med. 2009 Jan 13; 8:1. Doi: 10.1186/1476-5918-8-1.
9. Weight Training - Protecting You against Free Radical Damage. http://www.preventdisease.com/fitness/fitadults/ARTICLES/weighttraining_freeradicals.ht
10. http://www.ncbi.nlm.nih.gov/pubmed/22978553?dopt=AbstractPlus%20
11. http://www.ncbi.nlm.nih.gov/pubmed/22978553?dopt=AbstractPlus%20 Neubauer O, Reichhold S, Nersesyan A, et al. Exercise-induced DNA damage: is there a relationship with inflammatory responses? Exerc Immunol Rev. 2008; 14:51-72
12. http://www.poliquingroup.com/ArticlesMultimedia/Articles/Article/1138/Does_Cardio_Make_You_Fat.aspx
13. http://www.tabatatimes.com/crossfit-isnt-just-trademarked-hiit/

14. http://fitness.mercola.com/sites/fitness/archive/2012/01/25/cardio-may-damage-heart.aspx

15. http://running.competitor.com/2012/06/news/how-much-running-is-bad-for-your-heart_54331

16. http://www.theatlantic.com/health/archive/2011/12/distance-running-and-endurance-sports-can-be-hard-on-the-heart/250514/

17. Exercise-induced right ventricular dysfunction and structural remodeling in endurance athletes. André La Gerche , Andrew T. Burns , Don J. Mooney , Warrick J. Inder , Andrew J. Taylor , Jan Bogaert , Andrew I. MacIsaac , Hein Heidbüchel , David L. Prior

18. http://www.ncbi.nlm.nih.gov/m/pubmed/16421512/

19. http://www.ncbi.nlm.nih.gov/pmc/articles/PMC2077351/

20. Elwood P, Galante J, Pickering J, et al. Healthy Lifestyles Reduce the Incidence of Chronic Diseases and Dementia: Evidence from the Caerphilly Cohort Study. PLOS ONE. Retrieved 2013; 8(12)

21. Is the gut an athletic organ? Digestion, absorption and exercise. Brouns F[1], Beckers E Sports Med. Retreived 1993 Apr; 15(4):242-57

22. Exercise for depression". Cochrane Database Syst Rev 9: Cooney GM, Dwan K, Greig CA, Lawlor DA, Rimer J, Waugh FR et al. Retreived (2013). CD004366

23. http://sportsmedicine.about.com/od/injuryprevention/a/Ex_Immunity.htm

24. http://www.drwalt.com/blog/2015/03/17/high-intensity-cardio-workout-lower-blood-sugar-levels-better-than-lower-intensity-exercise/

25. http://www.peaktestosterone.com/Natural_Dopamine_Increasers.aspx

26. http://healthyliving.azcentral.com/exercise-its-effects-serotonin-dopamine-levels-2758.html

27. http://www.livestrong.com/article/413190-the-effects-of-exercises-on-the-circulatory-system/

28. http://www.eurekalert.org/pub_releases/2009-07/w-ehp070109.php

29. http://exercise.about.com/od/weightloss/ss/reducebellyfat_5.htm

30. http://www.huffingtonpost.com/richard-palmquist-dvm/signs-of-systemic-toxin-a_b_1214624.html

31. http://www.answers.com/Q/What_moves_lymph

32. http://www.ncbi.nlm.nih.gov/pubmed/22978553?dopt=AbstractPlus%20

33. http://www.mayoclinic.org/diseases-conditions/enlarged-heart/basics/prevention/CON-20034346

34. Kurosumi, Shibasaki & Ito 1984, p. 255

35. Randall 2012

36. Jameson, J. N. St C.; Dennis L. Kasper; Harrison, Tinsley Randolph; Braunwald, Eugene; Fauci, Anthony S.; Hauser, Stephen L; Longo, Dan L. (2005). Harrison's principles of internal medicine. New York: McGraw-Hill Medical Publishing Division

37. http://blogs.denverpost.com/fitness/2013/11/23/is-your-cardio-routine-making-you-fat/13461/

CHAPTER 8

How the Immune System Functions

1. http://www.ncbi.nlm.nih.gov/pmc/articles/PMC2515569/

2. http://www.medicalnewstoday.com/articles/282929.php

3. http://www.hightechhealth.com/enviromental-toxicity

4. Petersen, A. M.; Pedersen, B. K. (2005). "The anti-inflammatory effect of exercise". J Appl Physiol 98 (4): 1154–1162

5. http://physioage.com/about-hormones/men/when-do-i-start

6. Janeway C.A et al 2001. Basic concepts in immunology, Chapter 1 in Immunobiology, 5th ed, New York: Garland Science

7. Beck, Gregory; Gail S. Habicht (1996). "Immunity and the invertebrates" (PDF). Scientific American: 60–66. Retrieved 1 January 2007

8. Janeway C.A. 2001. Evolution of the immune system. In Immunobiology ed Janeway et al. 5th ed, 597–607. New York: Garland Science

9. http://en.wikipedia.org/wiki/Hematopoietic_stem_cell

10. http://healthmad.com/health/what-causes-a-weak-immune-system/

11. http://www.ucsf.edu/news/2014/07/116431/key-aging-immune-system-discovered

12. http://en.wikipedia.org/wiki/Immune_system

13. Rother KI (April 2007). "Diabetes treatment—bridging the divide". The New England Journal of Medicine 356 (15): 1499–501

14. Edwards JC, Cambridge G, Abrahams VM (1999). "Do self-perpetuating B lymphocytes drive human autoimmune disease?". Immunology 97 (2): 188–96

15. Finn AV, Nakano M, Narula J, Kolodgie FD, Virmani R (July 2010). "Concept of vulnerable/unstable plaque". Arterioscler. Thromb. Vasc. Biol. 30 (7): 1282–92

16. http://www.dailymail.co.uk/health/article-2324783/Women-live-longer-men-immune-systems-age-slowly.html

17. Firestein GS. Mechanisms of inflammation and tissue repair. In: Goldman L, Schafer AI, eds. Goldman's Cecil Medicine. 24th ed. Philadelphia, PA: Elsevier Saunders; 2012: chap

18. http://thechart.blogs.cnn.com/2012/01/11/15-top-killers-of-americans/

19. http://www.answers.com/Q/How_does_inhaling_carbon_monoxide_decrease_the_oxygen_level_in_your_blood

20. http://www.medicalnewstoday.com/articles/248423.php

21. Lecture on Inflammation and Innate Immunity

22. http://thechart.blogs.cnn.com/2012/01/11/15-top-killers-of-americans/

23. http://www.answers.com/Q/How_does_inhaling_carbon_monoxide_decrease_the_oxygen_level_in_your_blood

24. http://advancingyourhealth.org/cancer/2013/06/26/cigarette-smoking-cancer-risk/

25. http://en.wikipedia.org/wiki/Warburg_hypothesis

26. De Martel C. Lancet Oncol. 2012; doi: 10.1016/S1470-2045(12)70137-7

27. Coriolus Versicolor. Cancer.org. 2008-06-10. Retrieved 7 August 2012.

28. http://www.webmd.com/a-to-z-guides/autoimmune-diseases

29. http://labtestsonline.org/understanding/analytes/mercury/tab/test/

GMO and the Immune System

1. http://www.prnewswire.com/news-releases/studies-show-gmos-in-majority-of-us-processed-foods-58-percent-of-americans-unaware-of-issue-104510549.html

2. http://www.responsibletechnology.org/gmo-basics/gmos-in-food

3. http://en.wikipedia.org/wiki/Organic_farming

4. http://www.nongmoproject.org/learn-more/

5. http://whyfiles.org/062ag_gene_eng/4.html

6. http://www.foodsafetynews.com/2014/07/chinas-food-safety-issues-are-worse-than-you-thought/#.VV5yxEat5KA

7. http://www.globalanimal.org/2012/04/22/bp-oil-spill-deforms-sea-life/

8. http://chriskresser.com/why-grass-fed-trumps-grain-fed/

9. 2012 World of Conn, National Corn Growers Association (PDF). Retrieved 2012-12-29

10. http://www.nationofchange.org/first-long-term-study-released-pigs-cattle-who-eat-gmo-soy-and-corn-offers-frightening-results-13723

11. http://worldtruth.tv/alarming-new-study-of-monsanto-feed-on-pigs/

12. http://www.iher.org.au/content.php?pageID=3

13. http://www.bangmfood.org/stealth-gmos

14. http://www.huffingtonpost.com/2010/01/19/monsanto-gm-corn-causing_n_425195.html

15. http://www.highfructosecornsyrup.org/2009/02/guess-whats-lurking-in-your-food.html

16. http://www.sciencedaily.com/releases/2001/05/010511074623.htm

17. http://usatoday30.usatoday.com/news/health/story/2012-04-20/antibiotics-animals-human-meat/54434860/1

18. http://www.nationofchange.org/first-long-term-study-released-pigs-cattle-who-eat-gmo-soy-and-corn-offers-frightening-results-13723

19. http://uvamagazine.org/articles/the_hair_detective/

20. http://chemistry.about.com/cs/howthingswork/f/blbodyelements.htm

21. Aldai N, Dugan ME, Kramer JK, et al. Length of concentrate finishing affects the fatty acid composition of grass-fed and genetically lean beef: an emphasis on trans-18:1 and conjugated linoleic acid profiles. Animal: an international journal of animal bioscience. Aug 2011; 5(10):1643-1652

22. The debate over whether Monsanto is a corporate sinner or saint". The Economist. November 19, 2009

23. http://rationalwiki.org/wiki/Monsanto

24. http://www.memphisdailynews.com/editorial/Article.aspx?id=30496

25. http://modernfarmer.com/2014/03/monsantos-good-bad-pr-problem/

26. http://en.wikipedia.org/wiki/Monsanto

27. Maternal and fetal exposure to pesticides associated to genetically modified foods in Eastern Townships of Quebec, Canada. Reprod Toxicol (2011)

28. Scandanavian Journal of Immunology 49 (1999): 578–584Safety Assessment of the Bacillus thuringiensis Insecticidal Crystal Protein CRYIA

29. J Agric Food Chem, 16 November 2008

30. International Journal of Biological Sciences 2009; 5(7):706-726

31. Intragastric and intraperitoneal administration of Cry1Ac protoxin from Bacillus thuringiensis induces systemic and mucosal antibody responses in mice

32. Environmental Health Perspectives 107

33. Plant-Pesticides Risk and Benefits Assessments

34. Bacillus thuringiensis: An epidemiological study, Oregon, 1985-86

35. Safety Assessment of the Bacillus thuringiensis Insecticidal Crystal Protein CRYIA

36. Cry1Ac protoxin from Bacillus thuringiensis sp. Kurstak

37. http://beforeitsnews.com/health/2014/12/genetically-modified-crops-threaten-organic-farm-land-2558958.html

38. Pesticides in Mississippi air and rain: A comparison between 1995 and 2007. Michael S. Majewski[*], Richard H. Coupe[2], William T. Foreman[3] and Paul D. Capel[4]Article first published online: 4 APR 2014

39. http://www.examiner.com/article/stop-the-monsanto-rider-another-ploy-to-take-over-america-s-food

40. http://www.progressive.org/news/2007/07/5087/farmers-fight-save-organic-crops

41. http://rt.com/usa/monsanto-patents-sue-farmers-547/

42. Environ Toxicol Chem. 2014 Feb 19. Epub 2014 Feb 19. PMID: 24549493. [i] Michael S Majewski, Richard H Coupe, William T Foreman, Paul D Capel. Pesticides in Mississippi air and rain: A comparison between 1995 and 2007. Environ Toxicol Chem. 2014 Feb 19. Epub 2014 Feb 19. PMID: 24549493

43. http://www.collective-evolution.com/2014/07/15/new-study-links-gmos-to-cancer-liverkidney-damage-severe-hormonal-disruption/

44. GMO Food in the U.S. and the Biotechnology Industry's Power Sci Tech 4/29/2013 at 09:48:58 By Karl Grossman http://www.opednews.com/articles/GMO-Food-in-the-U-S-and-t-by-Karl-Grossman-130429-829.html

45. Swan SH, et al. Prenatal phthalate exposure and reduced masculine play in boys. Int J Androl. 2010 Apr; 33(2):259-69

46. Rudel RA, et al. Food packaging and bisphenol A and bis (2-ethyhexyl) phthalate exposure: findings from a dietary intervention. Environ Health Perspect. 2011 Jul; 119(7):914-20

47. http://www.collective-evolution.com/2014/07/15/new-study-links-gmos-to-cancer-liverkidney-damage-severe-hormonal-disruption/

48. http://www.governmentisgood.com/articles.php?aid=23&print=1

49. http://www.debate.org/opinions/is-lobbying-destroying-america

Hormones, Antibiotics, and the Immune System

1. Rudel RA, et al. Food packaging and bisphenol A and bis (2-ethyhexyl) phthalate exposure: findings from a dietary intervention. Environ Health Perspect. 2011 Jul; 119(7):914-20

2. Smith, MT. Advances in understanding benzene health effects and susceptibility. Ann Rev Pub Health. 2010; 31:133–48

3. Braun JM, et al. Impact of Early-Life Bisphenol A Exposure on Behavior and Executive Function in Children. Pediatrics. 2011; 128(5):873-882

4. Directorate General for Agriculture and Rural Development of the European Commission What is organic farming

5. http://www.care2.com/causes/food-animals-consume-80-percent-of-antibiotics-in-the-u-s.html

6. http://immunedisorders.homestead.com/antibiotics.html

7. http://immunedisorders.homestead.com/antibiotics.html

8. http://draxe.com/the-dangers-of-farmed-fish/

9. http://healthyeating.sfgate.com/fast-food-affects-nutrition-teens-4167.html

Pesticides, Fertilizers, and the Immune System

1. http://en.wikipedia.org/wiki/Organic_farming
2. http://www.appropedia.org/Conventional_farming
3. http://www.motherearthnews.com/nature-and-environment/environmental-policy/systemic-pesticides-zmaz10onzraw.aspx
4. http://www.nationofchange.org/omg-really-happens-truth-about-trying-wash-pesticides-produce-1362588509
5. Miller GT (2004), Sustaining the Earth, 6th edition. Thompson Learning, Inc. Pacific Grove, California. Chapter 9, Pages 211-216
6. Scott, JC, Stackelberg, PE, Thelin, GP, and Wolock, DM (February 15, 2007), The Quality of our nation's waters: Pesticides in the nation's streams and ground water, 1992–2001. Chapter 1, Page 4. US Geological Survey. Retrieved on September 13, 2007
7. Hetrick, J, R Parker, R Pisigan Jr, and N Thurman. 2000. Progress report on estimating pesticide concentration in drinking water and assessing water treatment effects on pesticide removal and transformation. Briefing Document for a Presentation to the FIFRA Scientific Advisory Panel (SAP)
8. http://organic.about.com/od/cropsfarming/f/Which-Pesticides-Can-Be-Used-For-Organic-Production.htm
9. http://www.thefarmersdaughterusa.com/2013/06/organic-pesticides.html
10. http://wimastergardener.org/?q=OrganicPesticides
11. http://www.greenfacts.org/en/arsenic/index.htm
12. PBS (2001), Pesticide resistance. Retrieved on September 15, 2007
13. Attention-Deficit/Hyperactivity Disorder and Urinary Metabolites of Organophosphate Pesticides. Maryse F. Bouchard, PhD, David C. Bellinger, PhD, Robert O. Wright, MD, MPH, and Marc G. Weisskopf, PhD
14. http://www.seattletimes.com/business/questions-remain-about-organic-foods-grown-in-china/
15. http://www.seattletimes.com/business/questions-remain-about-organic-foods-grown-in-china/
16. http://www.nbcnews.com/id/44701461/ns/health-food_safety/t/tainted-seafood-reaching-american-tables-experts-say/#.VSWmyJPeLh4
17. http://www.nytimes.com/2007/12/15/world/asia/15fish.html?pagewanted=all&_r=0
18. http://www.wnd.com/2007/06/41907/
19. http://abcnews.go.com/Health/Healthday/story?id=4507743&page=1
20. http://unitedstill.com/health/80-of-u-s-tilapia-comes-from-china-loaded-with-growth-hormones/
21. http://abcnews.go.com/Health/Healthday/story?id=4507743
22. http://www.wlf.louisiana.gov/sites/default/files/pdf/document/6582-Summary%20of%20the%20Imported%20Seafood%20Safety%20Act/Summary_of_the_Imported_Seafood_Safety_Act.pdf
23. http://www.nbcnews.com/id/44701461/ns/health-food_safety/t/tainted-seafood-reaching-american-tables-experts-say/#.VSWomTg-5CUk
24. http://www.nytimes.com/2007/06/29/business/29fish-web.html?_r=0
25. http://www.wlf.louisiana.gov/sites/default/files/pdf/document/6582-Summary%20of%20the%20Imported%20Seafood%20Safety%20Act/Summary_of_the_Imported_Seafood_Safety_Act.pdf
26. http://www.cnn.com/2007/LIVING/wayoflife/07/26/china.products/index.html?_s=PM:LIVING

27. http://www.cnn.com/2007/LIVING/wayoflife/07/26/china.products/index.html?_s=PM:LIVING

28. http://www.mexicocityvibes.com/air-pollution-in-mexico-city/

29. http://www.cnn.com/2014/01/20/health/pollution-china-pnas/index.html

30. http://ajed.assembly.ca.gov/sites/ajed.assembly.ca.gov/files/Fast%20Facts%20on%20California%27s%20Agricultural%20Economy.pdf

31. http://www.answers.com/Q/What_percentage_of_food_grown_in_United_States_is_grown_in_California

32. http://www.theguardian.com/environment/2014/mar/25/air-pollution-single-biggest-environmental-health-risk-who

33. http://www.allergiesguide.com/outdoor-allergies/air-pollution-may-significantly-worsen-respiratory-alle.html

34. http://www.allergyuk.org/why-is-allergy-increasing/why-is-allergy-increasing

35. http://archive.hhs.gov/news/press/2004pres/20040527a.html

36. http://rense.com/general/resi.htm

37. http://chefmom.sheknows.com/articles/3683/organic-potatoes-and-root-vegetables

38. http://www.cnn.com/2010/HEALTH/06/01/dirty.dozen.produce.pesticide/index.html

39. www.hindawi.com/journals/bmri/2013/151807/

40. http://www.motherearthnews.com/nature-and-environment/environmental-policy/systemic-pesticides-zmaz10onzraw.aspx

41. http://science.kqed.org/quest/2014/08/14/5-things-everyone-should-know-about-washing-food/

42. http://www.all-recycling-facts.com/fertilizer-pollution.html

43. http://www.health.state.mn.us/divs/eh/risk/studies/metals.html

44. http://www.turfprousa.com/health_effects_of_synthetic_fertilizer_3006a.html

45. https://www.organicconsumers.org/old_articles/foodsafety/sludge101403.php

46. http://www.nbcnews.com/id/23506826/ns/us_news-environment/t/did-pollutants-used-fertilizer-kill-cattle/#.VSagYpPeLh4

47. http://www.sourcewatch.org/index.php/Sewage_sludge

48. http://www.huffingtonpost.com/andrew-kimbrell/give-thanks-but-not-for-t_b_369698.html

49. http://environmentalhealthcollaborative.org/images/JimLazorchakPresentation.pdf

50. http://www.northumberlandtoday.com/2008/09/23/not-all-toxins-removed-from-biosolids

51. http://www.pccnaturalmarkets.com/sc/1203/biosolids_hit_the_fan.html

52. http://www.foodsafetynews.com/2010/10/sewage-sludge-as-fertilizer-safe/#.VSaxWJPeLh4

53. http://www.nbcnews.com/id/23506826/ns/us_news-environment/t/did-pollutants-used-fertilizer-kill-cattle/#.VSagYpPeLh4

54. http://www.sourcewatch.org/index.php/Sewage_sludge

55. http://www.huffingtonpost.com/andrew-kimbrell/give-thanks-but-not-for-t_b_369698.html

56. http://environmentalhealthcollaborative.org/images/JimLazorchakPresentation.pdf

57. http://www.northumberlandtoday.com/2008/09/23/not-all-toxins-removed-from-biosolids

58. http://www.pccnaturalmarkets.com/sc/1203/biosolids_hit_the_fan.html

59. http://www.foodsafetynews.com/2010/10/sewage-sludge-as-fertilizer-safe/#.VSaxWJPeLh4

60. https://sites.google.com/site/nosludgedumping/court-decision---200-dead-georgia-cattle/200-dead-cows-in-georgia

61. http://en.wikipedia.org/wiki/Organic_farming

62. http://www.appropedia.org/Conventional_farming

63. http://www.southlandorganics.com/blogs/news/17982096-health-effects-of-synthetic-fertilizer

64. http://www.creativewellnesscenter.com/index_htm_files/Heavy%20Metals%20article%20short%20version%20for%20website.pdf

65. Diabetes care, published online Feb. 19, 2013

66. http://blog.autismspeaks.org/2010/10/22/got-questions-answers-to-your-questions-from-the-autism-speaks%E2%80%99-science-staff-2/

67. http://articles.mercola.com/sites/articles/archive/2014/07/09/pregnant-women-environmental-toxin-exposure.aspx

Body-Fat Levels and the Immune System

1. https://fabfit4us.wordpress.com/2013/01/30/clear-out-your-bodys-toxins-for-more-energy-and-better-overall-health/

2. http://www.wileyprotocolsystems.com/component/content/article/81-articles/257-environmental-toxins.html

3. http://www.webmd.com/parkinsons-disease/guide/parkinsons-causes

4. http://www.thenaturalrecoveryplan.com/articles/symptoms-of-mercury-poisoning.html

5. http://www.mayoclinic.org/documents/mc5810-0311-pdf/DOC-20079194

6. http://www.drharryfisch.com/overweight-lower-testosterone-levels/

7. http://www.ncbi.nlm.nih.gov/pmc/articles/PMC4030042/

8. http://blog.naturalhealthyconcepts.com/2013/03/05/do-you-have-excessive-food-cravings-low-levels-of-dopamine-may-be-the-problem/

9. http://drhyman.com/downloads/Diabetes-and-Toxins.pdf

10. http://wellnessmama.com/5356/fix-your-leptin/

11. http://healthylivinghowto.com/1/post/2013/02/what-to-do-about-high-cortisol.html

12. http://fitnessblackbook.com/dieting_for_fat_loss/stubborn-body-fat-caused-by-excess-estrogen

13. http://www.wellnessresources.com/weight/articles/why_toxins_and_waste_products_impede_weight_loss_-_the_leptin_diet_weight_l/

14. The Inflammatory Syndrome: The Role of Adipose Tissue Cytokines in Metabolic Disorders Linked to Obesity. Brent E. Wisse. http://jasn.asnjournals.org/content/15/11/2792.abstract

15. http://www.ncbi.nlm.nih.gov/m/pubmed/9375771/

16. http://www.mdpi.com/1422-0067/12/5/3117/pdf

17. Inflammation, Oxidative Stress, and Obesity - MDPI.com

18. http://www.ncbi.nlm.nih.gov/pmc/articles/PMC2910551/

19. http://www.lymeneteurope.org/forum/viewtopic.php?f=6&t=85

20. Cytokine" in Stedman's Medical Dictionary, 28th ed. Wolters Kluwer Health, Lippincott, Williams & Wilkins (2006)

21. http://www.ncbi.nlm.nih.gov/pubmed/2555275

22. The Inflammatory Syndrome: The Role of Adipose Tissue Cytokines in Metabolic Disorders Linked to Obesity. Brent E. Wisse. http://jasn.asnjournals.org/content/15/11/2792.abstract

23. Inflammation in obesity related diseases. Robert, W. O'Rourke, MD,FACS http://www.ncbi.nlm.nih.gov/pmc/articles/PMC2749322/

24. Measures of adiposity predict interleukin-6 responses to repeated psychosocial stress. Christine M. McInnis, Miriam V. Thomas, Danielle Gianferante, Luke Hanlin, Xuejie Chen, Juliana G. Breines, Suzi Hong, Nicolas Rohleder

Dysfunction Junction

1. http://www.impactlab.net/2010/04/27/extraordinary-scans-reveal-what-being-fat-does-to-your-body/

2. http://www.myfitnesspal.com/blog/Tetonia/view/lymph-vessels-488512 127

3. http://www.healthcentral.com/obesity/c/276918/155337/obesity-blood?ap=831

4. Women and adipose tissue http://circ.ahajournals.org/content/105/7/804.full

5. http://www.nebido.com/en/hcp/research/testosterone-research/testosterone-reduces-visceral-fat-and-increases-muscle-mass-in-non-obese-men-aged-55-years-plus.php

6. http://www.webmd.com/diet/20050914/exercise-fights-hidden-body-fat

7. http://www.ncbi.nlm.nih.gov/pmc/articles/PMC3474619/

8. http://www.metaboliceffect.com/diet-to-lose-belly-fat/

9. http://www.researchgate.net/publication/6891103_Increased_subcutaneous_and_epicardial_adipose_tissue_production_of_proinflammatory_cytokines_in_cardiac_surgery_patients_Possible_role_in_postoperative_insulin_resistance

10. http://www.ncbi.nlm.nih.gov/pmc/articles/PMC1395476/

11. http://www.engg.ksu.edu/CHSR/outreach/resources/docs/15HumanHealthEffectsofHeavyMetals.pdf

12. http://www.nursingtimes.net/cellular-pathophysiology-part-2-responses-following-hypoxia/200091.article

13. http://www.ncbi.nlm.nih.gov/pmc/articles/PMC3576876/

14. Ungvari Z, Parrado-Fernandez C, Csiszar A, de Cabo R. Mechanisms underlying caloric restriction and lifespan regulation: implications for vascular aging" Circulation Research 2008;102(5) 519-28

15. Tannenbaum A, and Silverstone H. "Nutrition in relation to cancer. Adv. Cancer Res. 1 (1953): 451-501

16. http://www.researchgate.net/publication/8484315_Inflammatory_related_changes_in_bone_mineral_content_in_adults_with_cystic_fibrosis

17. http://www.womenshealthmag.com/health/chronic-inflammation

18. http://www.webmd.com/heart-disease/news/20100427/calcium-in-arteries-may-predict-heart-risk

19. http://www.webmd.com/lung/tc/pulmonary-embolism-topic-overview

20. http://www.nbcnews.com/id/18594089/ns/health-fitness/t/thin-people-can-be-fat-inside/#.VWSd1Uat5KA

21. http://nickburgraff.com/2013/06/06/skinny-fat-muffin-top-runner-pudge/

Yo-Yo Dieting and the Immune System

1. http://sportsmedicine.about.com/od/sportsnutrition/a/060304.htm
2. http://www.webmd.com/diet/20040603/yo-yo-dieting-may-hurt-immunity?page=2
3. http://www.newser.com/story/109961/weight-loss-may-unleash-bloodstream-toxins.html
4. http://www.roundkickgym.com/18metabolism.pdf
5. http://www.sheknows.com/health-and-wellness/articles/835443/hypothyroidism-dieting-can-damage-your-thyroid
6. http://heartdisease.about.com/od/lesscommonheartproblems/a/thyroidheart.htm
7. http://www.livestrong.com/article/353915-health-risks-of-yoyo-dieting/
8. http://www.webmd.com/a-to-z-guides/proteinuria-protein-in-urine
9. http://www.patient.co.uk/health/nephrotic-syndrome-leaflet
10. http://www.heart.org/HEARTORG/Conditions/HighBloodPressure/AboutHighBloodPressure/What-is-High-Blood-Pressure_UCM_301759_Article.jsp
11. Reddy JK, Rao MS (2006). "Lipid metabolism and liver inflammation. II. Fatty liver disease and fatty acid oxidation". Am. J. Physiol. Gastrointest. Liver Physiol. 290 (5): G852–8
12. http://www.wellnessresources.com/weight/articles/unclog_your_liver_lose_your_abdominal_fat_leptin_diet_weight_loss_challenge/

Fiber and the Immune System

1. http://bd.com/us/diabetes/page.aspx?cat=7001&id=7491
2. http://www.whfoods.com/genpage.php?tname=faq&dbid=16
3. http://www.alive.com/health/natural-products-for-detoxification/
4. http://cholesterol.about.com/od/cholesterolnutrition101/f/howfiberworks.htm
5. Fruits and Veggies, More Matters. What are phytochemicals? Produce for Better Health Foundation. 2014. Retrieved 18 June 2014
6. http://cspinet.org/new/pdf/special_report_-_label_makeover.pdf
7. http://www.arthritistoday.org/what-you-can-do/eating-well/arthritis-diet/fiber-inflammation.php
8. How Fiber Helps Control High Blood Sugar By Madeline Vann, MPH | medically reviewed by Pat F. Bass III, MD, MPH
9. Journal of Nutrition, 143:776-773, 2013
10. http://www.nationalfibercouncil.org/af_are.shtml

Probiotics, Prebiotics, and the Immune System

1. http://www.ncbi.nlm.nih.gov/pmc/articles/PMC3859913/
2. Gibson GR, Roberfroid MB (Jun 1995). "Dietary modulation of the human colonic microbiota: introducing the concept of prebiotics". J Nutr. 125 (6): 1401–1412. PMID 7782892
3. Food and Agricultural Organization of the United Nations and World Health Organization. 1 May 2002. Retrieved 6 January 2015
4. http://www.ehow.com/about_5553792_ph-level-blood.html
5. http://www.greenmedinfo.com/blog/probiotics-destroy-toxic-chemicals-our-gut-us
6. http://www.prevention.com/health/health-concerns/more-proof-probiotics-boost-immunity/
7. http://ajcn.nutrition.org/content/71/6/1682s.full
8. http://www.npr.org/2013/09/06/219669536/do-your-gut-bacteria-influence-your-metabolism
9. Slashinski MJ, McCurdy SA, Achenbaum LS, Whitney SN, McGuire AL; McCurdy; Achenbaum; Whitney; McGuire (2012). ""Snake-oil," "quack medicine," and "industrially cultured organisms:" biovalue and the commercialization of human microbiome research". BMC Medical Ethics 13: 28
10. http://www.livestrong.com/article/535648-does-stomach-acid-kill-probiotic-supplements/
11. http://www.healingwell.com/community/default.aspx?f=38&m=2023232
12. Ljungh A, Wadström T (2006). "Lactic acid bacteria as probiotics". Curr Issues Intest Microbiol 7 (2): 73–89. PMID 16875422
13. Anderson J, Gilliland S (1999). "Effect of fermented milk (yogurt) containing Lactobacillus acidophilus L1 on serum cholesterol in hypercholesterolemic humans". J Am Coll Nutr 18 (1): 43–50
14. http://womenshealthency.com/articles/lactobacillus-acidophilus/
15. http://wwwnc.cdc.gov/eid/article/19/10/pdfs/13-1092.pdf
16. http://www.slate.com/blogs/browbeat/2013/01/30/yogurt_vs_cultured_dairy_blend_what_s_the_difference.html
17. http://www.softdental.com/about_tech_lasergum_a5.html

Heavy Metals, Antibiotics, and the Immune System

1. http://www.ncbi.nlm.nih.gov/pmc/articles/PMC3760005/
2. http://www.healingdaily.com/conditions/free-radicals.htm
3. http://realtruth.org/news/141125-007.html
4. http://www.prevention.com/health/healthy-living/truth-about-antibiotics-your-meat
5. http://www.greenmedinfo.com/blog/probiotics-destroy-toxic-chemicals-our-gut-us
6. http://www.nutri-spec.net/articles/PDF/immuno-synbiotic.pdf
7. http://www.vivo.colostate.edu/hbooks/pathphys/digestion/basics/gi_immune.html
8. http://www.webmd.com/digestive-disorders/tc/probiotics-topic-overview
9. https://www.gutsense.org/gutsense/flora.html
10. ANTIBIOTIC RESISTANCE THREATS - Centers for Disease
11. Kiefer, D; Ali-Akbarian, L (2004). "A brief evidence-based review of two gastrointestinal illnesses: Irritable bowel and leaky gut syndromes

12. http://www.ncbi.nlm.nih.gov/pubmed/14970061

13. Svanström, et al. "Use of azithromycin and death from cardiovascular causes." New England Journal of Medicine, 2013; 368:1704-1712

14. http://www.dramyyasko.com/resources/autism-pathways-to-recovery/chapter-3/

15. Matsuzaki, T., and J. Chin. 2000. Modulating immune responses with probiotic bacteria. Immunol. Cell Biol. 78:67-73.

16. Gill, H. S., K. J. Rutherfurd, J. Prasad, and P. K. Gopal. 2000. Enhancement of natural and acquired immunity by Lactobacillus rhamnosus (HN001), Lactobacillus acidophilus (HN017) and Bifidobacterium lactis (HN019). Br J. Nutr. 83:167-176

17. http://en.wikipedia.org/wiki/Chelation

18. http://www.royalrife.com/aminos.html

Amino Acids and the Immune System

1. http://www.nlm.nih.gov/medlineplus/ency/article/002222.htm

2. http://www.cancer.org/acs/groups/cid/documents/webcontent/002903-pdf.pdf

3. Br J Nutr. 2007 Aug; 98(2):237-52. Epub 2007 Apr 3. Amino acids and immune function. Li P, Yin YL, Li D, Kim SW, Wu G

4. J Cardiovasc Pharmacol. 2010 Jun 7. [Epub ahead of print]. Effect of Long-Term L-Arginine Supplementation on Arterial Compliance and Metabolic Parameters in Patients with Multiple Cardiovascular risk Factors: Randomized, Placebo-Controlled Study. Guttman H[1], Zimlichman R, Boaz M, Matas Z, Shargorodsky M

5. http://www.livestrong.com/article/542316-can-amino-acids-boost-brain-function/

6. http://www.livestrong.com/article/529493-tyrosine-brain-function/

7. http://www.ncbi.nlm.nih.gov/pubmed/19022976

8. Pompella, A; Visvikis, A; Paolicchi, A; Tata, V; Casini, AF (2003). "The changing faces of glutathione, a cellular protagonist". Biochemical Pharmacology 66 (8): 1499–503

9. White, C. C.; Viernes, H.; Krejsa, C. M.; Botta, D.; Kavanagh, T. J. (2003). "Fluorescence-based microtiter plate assay for glutamate–cysteine ligase activity". Analytical Biochemistry 318 (2): 175–180

10. http://aminoacidstudies.org/l-glutathione/

11. http://articles.mercola.com/sites/articles/archive/2013/01/13/mercury-detoxification-protocol.aspx

12. http://www.precisionnutrition.com/whey-protein-allergies-intolerances-bloating

13. http://drhyman.com/blog/2010/05/19/glutathione-the-mother-of-all-antioxidants/

14. http://www.ncbi.nlm.nih.gov/pmc/articles/PMC3140215/

15. Litman GW, Cannon JP, Dishaw LJ (November 2005). "Reconstructing immune phylogeny: new perspectives". Nature Reviews Immunology 5 (11): 866–79

16. http://en.wikipedia.org/wiki/Blood_proteins

17. http://emedicine.medscape.com/article/166724-overview

18. http://www.nature.com/ki/journal/v61/n6/full/4493004a.html

Protein, Bone Density, and Kidney Function

1. Kerstettner, J.E., O'Brien, K.O., Insogna, K.L. "Dietary Protein Affects Intestinal Calcium Absorption," American Journal of Clinical Nutrition, 68(4), 1998, pages 859-865

2. Leibson CL, Toteson ANA, Gabriel SE, Ransom JE, Melton JL III. Mortality, disability, and nursing home use for persons with and without hip fracture: a population-based study. Journal of the American Geriatrics Society 2002; 50:1644–50

3. Walser M: Effects of protein intake on renal function and on the development of renal disease. In The Role of Protein and Amino Acids in Sustaining and Enhancing Performance. Committee on Military Nutrition Research, Institute of Medicine. Washington, DC: National Academies Press; 1999:137-154

4. http://www.sciencedirect.com/science/article/pii/B9780123919342000138

5. http://www.diabetes.org/living-with-diabetes/complications/kidney-disease-nephropathy.html

6. http://www.bovinevetonline.com/news/industry/Importance-of-calcium-and-phosphorus-in-the-ruminant-diet-242403561.html

7. http://undergroundhealthreporter.com/cutting-back-belly-fat-and-processed-foods-can-reduce-kidney-disease-risk/#axzz3XP5xVZQW

8. http://www.ncbi.nlm.nih.gov/pubmed/18721742

9. http://www.medicalnewstoday.com/articles/268144.php

10. http://www.cspinet.org/new/201203051.html

11. http://www.medicalnewstoday.com/articles/289687.php

12. http://www.ncbi.nlm.nih.gov/pubmed/15660573

13. http://www.davita.com/kidney-disease/diet-and-nutrition/diet-basics/what-is-albumin?/e/5317

14. http://www.ncbi.nlm.nih.gov/pubmed/21288313

Blood Sugar, Insulin, and the Immune System

1. http://immunedisorders.homestead.com/Sugar.html

2. http://www.buffalo.edu/news/releases/2000/08/4839.html

3. http://www.ncbi.nlm.nih.gov/pmc/articles/PMC2868080/

4. http://www.diabetes.co.uk/Diabetes-and-Hyperglycaemia.html

5. Stedman, Thomas Lathrop (December 2005) [1911]. "Stedman's Medical Dictionary" (28th ed.). Baltimore: Lippincott Williams & Wilkins. p. 2100. ISBN 0-7817-3390-1

6. http://en.wikipedia.org/wiki/Hyperinsulinemia

7. "Equivalent insulin resistance". PubMed. PMID 17234296. Retrieved May 30, 2014

8. New evidence of how high glucose damages blood vessels could lead to new treatments. (2009, May 11). Retrieved from http://news.mcg.edu/archives/1930

9. http://www.ncbi.nlm.nih.gov/pmc/articles/PMC3762736/

10. http://no-more-heart-disease.com/endothelial-cells/

11. http://www.sharecare.com/health/vascular-disease/what-complications-peripheral-vascular-disease

12. Richard A C Hughes (23 February 2002). "Clinical review: Peripheral neuropathy". British Medical Journal 324: 466

13. http://www.mayoclinic.org/diseases-conditions/autonomic-neuropathy/basics/definition/con-20029053

14. http://www.ncbi.nlm.nih.gov/pmc/articles/PMC2756154/

15. http://www.ncbi.nlm.nih.gov/pmc/articles/PMC2705866/

16. http://www.ncbi.nlm.nih.gov/pmc/articles/PMC3955123/

17. http://care.diabetesjournals.org/content/25/3/620.full

18. http://www.ncbi.nlm.nih.gov/pmc/articles/PMC2705866/

19. http://www.keratin.com/am/am023.shtm

20. Acute and chronic inflammation - Johns Hopkins Medicine

21. Boyle JJ (January 2005). "Macrophage activation in atherosclerosis: pathogenesis and pharmacology of plaque rupture". Curr Vasc Pharmacol 3 (1): 63–8

22. http://www.nature.com/onc/journal/v23/n12/pdf/1207332a.pdf?origin=publication_detail

23. http://en.wikipedia.org/wiki/Endocrine_system

24. Murray, Michael, ND. Pizzorno, Joseph, ND, and Pizzorno, Lara, MA, LMT. The Encyclopedia of Healing Foods. New York, NY: Atria Books, 2005

25. Murray, Michael, ND, and Pizzorno, Joseph, ND. Encyclopedia of Natural Medicine. 2nd ed. New York, NY: Three Rivers Press, 1998

26. Diabetes Care, April 2013

27. http://en.wikipedia.org/wiki/Insulin

28. http://diabetes.about.com/od/whatisdiabetes/a/How-Insulin-Works-In-The-Body.htm

Cholesterol and the Immune System

1. http://www.ncbi.nlm.nih.gov/pubmed/9101427

2. http://www.medindia.net/news/Why-Saturated-and-Unsaturated-Fats-Are-Different-For-Your-Health-91771-1.htm

3. http://www.ncbi.nlm.nih.gov/pmc/articles/PMC3315351/

4. http://en.wikipedia.org/wiki/Atherosclerosis

5. https://news.usc.edu/74887/immune-system-can-wipe-brain-of-alzheimers-indicator/

6. https://www.insidetracker.com/blog/post/56921504250/45247913486-high-white-blood-cell-count-what-you-should

7. http://www.medicalnewstoday.com/articles/253507.php

8. http://en.wikipedia.org/wiki/High-density_lipoprotein

9. Peterson MM, Mack JL, Hall PR et al. (December 2008). "Apolipoprotein B Is an innate barrier against invasive Staphylococcus aureus infection". Cell Host & Microbe 4 (6): 555–66

10. http://circres.ahajournals.org/content/95/8/764.long

11. http://www.sharecare.com/health/high-cholesterol/health-guide/heart-health-improve-cholesterol/good-and-bad-cholesterol

12. http://heartdisease.about.com/od/cholesteroltriglyceride1/a/Cholesterol-And-Triglycerides.htm

13. http://my.clevelandclinic.org/services/heart/prevention/risk-factors/cholesterol/triglycerides

14. http://www.ext.colostate.edu/pubs/foodnut/09319.html
15. http://www.healthline.com/health/high-cholesterol/lipid-disorder#Overview1
16. www.ihs.gov/healthcommunications/pe/documents/LipidsAnatomy
17. http://www.acaloriecounter.com/diet/monounsaturated-fat-polyunsaturated-fat/
18. http://www.health.harvard.edu/staying-healthy/the-truth-about-fats-bad-and-good
19. http://saveyourarteries.com/frames/subframes/howNitricOxideWorks/How%20Nitric%20Oxide%20Works.htm
20. http://www.mayoclinic.org/diseases-conditions/high-blood-cholesterol/in-depth/trans-fat/art-20046114
21. http://www.cleveland.com/healthfit/index.ssf/2008/07/no_trans_fats_may_actually_mea.html
22. http://drhyman.com/blog/2013/12/05/never-eat-frankenfats/#openModal
23. http://en.wikipedia.org/wiki/Glycemic_index
24. http://vancouver.healthcastle.com/sugar-startling-facts-about-how-its-made
25. http://www.rodalenews.com/sugar-and-health
26. http://www.ncsf.org/enew/articles/articles-convertingcarbs.aspx
27. http://non-gmoreport.com/articles/jun08/sugar_beet_industry_converts_to_gmo.php
28. http://en.wikipedia.org/wiki/Carbohydrate#Classification
29. http://en.wikipedia.org/wiki/High_fructose_corn_syrup
30. http://ajcn.nutrition.org/content/88/6/1716S.full
31. http://www.relfe.com/07/fructose_corn_syrup_sugar_comparison.html
32. http://www.health.harvard.edu/heart-health/abundance-of-fructose-not-good-for-the-liver-heart
33. http://healthyeating.sfgate.com/eating-protein-carbs-lower-glucose-readings-11738.htm

Cholesterol

1. Cholesterol at the US National Library of Medicine Medical Subject Headings (MeSH)
2. http://www.johnmuirhealth.com/health-education/health-wellness/heart-disease-risk-factors/cholesterol-lipids.html
3. http://www.livestrong.com/article/31887-function-cholesterol-body/
4. http://www.ehow.com/how-does_5128464_body-produce-cholesterol.html
5. http://www.hamsnetwork.org/metabolism/
6. http://courses.washington.edu/conj/bess/fats/fats.html
7. http://www.ncbi.nlm.nih.gov/pubmed/9519340
8. http://medical-dictionary.thefreedictionary.com/lipoprotein
9. http://www.greenmedinfo.com/blog/there-only-one-type-cholesterol-heres-why
10. http://courses.washington.edu/conj/bess/cholesterol/liver.html
11. http://www.ncbi.nlm.nih.gov/pmc/articles/PMC21484/

LDL and HDL Cholesterol

1. http://en.wikipedia.org/wiki/Cholesterol
2. http://health.usnews.com/health-news/blogs/eat-run/2013/03/27/new-ways-to-lower-cholesterol-with-diet
3. http://www.peakhealthadvocate.com/1658/probiotic-yogurt-shown-to-help-lower-cholesterol-naturally/
4. http://www.ncbi.nlm.nih.gov/pubmed/10497712

The Causes of Heart Disease

1. http://www.ncbi.nlm.nih.gov/pmc/articles/PMC2869506/
2. http://healthyeating.sfgate.com/can-carbohydrates-raise-cholesterol-5983.html
3. http://www.medicalnewstoday.com/articles/270710.php
4. http://newsroom.ucla.edu/releases/majority-of-hospitalized-heart-75668
5. http://en.wikipedia.org/wiki/Endothelial_dysfunction
6. http://en.wikipedia.org/wiki/Endothelium
7. http://www.sciencedirect.com/science/article/pii/S0925443913002
8. http://circ.ahajournals.org/content/105/5/576.full
9. http://www.progressivehealth.com/sugar-may-be-the-cause-of-your-elevated-cholestero.htm
10. http://www.its.caltech.edu/~bich113/PDFs/Lectures/2015_endocytosis.pdf
11. http://press.endocrine.org/doi/abs/10.1210/jcem.84.9.5959
12. http://www.livescience.com/6356-sugar-diet-hurts-cholesterol-levels.html
13. http://www.doctoroz.com/videos/cholesterol-facts-vs-myths
14. http://www.health24.com/Diet-and-nutrition/Nutrition-basics/Sugars-effect-on-cholesterol-20120721
15. http://www.webmd.com/food-recipes/features/health-effects-of-sugar
16. http://colebradburn.com/2011/10/19/sugar-cholesterol-and-plaque-explained/
17. http://www.webmd.com/heart-disease/news/20100420/high-sugar-diet-linked-lower-good-cholesterol
18. http://healthyeating.sfgate.com/sugar-intake-raise-cholesterol-levels-4101.html
19. http://www.cbn.com/cbnnews/healthscience/2012/october/cholesterol-myth-what-really-causes-heart-disease/
20. http://chriskresser.com/the-most-important-thing-you-probably-dont-know-about-cholesterol
21. http://healthyeating.sfgate.com/can-sweets-increase-ldl-2244.html
22. http://www.examiner.com/article/sugar-increases-risk-for-heart-attack-size-of-ldl-cholesterol-smaller
23. http://www.naturalnews.com/036553_sugar_inflammation_longevity.html

24. http://www.lowcarbmonthly.com/general-health/the-relationship-between-sugar-and-inflammation.html

25. http://www.ncbi.nlm.nih.gov/pubmed/1235145

26. http://www.ncbi.nlm.nih.gov/pubmed/21262005

27. http://www.ncbi.nlm.nih.gov/pubmed/2423348

28. http://www.marksdailyapple.com/the-straight-dope-on-cholesterol-10-things-you-need-to-know-part-2/#axzz3XmPTppn6

29. http://medical-dictionary.thefreedictionary.com/oxLDL

30. Bile at end http://www.jci.org/articles/view/61758

31. https://books.google.com/books?id=ywvSBQAAQBAJ&pg=PA490&lpg=PA490&dq=not+having+enough+hdl+to+remove+foam+cells&source=bl&ots=Xrv5CW77Tu&sig=ZsnI_GAaOIwB4RksuatFuxz3ZXI&hl=en&sa=X&ei=CBBrVarlO4iSyQTvvIOYAg&ved=0CDUQ6AEwAw#v=onepage&q=not%20having%20enough%20hdl%20to%20remove%20foam%20cells&f=false

32. http://www.researchgate.net/profile/Akif_Ibragimov/publication/259528947_Foam_Cell_1/links/00b7d52c6393cd8793000000.pdf

33. http://www.ncbi.nlm.nih.gov/pmc/articles/PMC4167628/

34. http://www.webmd.com/heart-disease/guide/heart-disease-c-reactive-protein-crp-testing

35. http://www.laddmcnamara.net/2012/03/oxidized-ldl-cholesterol-testing/

36. Aneurysm" at Dorland's Medical Dictionary

Hormones and Cholesterol

1. https://books.google.com/books?id=BqJ0Yj-IZyQC&pg=PA31&lpg=PA31&dq=Estrogen+lowers+LDL+%28bad%29+cholesterol+and+increase+HDL+%28good%29+cholesterol&source=bl&ots=Hu3OCK4SGX&sig=ezh35eqcTLGz3GwCvfoPzImPPzI&hl=en&sa=X&ei=L-C1rVYr_CYWFyQTa2YO4DA&ved=0CFEQ6AEwCA#v=onepage&q=Estrogen%20lowers%20LDL%20%28bad%29%20cholesterol%20and%20increase%20HDL%20%28good%22%20cholesterol&f=false

2. http://www.livestrong.com/article/376574-estrogen-high-cholesterol/

3. http://www.ncbi.nlm.nih.gov/pmc/articles/PMC2656393/

4. http://circ.ahajournals.org/content/113/13/1708.full

5. http://www.livestrong.com/article/542385-does-progesterone-affect-cholesterol/

6. http://www.themenshealthblog.com/2009/06/testosterone-replacement-improvesmens-liver-function

7. http://onlinelibrary.wiley.com/doi/10.1002/hep.21060/pdf

8. http://cholesterol.about.com/lw/Health-Medicine/Conditions-and-diseases/Cholesterol-and-Your-Thyroid.htm

9. http://www.newswise.com/articles/testosterone-replacement-for-men-with-low-testosterone-improves-liver-function-metabolic-syndrome

10. http://www.ncbi.nlm.nih.gov/pmc/articles/PMC2954460/

11. http://joe.endocrinology-journals.org/content/206/2/217.full.pdf

12. http://www.bbc.com/news/business-28212223

13. http://articles.mercola.com/sites/articles/archive/2012/02/01/29-billion-reasons-to-lie-about-cholesterol.aspx

14. http://www.telegraph.co.uk/news/health/news/8267876/Statins-the-drug-firms-goldmine.html

15. http://www.cbsnews.com/news/with-drug-prices-doubling-are-americans-getting-bilked/

16. GreenMedInfo August 11, 2012

17. Atherosclerosis August 24, 2012

18. Activist Post September 27, 2012

19. Atherosclerosis August 24, 2012

20. Diabetes Care. 2012 Aug 8. [Epub ahead of print]

21. FDA.gov FDA Expands Advice on Statin Risks

22. Greenmedinfo.com May 1, 2012

23. American Journal of Cardiovascular Drugs 2008;8(6):373-418

24. Greenmedinfo.com April 2, 2012 Adverse Health Effects of Statins

25. http://www.wellnessresources.com/freedom/articles/antidepressants_strongly_linked_to_heart_disease

Functional Training, Muscle Tone, and the Immune System

1. http://chemistry.about.com/od/waterchemistry/f/How-Much-Of-Your-Body-Is-Water.htm

2. http://en.wikipedia.org/wiki/Body_water

3. https://www.reddit.com/r/askscience/comments/277l99/when_you_drink_water_how_is_it_distributed_around/

4. http://www.sciencedaily.com/releases/2007/12/071218105414.htm

5. http://www.hindawi.com/journals/mi/2010/171023/

6. http://g-se.com/uploads/biblioteca/aminoacids_immune_system.pdf

7. http://www.digitalnaturopath.com/treat/T73593.html

8. http://thinkmuscle.com/supplement-profiles/glutamine/

9. http://www.biomedcentral.com/1471-2466/14/115

10. http://www.nature.com/pr/journal/v63/n3/full/pr200852a.html

11. https://books.google.com/books?id=AbmXeprR82sC&pg=PA156&lpg=PA156&dq=glutamine+lowers+free+radical+damage&source=bl&ots=Tp3-pkt3Pj&sig=WnyV4gTgAzZcpJ9KVvb0E8MfYqY&hl=en&sa=X&ei=UqZrVYuRHsuCyQTLoIPgCg&ved=0CEIQ6AEwBw#v=onepage&q=glutamine%20lowers%20free%20radical%20damage&f=false

12. http://www.webmd.com/vitamins-supplements/ingredientmono-878-GLUTAMINE.aspx?activeIngredientId=878&activeIngredientName=GLUTAMINE

13. Lacey JM, Wilmore DW. Nutr Rev. 1990; 48:297-309

14. http://www.ncbi.nlm.nih.gov/pmc/articles/PMC3750756/

15. http://www.itmonline.org/arts/glutamine.htm

16. http://www.bodybuilding.com/fun/diane3.htm

17. Suarez I, Bodega G, Fernandez B (Aug–Sep 2002). "Glutamine synthetase in brain: effect of ammonia". Neurochem Int. 41 (2-3): 123–42

18. http://www.ncbi.nlm.nih.gov/pubmed/10356308

19. http://missinglink.ucsf.edu/lm/immunology_module/prologue/objectives/obj04.html

20. http://www.webmd.com/vitamins-supplements/ingredientmono-878-GLUTAMINE.aspx?activeIngredientId=878&activeIngredientName=GLUTAMINE

21. http://www.ncbi.nlm.nih.gov/pubmed/24965526

Dehydration and the Immune System

1. http://en.wikipedia.org/wiki/Kidney

2. http://www.fatigueanswers.com/dehydration.html

3. http://www.menshealth.com/mhlists/stroke_prevention/printer.php

4. http://www.livestrong.com/article/461122-does-drinking-water-keep-my-metabolism-going/

5. http://www.boost-immune-health.com/malfunction-or-disorders.html

6. http://easacademy.org/research-news/article/exercise-induced-dehydration-with-and-without-environmental-heat-stress-results-in-increased-oxidation

7. http://en.wikipedia.org/wiki/Mucus

8. http://en.wikipedia.org/wiki/Lung

9. http://www.answers.com/Q/What_is_the_carbon_dioxide-oxygen_cycle

10. http://metabolichealing.com/kidney-function-dehydration-the-elderly/

11. http://www.bodybuilding.com/fun/behar12.htm

12. http://bharatsangani.com/ask-the-doctor/miscellaneous/headaches-the-most-common-medical-complaint/

13. http://www.redcrossblood.org/learn-about-blood/blood-components/plasma

14. http://en.wikipedia.org/wiki/Body_water

15. http://water.usgs.gov/edu/propertyyou.html

16. http://www.theiflife.com/speed-up-your-metabolism-fatty-liver-disease/

17. http://www.aplaceformom.com/senior-care-resources/articles/elderly-dehydration

Water and the Immune System

1. http://www.beaconlearningcenter.com/documents/1966_3269.pdf

2. http://en.wikipedia.org/wiki/Extracellular_fluid

3. http://www.virology.ws/2009/07/01/the-inflammatory-response/

4. https://answers.yahoo.com/question/index;_ylt=A0LEVr8AvztVl6EAEosPxQt.;_ylu=X3oDMTByOHZyb21tBGNvbG8DYmYxBHBvcwMxBHZoaWQDBHNlYwNzcg--?qid=20080225170605AAdOwdf

5. Klaassen, C.D., Ed.: Casarett and Doull's Toxicology: The Basic Science of Poisons. Sixth Edition, McGraw-Hill, 2007 [2001]

6. https://answers.yahoo.com/question/index?qid=20080225170605AAdOwdf

7. http://www.waterbenefitshealth.com/water-and-brain.html

8. http://www.ncbi.nlm.nih.gov/pmc/articles/PMC3313737/

9. http://www.thyroid.org/iodine-deficiency/

10. http://chriskresser.com/thyroid-blood-sugar-metabolic-syndrome/

11. http://www.khaleejtimes.com/kt-article-display-1.asp?section=health&xfile=/data/health/2012/May/health_May36.xml

12. http://en.wikipedia.org/wiki/Intracellular

13. http://health.blurtit.com/608856/what-happens-when-your-body-gets-too-cold

14. http://health.blurtit.com/29968/what-happens-to-the-human-body-when-it-gets-too-hot

15. http://www.i-sis.org.uk/TIOCW.php

16. http://www.pelicanwater.com/blog/health-risks-from-drinking-demineralized-water/

17. http://www.ncbi.nlm.nih.gov/pubmed/18946667

Excess Water Consumption

1. http://en.wikipedia.org/wiki/Hyponatremia

2. Schrier, Robert W. (2010). "Does 'asymptomatic hyponatremia' exist?" Nature Reviews Nephrology 6 (4): 185

3. http://www.webmd.com/osteoporosis/features/soda-osteoporosis

4. http://www.livestrong.com/article/501796-does-soda-cause-kidney-stones/

5. http://gastrolyte.com.au/dehydration/dehydration-and-alcohol/

6. http://phys.org/news6067.html

7. http://www.collective-evolution.com/2013/10/26/whats-in-your-mug-the-toxic-truth-about-tea/

8. Coffee- http://www.cofei.com/history/where-does-coffee-come-from.html

9. Coffee/pesticides- http://camanoislandcoffee.com/clean-your-nose-with-coffee/

10. http://www.alternet.org/food/tea-pesticides-3

11. http://www.ncbi.nlm.nih.gov/pmc/articles/PMC2022666/

12. http://www.peoplespharmacy.com/2009/07/06/caffeine-helps/

Water Sources

1. http://www.naturalnews.com/036978_water_treatment_filters_bacteria.html

2. http://en.wikipedia.org/wiki/Water_supply_and_sanitation_in_the_United_State

3. http://www.webmd.com/a-to-z-guides/features/drugs-in-our-drinking-water

4. http://water.epa.gov/drink/local/

5. http://www.news-press.com/story/opinion/contributors/2014/04/13/beware-water-purification-scams/7655569/

Electrolytes and the Immune System

1. http://en.wikipedia.org/wiki/Salt
2. http://etasr.com/index.php/ETASR/article/view/174
3. http://www.texasoncology.com/cancer-treatment/side-effects-of-cancer-treatment/less-common-side-effects/blood-test-abnormalities/electrolyte-imbalance/
4. http://www.builtlean.com/2012/11/28/electrolytes/
5. http://www.livestrong.com/article/518878-salt-sodium-inflammation/
6. http://www.latimes.com/science/sciencenow/la-sci-sn-excess-sodium-intake-20140813-story.html
7. http://www.mayoclinic.org/diseases-conditions/hyponatremia/expert-answers/low-blood-sodium/FAQ-20058465
8. http://www.mayoclinic.org/healthy-lifestyle/nutrition-and-healthy-eating/expert-answers/sea-salt/faq-20058512
9. http://www.peoplespharmacy.com/2012/09/20/furosemide-lasix-side-effects-generic-troubles/
10. http://waterimportance.com/
11. Gutierrez-Cuesta J, Sureda FX, Romeu M, et al. Chronic administration of melatonin reduces cerebral injury biomarkers in SAMP8. J Pineal Res. 2007 Apr;42(4):394-402

Functional Sex Improves Immune Functions

1. http://www.dailymail.co.uk/health/article-2031498/Sex-Why-makes-women-fall-love--just-makes-men-want-MORE.html
2. http://www.mirror.co.uk/lifestyle/sex-relationships/sex/how-great-sex-can-help-150806
3. http://timesofindia.indiatimes.com/life-style/relationships/man-woman/How-sex-can-help-you-live-longer/articleshow/10245026.cms
4. http://www.mirror.co.uk/lifestyle/sex-relationships/sex/how-great-sex-can-help-150806
5. http://www.harvardprostateknowledge.org/does-frequent-ejaculation-help-ward-off-prostate-cancer
6. http://www.everydayhealth.com/heart-health/why-you-should-have-more-sex-for-heart-health.aspx
7. http://breastcancerconqueror.com/sex-may-help-prevent-breast-cancer/
8. http://www3.scienceblog.com/community/older/1999/C/199902516.html
9. AJ Macpherson and E Slack. (2007). "The functional interactions of commensal bacteria with intestinal secretory IgA." Current Opinion in Gastroenterology 23 (6): 673–678
10. http://www.medicalnewstoday.com/articles/275795.php
11. http://www.zenlama.com/oxytocin-the-love-hormone-vs-cortisol-the-stress-hormone-a-complete-comparison/
12. Acta Psychological Sinica, 2007, 39(3):502-512
13. Endocrinology, 1992 Jul, 131(1):395-9, "Role of dopamine in the regulation of gonadotropin-releasing hormone in the male rat brain as studied by in situ hybridization"

14. http://blog.lef.org/2011/10/how-to-naturally-enhance-libido-through.html
15. http://www.ncbi.nlm.nih.gov/pubmed/19896530
16. New York Post, March 6, 2013

Sleep and the Immune System

1. http://www.ncbi.nlm.nih.gov/pmc/articles/PMC4117056/
2. http://www.webmd.com/sleep-disorders/excessive-sleepiness-10/immune-system-lack-of-sleep
3. http://beyond-health.co.uk/importance-of-a-good-nights-sleep/
4. http://www.vcmedicine.com/newsletter-archives/adrenal-glands.pdf

Drugs and the Immune System

1. http://www.livestrong.com/article/234411-harmful-effects-of-prescription-drugs/
2. http://www.ehow.com/facts_5747349_prescription-metabolism-increase-weight-gain_.html
3. http://www.foxnews.com/health/2014/03/11/low-libido-6-drugs-that-affect-your-sex-drive/
4. http://senior-health.emedtv.com/beta-blockers/beta-blocker-sexual-side-effects.html
5. http://www.lifescript.com/health/centers/diabetes/articles/
6. http://www.health.com/health/condition-article/0,,20188113_2,00.html
7. http://www.webmd.com/erectile-dysfunction/guide/drugs-linked-erectile-dysfunction
8. http://www.builtlean.com/2013/06/24/drugs-weight-gain/

Vitamins, Minerals, and the Immune System

1. http://www.whfoods.com/genpage.php?tname=faq&dbid=24
2. http://www.orthomolecular.org/resources/omns/v08n09.shtml
3. http://www.livestrong.com/article/282513-a-list-of-fat-soluble-vitamins/
4. http://en.wikipedia.org/wiki/United_States_Pharmacopeia
5. http://en.wikipedia.org/wiki/Carotenoid
6. http://en.wikipedia.org/wiki/Phytochemical
7. http://www.andjrnl.org/article/S2212-2672%2814%2901633-5/abstract

CHAPTER 9

Functional Hormone Replacement

1. Low test cause death http://www.ncbi.nlm.nih.gov/pmc/articles/PMC2834340/
2. http://www.lifescript.com/health/centers/menopause/articles/is_it_time_to_try_hormone_therapy.aspx
3. http://www.webmd.com/menopause/menopause-information
4. http://www.healthline.com/health-slideshow/warning-signs-male-menopause#2
5. http://www.webmd.com/depression/news/20030103/testosterone-may-help-depressed-men
6. http://en.wikipedia.org/wiki/Human_vertebral_column
7. http://www.peaktestosterone.com/Testosterone_Insulin.aspx
8. http://www.predatornutrition.com/blog/2012/03/15/testosterone-leptin-body-fat-levels-and-how-they-correlate/
9. http://douglassreport.com/2013/05/17/low-testosterone-joint-pain/
10. http://www.dummies.com/how-to/content/what-happens-to-aging-muscles.html
11. http://www.healthline.com/health/low-testosterone/testosterone-levels-by-age#Adolescence3
12. http://marnieclark.com/fat-cells-make-estrogen-and-what-you-can-do-about-that/
13. http://www.peaktestosterone.com/Testosterone_Body_Fat.aspx
14. http://www.medscape.com/viewarticle/722328_4
15. http://www.ncbi.nlm.nih.gov/pubmed/12843144
16. http://jap.physiology.org/content/101/4/1252
17. Stem cells produce less as we age- http://www.ucsf.edu/news/2014/07/116431/key-aging-immune-system-discovered
18. http://www.ncbi.nlm.nih.gov/pmc/articles/PMC3474619/
19. http://www.livestrong.com/article/466495-harmful-stimulants-in-diet-pills/
20. http://www.huffingtonpost.com/dr-peter-breggin/stimulants-for-adhd-shown_b_216912.html
21. http://www.sharecare.com/health/sex-and-relationships/article/testosterone-boosts-sex-drive
22. http://www.menshealth.com/health/testosterone-side-effects
23. New York Post, March 6, 2013
24. http://www.brownandmccool.com/Top%2010%20Myths%20About%20Testosterone%20in%20Women.pdf
25. http://www.health.harvard.edu/newsweek/Hot-flashes-in-men-An-update.htm
26. http://www.livestrong.com/article/68797-testosterone-muscle-growth/
27. http://www.ncbi.nlm.nih.gov/pmc/articles/PMC150875/
28. http://www.healthafter50.com/alerts/arthritis/JohnsHopkinsArthritisHealthAlert_1984-1.html
29. http://www.livestrong.com/article/230789-the-effects-of-testosterone-on-metabolism
30. http://www.livestrong.com/article/376574-estrogen-high-cholesterol/
31. http://www.ncbi.nlm.nih.gov/pubmed/11842998

32. http://onlinelibrary.wiley.com/doi/10.1111/j.1365-2796.2008.02010.x/full

33. http://www.ccjm.org/index.php?id=107937&tx_ttnews[tt_news]=362281&cHash=b40a5591f4fb9b2a3ae5ac576a32fd82

34. http://breakthroughs.cityofhope.org/testosterone-prostate-cancer-risk

35. http://www.sciencedaily.com/releases/2011/04/110419121353.htm

36. http://runels.com/testosteronetreatsautoimmune.html

37. http://www.ncbi.nlm.nih.gov/pubmed/25128861

38. http://www.researchgate.net/profile/Martin_Feelisch/publication/11944012_Mechanisms_of_the_antioxidant_effects_of_nitric_oxide/links/00b7d5228879022fd3000000.pdf

39. http://www.ncbi.nlm.nih.gov/pubmed/15240608

40. http://runels.com/testosteronetreatsautoimmune.html

41. http://www.ncbi.nlm.nih.gov/pubmed/2917954

42. Rebuffe-Sevia, M. Marin, P. Bjorntorp, P. Effect of testosterone on abdominal adipose tissue in men. Int. J. Obes. Novemeber 1991. Vol. 15(11);pp. 791-795

43. http://www.peaktestosterone.com/Testosterone_Mood.aspx

44. http://www.doctorbreen.com/bioidentical-hormone-replacement/learn-about-hormones/testosterone/

45. https://www.hgh1.com/testosterone/low-energy/

46. Boyanor, MA. Boneva, Z. Christove, VG. Testosterone supplementation in men with type 2 Diabetes, visceral obesity and partial androgen deficiency. The Aging Male. 2003. Vol. 6(1); pp.1-7

47. http://www.news-medical.net/news/20150309/Testosterone-estrogen-raise-mens-risk-of-heart-disease.aspx

48. http://www.webmd.com/alzheimers/news/20101008/low-testosterone-linked-to-alzheimers-risk

49. http://www.everydayhealth.com/erectile-dysfunction/causes-of-low-libido.aspx

50. http://timesofindia.indiatimes.com/life-style/health-fitness/health-news/Low-testosterone-linked-to-prostate-cancer/articleshow/34692431.cms

51. http://www.health.harvard.edu/newsweek/Hormone-replacement-the-male-version.htm

52. http://www.thebodywellusa.com/blog/is-testosterone-going-to-give-me-a-heart-attack/

53. http://www.hivehealthmedia.com/deadly-tag-team-of-belly-fat-and-high-blood-pressure/

54. http://www.webmd.com/men/news/20030527/low-testosterone-linked-to-heart-disease

55. http://www.sharecare.com/health/endocrine-system/how-testosterone-affect-heart-health

56. http://www.huffingtonpost.com/2013/07/30/testosterone-women-hormone-therapy_n_3634847.html

57. http://www.healthline.com/health/low-testosterone/depression

58. http://kidneysteps.com/2013/01/kidney-disease-and-testosterone/

59. International Journal of Obesity and Related Metabolic Disorders : Journal of the International Association for the Study of Obesity, 2000, 24(4):485-491, "Low serum testosterone level as a predictor of increased visceral fat in Japanese-American men"

60. http://en.wikipedia.org/wiki/Abdominal_obesity

61. http://www.ncbi.nlm.nih.gov/pmc/articles/PMC3045758/

62. http://www.headaches.org/education/Headache_Topic_Sheets/Hormones_and_Migraine

63. http://migraine.com/stories/bio-identical-progesterone-and-estrogen/
64. http://www.mdjunction.com/forums/migraine-headaches-discussions/general-support/1896392-low-testosterone-caused-daily-headaches
65. http://www.sciencedaily.com/releases/2008/01/080109111320.htm
66. http://www.practicalpainmanagement.com/treatments/hormone-therapy/testosterone-replacement-chronic-pain-patients
67. http://en.wikipedia.org/wiki/Opioid_receptor
68. http://www.doctoroz.com/blog/jacob-teitelbaum-md/depressed-and-craving-carbs-type-4-sugar-addiction
69. http://www.calmclinic.com/anxiety/causes/hormones
70. http://www.webmd.com/men/news/20030527/low-testosterone-linked-to-heart-disease
71. http://www.ncbi.nlm.nih.gov/pubmed/15240608

Hematocrit and Estrogen Levels for Males and Females

1. http://en.wikipedia.org/wiki/Hematocrit
2. http://www.ncbi.nlm.nih.gov/pmc/articles/PMC2817018/
3. https://docs.google.com/document/preview?hgd=1&id=1HkuvvA_sIlShM4EDak9vGla0M0KTZ07v_tUoFZKzqm0
4. https://www.healthtap.com/topics/aspirin-hematocrit
5. http://www.chemocare.com/docs/self-help/cbc.pdf
6. http://scholar.harvard.edu/mamontano/publications/effects-short-term-and-long-term-testosterone-supplementation-blood-viscosity
7. http://www.hindawi.com/journals/mi/2014/615917/
8. http://www.sciencedaily.com/releases/2009/10/091001163724.htm
9. http://www.huffingtonpost.com/2011/04/06/stroke-risks-fade-when-wo_n_845469.html
10. http://www.natural-progesterone-advisory-network.com/estrogen-dominance-linked-to-cancer/

Synthetic vs. Bioidentical Hormones

1. http://www.mayoclinic.org/diseases-conditions/menopause/expert-answers/bioidentical-hormones/FAQ-20058460
2. http://pcos.about.com/od/glossary/g/Bioidentical-Hormones.htm
3. http://www.doctoroz.com/blog/lauren-streicher-md/buyer-beware-bioidentical-hormones-myths
4. http://womensvoicesforchange.org/ten-myths-about-bio-identical-hormones.htm
5. https://www.womentowomen.com/bioidenticals-and-hrt/history-of-hormone-replacement-therapy-hrt/
6. http://www.health.harvard.edu/press_releases/myths-and-truths-about-bioidentical-hormones
7. http://www.herplace.com/hormone-info/natural-vs-synthetic.htm
8. http://en.wikipedia.org/wiki/Bioidentical_hormone_replacement_therapy
9. http://www.drholly.typepad.com/natural_vs_synthetic/
10. http://www.holtorfmed.com/the-bioidentical-hormone-debate-are-bioidentical-hormones-estradiol-estriol-and-progesterone-safer-or-more-efficacious-than-commonly-used-synthetic-versions-in-hormone-replacement-therapy/

11. http://www.smart-publications.com/articles/progestin-drugs-more-side-effects-and-risks
12. http://www.aestheticsolutionsinc.com/pdf/Hormones-Controversy.pdf
13. Stanczyk FZ. All progestins are not created equal.Steroids 2003; 68:879-90
14. Ylikorkala O, Evio S, Effects of hormone therapy and alendronate on C-reactive protein, E-selectin, and sex hormone-binding globulin in osteoporotic women, Fertil Steril. 2003 Sep; 80(3):541-5
15. http://womeninbalance.org/wp-content/uploads/2012/10/WinB_ProgBro_English_2008.pdf
16. http://americannutritionassociation.org/newsletter/synthetic-hormone-replacement-therapy-unavoidably-dangerous-answer
17. http://www.natural-progesterone-advisory-network.com/synthetic-hormones-are-dangerous-monster-hormones/
18. http://sites.silaspartners.com/partner/Article_Display_Page/0,,PTID40961_CHID146404_CIID144382,00.html
19. http://www.menshealth.com/nutrition/muscles-bottle
20. http://www.livestrong.com/article/280443-does-dhea-raise-testosterone-levels-in-men/
21. http://www.huffingtonpost.com/julie-chen-md/saliva-tests_b_4366310.html
22. http://www.ncbi.nlm.nih.gov/pubmed/11844745
23. http://www.ncbi.nlm.nih.gov/pubmed/850146
24. http://www.sciencedaily.com/releases/2010/10/101019212921.htm
25. http://abcnews.go.com/Health/HeartFailureTreatment/testosterone-heart-failure/story?id=16155591
26. http://www.news-medical.net/news/20140702/Testosterone-therapy-does-not-increase-mens-risk-for-heart-attack-shows-UTMB-study.aspx
27. http://www.bestnaturaltestosteronesupplements.com/low-testosterone-causes-heart-disease-and-type-2-diabetes/
28. http://www.nature.com/nrendo/journal/v9/n8/full/nrendo.2013.122.html
29. http://www.ncbi.nlm.nih.gov/pmc/articles/PMC3832228/
30. Suarez, M., et al., "Biometric Analysis of Controlled Clinical Study For Growth Factor Formulation on Multiple Parameters of Aging-Related Dysfunctions", High Tech Research Institute, 2002
31. http://www.ncbi.nlm.nih.gov/pmc/articles/PMC3179330/
32. http://www.ncbi.nlm.nih.gov/pubmed/24706014
33. http://www.ncbi.nlm.nih.gov/pmc/articles/PMC3348495
34. http://www.lifeextension.com/Magazine/2007/7/report_diabetes/Page-01
35. http://www.webmd.com/fibromyalgia/news/20020627/growth-hormone-eases-fibromyalgia-pain
36. http://www.ncbi.nlm.nih.gov/m/pubmed/7690364/
37. http://www.smh.com.au/sport/riding-hgh-the-costly-pursuit-of-performance-20130209-2e5di.html
38. http://www.somatropin.cn/effects.html
39. http://joe.endocrinology-journals.org/content/118/3/353.abstract
40. http://www.urmc.rochester.edu/encyclopedia/content.aspx?ContentTypeID=167&ContentID=testosterone_free

How to Properly Balance Female Hormones

1. http://www.4hourlife.com/2012/03/11/female-sexual-desire-testosterone-and-the-menstrual-cycle-for-dummies/
2. http://www.urmc.rochester.edu/encyclopedia/content.aspx?ContentTypeID=167&ContentID=testosterone_free
3. http://www.ncbi.nlm.nih.gov/pmc/articles/PMC3252029/
4. http://www.ncbi.nlm.nih.gov/pmc/articles/PMC3902234/
5. http://www.obesityaction.org/educational-resources/resource-articles-2/obesity-related-diseases/polycystic-ovarian-syndrome-pcos-and-obesity
6. http://www.heart.org/HEARTORG/Conditions/More/MyHeartandStrokeNews/Menopause-and-Heart-Disease_UCM_448432_Article.jsp
7. http://awaremed.com/addictioneducation/low-estrogen-progesterone-causes-sugar-craving-addiction/
8. http://www.diagnose-me.com/symptoms-of/progesterone-excess.html
9. http://www.livestrong.com/article/290116-the-effects-of-progesterone-on-endometriosis/
10. http://www.icnr.com/articles/natural-progesterone.html
11. http://www.kettlebyherbfarms.com/pdfs/Wild%20Yam%20Cream.pdf
12. http://www.zoominfo.com/p/Jerilyn-Pryor/30026779
13. http://boulderintegrativehealth.com/files/women-and-testosterone1.pdf

Women's Health Initiative Study

1. http://en.wikipedia.org/wiki/Women%27s_Health_Initiative
2. http://www.womensinternational.com/connections/inflammation.html
3. http://yourhormonebalance.com/hormone-balance-basics/know-your-hormones/
4. http://www.a4m.com/assets/pdf/bookstore/aamt_vol7_41_smith.pdf
5. http://www.ncbi.nlm.nih.gov/pubmed/1102551
6. http://yourhormonebalance.com/hormone-balance-basics/know-your-hormones/
7. http://doctortaz.com/health-tips-2/estrogen-dominance-is-linked-to-increased-risk-of-breast-cancer-preventing-estrogen-dominance-is-the-first-step-in-preventing-breast-cancer/
8. http://www.today.com/id/10034785/ns/today-today_health/t/estrogen-your-heart-does-it-help-or-hurt/#.VXn8BEat5KA
9. http://www.drugs.com/cdi/provera.html
10. http://www.wsj.com/articles/SB10001424052970204528204577009741133297800
11. http://hormonebalance.org/pdf/Glaser%202013%20Myths%20and%20Misconceptions.pdf
12. http://www.life-enhancement.com/magazine/article/498-what-women-want-to-know-about-natural-progesterone
13. http://en.wikipedia.org/wiki/Women%27s_Health_Initiative
14. http://www.ncbi.nlm.nih.gov/pubmed/17640158
15. http://www.ncbi.nlm.nih.gov/pmc/articles/PMC4025915/
16. https://en.wikipedia.org/wiki/Xenoestrogen
17. https://www.psychologytoday.com/blog/attention-please/201310/hormone-imbalance-not-bipolar-disorder

18. http://hormonebalance.org/pdf/Glaser%202013%20Myths%20and%20Misconceptions.pdf

19. https://en.wikipedia.org/wiki/Xenoestrogen

20. Roy JR, Chakraborty S, Chakraborty TR (June 2009). "Estrogen-like endocrine disrupting chemicals affecting puberty in humans--a review". Med. Sci. Monit. 15 (6): RA137–45

21. https://www.nrdc.org/health/atrazine/files/atrazine.pdf

Birth Control Pills

1. http://www.modernmom.com/c210d8e4-3b45-11e3-8407-bc764e04a41e.html
2. http://www.breastcancer.org/research-news/study-questions-birth-control-and-risk
3. https://en.wikipedia.org/wiki/Combined_oral_contraceptive_pill
4. https://en.wikipedia.org/wiki/Norplant
5. https://en.wikipedia.org/wiki/Vaginal_ring
6. http://www.drugs.com/news/oral-contraceptives-may-affect-testosterone-levels-long-term-1675.html
7. http://time.com/the-best-form-of-birth-control-is-the-one-no-one-is-using/

Preventing Hair Loss in Females

1. http://www.webmd.com/skin-problems-and-treatments/hair-loss/features/women-hair-loss-causes?page=2
2. http://www.huffingtonpost.com/alan-j-bauman/hair-loss-during-menopause_b_3873608.html
3. http://www.americanhairloss.org/women_hair_loss/causes_of_hair_loss.asp
4. https://en.wikipedia.org/wiki/Dihydrotestosterone
5. http://www.hair-sg.com/alpha-5-reductase-enzyme-and-its-role-in-causing-hair-loss/
6. http://hormonebalance.org/pdf/Glaser%202013%20Myths%20and%20Misconceptions.pdf\
7. https://en.wikipedia.org/wiki/Sex_hormone-binding_globulin
8. http://www.ncbi.nlm.nih.gov/pubmed/11788176
9. http://www.drkarlisullis.com/Karlis_Ullis,_M.D./ARTICLES/Entries/2010/8/2_ROLE_OF_ESTRADIOL_AND_SEX_HORMONE_BINDING_GLOBULIN_FOR_MALE_FITNESS_AND_HEALTH_%5BPART_I%5D%26LOW_SEX_HORMONE_BINDING_GLOBULINE_%28SHBG%29_POSITIVE_AND_NEGATIVE_EFFECTS_%5BPART_II%5D.html
10. http://www.ncbi.nlm.nih.gov/pubmed/2591057
11. http://www.ncbi.nlm.nih.gov/pubmed/561671
12. http://www.ncbi.nlm.nih.gov/pubmed/1828548
13. http://www.hairsentinel.com/estrogen-and-hair-loss.html
14. https://en.wikipedia.org/wiki/Spironolactone
15. http://www.realself.com/question/effective-spironolactone-for-female-hair-loss
16. http://www.hairlosstalk.com/hair-loss-treatments/women-spironolactone-topical/index.php
17. http://www.rxlist.com/propecia-side-effects-drug-center.htm

18. http://www.drugwatch.com/propecia/side-effects/

19. http://www.raysahelian.com/finasteride.html

20. http://www.nytimes.com/2015/04/16/fashion/new-hair-thinning-treatments-for-women.html?ref=fashion&smid=tw-nytfashion&_r=0

21. http://www.everydayhealth.com/skin-and-beauty/thyroid-disease-and-hair-loss.aspx

Testosterone and Breast Cancer

1. http://en.wikipedia.org/wiki/Warburg_hypothesis

2. http://www.medicalnewstoday.com/articles/270660.php

3. http://www.ncbi.nlm.nih.gov/pmc/articles/PMC2990475/

4. http://www.researchgate.net/profile/Dominique_Singer/publication/23554695_Respiratory_response_of_malignant_and_placental_cells_to_changes_in_oxygen_concentration/links/0deec52cb1013c6d48000000.pdf

5. http://www.ncbi.nlm.nih.gov/pubmed/15240608

6. https://books.google.com/books?id=2GsgBAAAQBAJ&pg=PA237&lpg=PA237&dq=Inappropriate+expression+of+cytokines+can+create+an+immune+response+that+causes+cell+proliferation&source=bl&ots=-

7. http://press.endocrine.org/doi/full/10.1210/jc.2005-1097 zqhZo97Ax&sig=Dqg544idooqmTZ2NX_ufprmqUeM&hl=en&sa=X&ved=0CFAQ6AEwB2oVChMI6rqExaKPxgIVEX6SCh3gtABu#v=onepage&q=Inappropriate%20expression%20of%20cytokines%20can%20create%20an%20immune%20response%20that%20causes%20cell%20proliferation&f=false

8. http://www.medpagetoday.com/MeetingCoverage/ENDO/39965

9. http://cdn.intechopen.com/pdfs-wm/22058.pdf

10. http://www.researchgate.net/profile/Martin_Feelisch/publication/11944012_Mechanisms_of_the_antioxidant_effects_of_nitric_oxide/links/00b7d5228879022fd3000000.pdf

11. http://www.ncbi.nlm.nih.gov/pubmed/11955793

12. http://www.ncbi.nlm.nih.gov/m/pubmed/22681168/

13. http://www.ncbi.nlm.nih.gov/pmc/articles/PMC3002174/

14. http://evolutionarypsychiatry.blogspot.com/2012/11/inflammation-and-depression-cause-or.html

15. http://www.ncbi.nlm.nih.gov/pmc/articles/PMC3992230/

16. http://www.researchgate.net/publication/256539435_Reduced_breast_cancer_incidence_in_women_treated_with_subcutaneous_testosterone_or_testosterone_with_anastrozole_A_prospective_observational_study

17. http://www.ascopost.com/issues/october-15,-2014/testosteroneanastrozole-implants-relieve-menopausal-symptoms-in-breast-cancer-survivors.aspx

18. https://en.wikipedia.org/wiki/Hormone_receptor_positive_breast_tumor

19. http://www.webmd.com/breast-cancer/breast-cancer-types-er-positive-her2-positive

20. http://www.nature.com/nrendo/journal/v9/n12/full/nrendo.2013.179.html

21. http://www.huffingtonpost.ca/2013/09/12/men-low-sex-drive_n_3914690.html

22. Donaldson C, Eder S, et al. Estrogen attenuates left ventricular and cardiomyocyte hypertrophy by an estrogen receptor-dependent pathway that increases calcineurin degradation. Circ Res, 2009 Jan 30;104(2):265-75

23. Atsma F, van der Schouw YT, et al. Lifetime endogenous estrogen exposure and electrocardiographic frontal T axis changes in postmenopausal women. Maturitas, 2009 Aug 20;63(4):347-51

24. http://www.ncbi.nlm.nih.gov/pubmed/11844745

25. Hong S, Didwania A, et al. The expanding use of third-generation aromatase inhibitors: what the general internist needs to know. J Gen Intern Med, 2009 Nov; 24 Suppl 2:S383-8.

26. Cella D, Fallowfield L, et al. Quality of life of postmenopausal women in the ATAC ("Arimidex", tamoxifen, alone or in combination) trial after completion of 5 years' adjuvant treatment for early breast cancer. Breast Cancer Res Treat, 2006 Dec;100(3):273-84

27. Burnett-Bowie SA, McKay EA, et al. Effects of aromatase inhibition on bone mineral density and bone turnover in older men with low testosterone levels. J Clin Endocrinol Metab, 2009 Dec;94(12):4785-92

28. Winters L, Habin K, et al. Aromatase inhibitors and musculoskeletal pain in patients with breast cancer. Clin J Oncol Nurs, 2007;11(3):433-9

29. http://www.huffingtonpost.ca/2013/09/12/men-low-sex-drive_n_3914690.html

30. http://stpetehw.com/testosterone-replacement-therapy-how-it-affects-your-heart-health/

31. http://www.pm360online.com/aromatase-inhibitors-linked-to-cardiovascular-disease/

32. http://www.webmd.com/breast-cancer/news/20101209/aromatase-inhibitors-may-raise-heart-risks

33. http://www.naturalnews.com/033409_breast_cancer_toxic.html

34. http://jnci.oxfordjournals.org/content/103/17/NP.6.full

35. http://nancyspoint.com/the-dark-side-of-aromatase-inhibitors-part-1/comment-page-1/#comments

Testosterone and Prostate Cancer

1. http://lomalindahealth.org/medical-center/our-services/cancer-center/prostate-cancer-center/general-info/prostate-cancer-nutrition.page

2. http://en.wikipedia.org/wiki/Warburg_hypothesis

3. http://www.medicalnewstoday.com/articles/270660.php

4. http://www.ncbi.nlm.nih.gov/pmc/articles/PMC2990475/

5. http://www.researchgate.net/profile/Dominique_Singer/publication/23554695_Respiratory_response_of_malignant_and_placental_cells_to_changes_in_oxygen_concentration/links/0deec52cb1013c6d48000000.pdf

6. http://www.ncbi.nlm.nih.gov/pubmed/15240608

7. https://books.google.com/books?id=2GsgBAAAQBAJ&pg=PA237&lpg=PA237&dq=Inappropriate+expression+of+cytokines+can+create+an+immune+response+that+causes+cell+proliferation&source=bl&ots=-

8. http://press.endocrine.org/doi/full/10.1210/jc.2005-1097zqhZ097Ax&sig=Dqg544ido0qmTZ2NX_ufprmqUeM&hl=en&sa=X&ved=0CFAQ6AEwB2oVChMI6rqExaKPxgIVEX6SCh3gtABu#v=onepage&q=Inappropriate%20expression%20of%20cytokines%20can%20create%20an%20immune%20response%20that%20causes%20cell%20proliferation&f=false

9. http://www.medpagetoday.com/MeetingCoverage/ENDO/39965

10. http://cdn.intechopen.com/pdfs-wm/22058.pdf

11. http://www.ncbi.nlm.nih.gov/pubmed/11955793

12. http://www.ncbi.nlm.nih.gov/m/pubmed/22681168/

13. http://www.ncbi.nlm.nih.gov/pmc/articles/PMC3002174/

14. http://evolutionarypsychiatry.blogspot.com/2012/11/inflammation-and-depression-cause-or.html

15. http://www.ncbi.nlm.nih.gov/pmc/articles/PMC3992230/

16. http://www.lef.org/Magazine/2008/12/Destroying-the-Myth-about-Testosterone-Replacement-Prostate-Cancer/Page-01?p=1

17. http://www.midwestmensclinic.com/whats-the-connection-between-prostate-cancer-and-testosterone/

18. http://www.lifeextension.com/Magazine/2010/6/Abraham-Morgentaler-Testosterone-Therapy-for-Life/Page-01

19. http://area1255.blogspot.com/2014/05/debunking-hoax-testosterone-gels-and.html

20. http://www.harvardprostateknowledge.org/testosterone-supplementation-after-prostate-cancer

21. http://innovativemedicine.org/wp-content/uploads/sites/15/2013/07/test+prostatecancer.pdf

22. http://www.medscape.com/viewarticle/808065

23. http://www.jurology.com/article/S0022-5347%2813%2900259-0/abstract

24. http://onlinelibrary.wiley.com/doi/10.1002/tre.178/pdf

25. https://books.google.com/books?id=12JKCAAAQBAJ&pg=PT51&lpg=PT51&dq=anabolic+tissues+in+the+brain&source=bl&ots=ujmzmey-ky_&sig=QFFVVDA1yGdk1oTO6OrF38wtFhA&hl=en&sa=X&ved=0CEAQ6AEwBWoVChMIqKSSjJKVxgIVRSqsCh1h3wAP#v=onepage&q=anabolic%20tissues%20in%20the%20brain&f=false

26. http://www.businessinsider.com/america-has-way-too-many-lawyers-and-the-bubble-is-growing-2013-7

27. https://www.t-nation.com/training/steroids-the-birth-of-a-demon

28. https://en.wikipedia.org/wiki/DEA_number

29. http://www.deadiversion.usdoj.gov/schedules/orangebook/c_cs_alpha.pdf

30. https://www.drugpolicy.org/sites/default/files/DPA-MAPS_DEA_Science_Final.pdf

31. http://www.medicalnewstoday.com/articles/236688.php

32. http://www.petition2congress.com/5202/first-do-no-harm-dea-targets-physicians-who-treat-their-patients/view/

33. http://commonhealth.wbur.org/2013/10/fda-opioid-control-tightens

34. http://www.endocrinologyadvisor.com/androgen-and-reproductive-disorders/fda-panel-calls-for-tighter-restrictions-on-testosterone-therapy/article/372352/

35. http://www.newsmax.com/Stossel/Stossel-medicine-doctors-FDA/2010/02/24/id/350765/

36. THE SECRET FEMALE HORMONE-How Testosterone Replacement Can Change Your Life. Kathy, C. Maupin, M.D. Brett Newcomb, M.A., L.P.C.

37. http://www.m.webmd.com/men/news/20140918/fda-panel-limit-testosterone-drug-use

38. http://www.mensjournal.com/health-fitness/health/fda-to-middle-aged-men-you-probably-don-t-need-testosterone-therapy-20140919

39. http://www.fda.gov/Drugs/DrugSafety/ucm436259.htm

40. http://www.naturalnews.com/035641_corruption_FDA_Big_Pharma.html

41. http://blogs.plos.org/workinprogress/2012/01/25/how-much-money-do-drug-companies-pay-the-fda/

42. Morgentaler, Abraham. 2015. "Testosterone deficiency and cardiovascular mortality." Asian Journal of Andrology 17 (1): 26-31. doi:10.4103/1008-682X.143248.http://dx.doi.org/10.4103/1008-682X.143248

43. http://www.dailymail.co.uk/news/article-2555950/70-MILLION-Americans-mind-altering-drugs-shock-statistic-shows-extent-use-illegal-legal-narcotics.html

44. http://www.medicalnewstoday.com/articles/262352.php

45. http://www.jabfm.org/content/21/1/45.full

46. http://articles.latimes.com/2009/jun/08/health/he-lying8

47. http://www.alternet.org/story/156232/take_a_pill,_kill_your_sex_drive_6_reasons_antidepressants_are_misnamed
48. http://painphysicianjournal.com/2012/july/2012;15;ES145-ES156.pdf
49. http://www.ncbi.nlm.nih.gov/pubmed/23801566
50. http://www.stoppain.org/pcd/_pdf/OpioidChapter2.pdf
51. http://biology.stackexchange.com/questions/10446/which-hormones-can-cross-the-blood-brain-barrier
52. https://en.wikipedia.org/wiki/Blood%E2%80%93brain_barrier
53. http://www.ncbi.nlm.nih.gov/pmc/articles/PMC3480182/
54. http://www.eurekalert.org/pub_releases/2014-06/tes-trm062214.php

CHAPTER 10

Chronic Pain

1. Adrenal gland. Medline Plus/Merriam-Webster Dictionary. Retrieved 11 February 2015
2. http://en.wikipedia.org/wiki/Cortisol
3. The Immune System and the Nervous System. Retrieved February 25, 2009
4. Adrenal gland symptoms and Pain. Retreived March 26,2015 http://symptoms.rightdiagnosis.com/cosymptoms/adrenal-gland-symptoms/pain.htm
5. Palacios R, Sugawara I (January 1982). "Hydrocortisone abrogates proliferation of T cells in autologous mixed lymphocyte reaction by rendering the interleukin-2 Producer T cells unresponsive to interleukin-1 and unable to synthesize the T-cell growth factor". Scand. Journal of Immunology 15 (1): 25–31
6. http://emedicine.medscape.com/article/765753-overview
7. http://psychologytoday.psychtests.com/articles/mentalhealth/card_cat.htm
8. http://www.livestrong.com/article/396871-low-dopamine-anxiety/
9. http://en.wikipedia.org/wiki/Adrenal_cortex
10. Perceived stress and cortisol levels predict speed of wound healing in healthy male adults". Ebrecht M, Hextall J, Kirtley LG, Taylor A, Dyson M, Weinman J (2004). Psychoneuroendocrinology 29 (6): 798–809
11. http://www.drpamelaowens.com/262/
12. http://cortisolconnection.com/ch6_6.php
13. https://www.psychologytoday.com/blog/the-athletes-way/201402/chronic-stress-can-damage-brain-structure-and-connectivit
14. Cabergoline, a dopamine receptor agonist, has an antidepressant-like property and enhances brain-derived neurotrophic factor signaling. Psychopharmacology (Berl). 2010 Aug; 211(3):291-301
15. http://www.ncbi.nlm.nih.gov/pmc/articles/PMC3257832/
16. http://www.practicalpainmanagement.com/pain/cortisol-screening-chronic-pain-patients

17. Cortisol and immunity. W.McK. Jefferies. 2423 Newbury Drive, Cleveland, Ohio 44118, USA Retreived March, 22, 2004

18. Role of serum cortisol levels in children with asthma. Am J Respir Crit Care Med. 2002 Mar 1; 165(5):708-12.Landstra AM[1], Postma DS, Boezen HM, van Aalderen WM

19. http://www.aafa.org/display.cfm?id=8&sub=42

20. http://www.sharecare.com/health/chronic-pain/chronic-pain-affect-immune-system

21. http://americannutritionassociation.org/newsletter/deadly-nsaids

22. http://en.wikipedia.org/wiki/Platelet

23. http://www.rightdiagnosis.com/k/kidney_damage_nonsteroidal_anti_inflammatory_drugs/intro.htm

24. http://health.usnews.com/health-news/family-health/cancer/articles/2011/09/12/nsaid-painkillers-linked-to-risk-of-kidney-cancer

25. Cho E, Curhan G, Hankinson SE, et al. Prospective evaluation of analgesic use and risk of renal cell cancer. Archives of Internal Medicine. 2011;171(16):1487-149

26. http://www.minddisorders.com/Flu-Inv/Hypochondriasis.html

27. http://www.wisegeek.org/what-is-a-soft-tissue-injury-in-a-car-accident.htm

28. http://www.healthimaging.com/topics/diagnostic-imaging/radiology-mri-not-helpful-whiplash-diagnosis

29. http://nationalpainreport.com/researchers-claim-breakthrough-in-fibromyalgia-study-8820525.html

30. http://news.harvard.edu/gazette/story/2013/07/nerve-damage-and-fibromyalgia/

31. http://www.medicaldaily.com/breakthrough-fibromyalgia-research-pain-your-skin-not-your-head-246925

32. Role of the immune system in chronic pain Nat Rev Neurosci. 2005 Jul; 6(7):521-32. Marchand F[1], Perretti M, McMahon SB. http://www.ncbi.nlm.nih.gov/pubmed/15995723

33. Immune dysfunction may result in chronic pain syndrome. Retreived July 3, 2014 http://zeenews.india.com/news/health/health-news/immune-dysfunction-may-result-in-chronic-pain-syndrome_28622.html

34. http://www.natap.org/2008/HIV/101708_01.htm

35. Goldstein A, Lowery PJ (September 1975). "Effect of the opiate antagonist naloxone on body temperature in rats". Life Sciences 17 (6): 927–31

36. Harrison S, Geppetti P (Jun 2001). "Substance p". The International Journal of Biochemistry & Cell Biology 33 (6): 555–76

37. http://en.wikipedia.org/wiki/Autoantibody

38. http://www.healthimaging.com/topics/diagnostic-imaging/radiology-mri-not-helpful-whiplash-diagnosis

39. http://arachnoiditisnz.org/about-arachnoiditis/

40. American Journal of Clinical Nutrition; Dietary intake of trans fatty acids and systemic inflammation in women; D Mozaffarian et al.; April 2004

41. Torrance N, Elliott AM, Lee AJ, Smith BH. Severe chronic pain is associated with increased 10 year mortality. A cohort record linkage study. Eur J Pain. 2010(Apr);14(4):380-386

CHAPTER 12

How to Become a Functional Personal Trainer

1. http://blogs.findlaw.com/injured/2012/11/nba-star-francisco-garcia-settles-exercise-ball-lawsuit.html

2. http://www.argusleader.com/story/news/2014/04/17/exercise-ball-explosion-leads-injuries-lawsuit/7810807/

3. http://www.law360.com/articles/212581/nba-team-sues-exercise-ball-cos-over-4m-injury

4. http://theathleteslawyer.com/2014/04/

5. http://nicktumminello.com/2010/03/rethink-all-of-your-stability-ball-exercises/

www.ingramcontent.com/pod-product-compliance
Lightning Source LLC
Chambersburg PA
CBHW080212040426
42333CB00043B/2488